20 Nov 83

To Erica —
Many Thanks for the Super
Effort & help
in making This book possible
— With

Warmest
Regards

Appreciation

CAN YOU PREVENT
CANCER?
**REALISTIC GUIDELINES
FOR DEVELOPING
CANCER-PREVENTIVE
LIFE HABITS**

Prior Books by **Dr. Rosenbaum**

LIVING WITH CANCER, New York, 1975, Praeger Publishers

MIND AND BODY, San Francisco, 1977, Life Mind & Body

HEALTH THROUGH NUTRITION, San Francisco, 1978, Alchemy Books

UP AND AROUND REHABILITATION EXERCISES FOR CANCER PATIENTS, San Francisco, 1978, Life Mind & Body

COMPREHENSIVE GUIDE FOR CANCER PATIENTS, Palo Alto, Calif., 1980, Bull Publishing Co.

DECISION FOR LIFE, Palo Alto, Calif., 1980, Bull Publishing Co.

NUTRITION FOR THE CANCER PATIENT, Palo Alto, Calif., 1980, Bull Publishing Co.

REHABILITATION FOR CANCER PATIENTS, Palo Alto, Calif., 1980, Bull Publishing Co.

SEXUALITY AND CANCER, Palo Alto, Calif., 1980, Bull Publishing Co.

LIVING WITH CANCER, St. Louis, 1982, The Mosby Medical Library, The C.V. Mosby Co.

About the Author

Dr. Rosenbaum, a hematologist and oncologist, is in private practice in San Francisco. At the Mount Zion Hospital and Medical Center, he is Associate Chief of Medicine and Hematologist, Department of Pathology and Laboratory Medicine. He is director of the Tumor Immunology Program at the Claire Zellerbach Saroni Tumor Institute of Mount Zion Hospital and Medical Center and Associate Clinical Professor of Medicine at the University of California Medical School, San Francisco. He is also Chief of Oncology at French Hospital and Medical Center and Medical Director for the Regional Cancer Foundation of San Francisco and Marin.

CAN YOU PREVENT

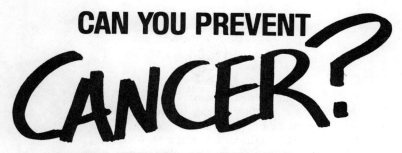

CANCER?

REALISTIC GUIDELINES FOR DEVELOPING CANCER-PREVENTIVE LIFE HABITS

**The Claire Zellerbach Saroni Tumor Institute of
Mount Zion Hospital and Medical Center, San Francisco**

ERNEST H. ROSENBAUM, M.D.

Associate Chief of Medicine, Mount Zion Hospital and Medical Center;
Associate Clinical Professor of Medicine, University of California Medical School, San Francisco;
Chief of Oncology, French Hospital and Medical Center, San Francisco;
Medical Director, Regional Cancer Foundation of San Francisco and Marin, California

Foreword by
GUY R. NEWELL, M.D.

Director of Cancer Prevention,
University of Texas M.D. Anderson Hospital
and Tumor Institute at Houston

The C. V. Mosby Company

ST. LOUIS   TORONTO   1983

Publisher: Thomas A. Manning
Editor: Nancy L. Mullins
Editing supervisor: Peggy Fagen
Manuscript editor: Roger McWilliams
Book design: Nancy Steinmeyer
Cover design: Diane Beasley
Production: Carol O'Leary, Barbara Merritt

THE MOSBY PRESS
The C.V. Mosby Company
11830 Westline Industrial Drive, St. Louis, Missouri 63146

Library of Congress Cataloging in Publication Data

Main entry under title:

Can you prevent cancer?

Bibliography: p.
Includes index.
1. Cancer—Prevention. 2. Self-care, Health.
3. Habit. I. Rosenbaum, Ernest H. II. Claire Zellerbach
Saroni Tumor Institute. [DNLM: 1. Attitude to health.
2. Health education. 3. Neoplasms—Prevention and control.
QZ 200 C2085]
RC268.C33 1983   616.99′405   83-11387
ISBN 0-8016-4198-5

F/VH/VH 9 8 7 6 5 4 3 2 1   02/D/248

Contributors

ERICA T. GOODE, M.D., M.P.H.

Private practice, Internal Medicine;
Attending Physician, Children's Hospital;
Instructor of Medicine, University of California,
San Francisco; Director, Eating Disorders Clinic,
San Francisco, California

PATRICIA T. KELLY, Ph.D.

Director, Stanton and Corinne Sobel Genetic Counseling Service,
Mount Zion Hospital and Medical Center;
Director, Cancer Risk Analysis Service, Regional
Cancer Foundation of San Francisco and Marin, California

STEVEN E. LOCKE, M.D.

Research Psychiatrist, Beth Israel Hospital;
Instructor in Psychiatry, Harvard Medical School,
Boston, Massachusetts

NICHOLAS L. PETRAKIS, M.D.

Professor of Preventive Medicine,
Chairman, Department of Epidemiology and International Health,
University of California, San Francisco,
San Francisco, California

PHILLIP L. POLAKOFF, M.D., M.P.H.

Medical Director, Western Institute of Occupational and Environmental
Sciences; Assistant Clinical Professor of Social and Family Medicine,
Stanford University Medical School, Stanford, California;
Assistant Clinical Professor of Physical Medicine,
University of California, Irvine,
Irvine, California

MARY E. WHEAT, M.D.

Assistant Director Ambulatory Medicine, Mount
Zion Hospital and Medical Center; Instructor of
Medicine, University of California, San Francisco,
San Francisco, California

To

Those individuals whose goal is to preserve life
through the prevention and cure of disease

To

The epidemiologists — the "medical detectives" — and
the physicians who advise and treat patients

And to

The patients and their families
who strive with the medical team to improve
their health to live and enjoy life

Foreword

Hippocrates (ca. 460–370 BC) first described cancer with the terms "carcinos" and "carcinoma" and noted its grave prognosis. He also was the first to describe the general concept of environmental influences on disease by relating what he knew as the four basic elements of fire, air, water, and earth to biologic counterparts that produced the qualities of heat, cold, wetness, and dryness. The first link between cancer and occupational exposure has been ascribed to the observation of scrotal cancer in British chimney sweeps in 1775 by Sir Percival Pott, a practicing English surgeon. Another practicing surgeon, Alton Ochsner, noted the association between cigarette consumption and squamous cell cancer of the lung in men who had served in World War I. Until then, lung cancer was a medical curiosity. A great leap in revealing how the environment relates to cancer took place about two decades ago, when studies of Japanese migrants to the United States were initiated by William Haenszel. The modern recognition that common fatal cancers occur in large part as a result of life-style and other environmental factors and are therefore, in principle, preventable, came in the form of a World Health Organization report by an expert committee in 1964. Much fine tuning of the concept has been done, and much more attempted, in the almost 20 years since that report, but all of the major elements were presented then.

So much for the past. The contributions of environmental factors to cancer causation are well established. Controlling those factors is now the problem at hand, and this book focuses on the two most important persons in the process of controlling cancer: the primary care physician and the person who wants to do everything he or she can to avoid cancer. The primary care physician, through providing services and encouraging behavior modification, can offer first-line cancer control. In addition, there is a broadening public awareness of the role of prevention in determining health outcomes. The public is examining health alternatives and seems willing to assume greater responsibility for individual health care decisions, and the news media are replete with health-related issues.

Traditionally, the clinician's training has been oriented toward the symptomatic patient rather than to the care of well people. Only in the relatively recent past has the concept of disease prevention, as practiced by the public health specialist, been adopted by the clinical practitioner and incorporated into comprehensive patient care. The reason for the change is simple: the primary care physician now assumes responsibility for maintaining the health of his or her patients as well as the responsibility for treating their diseases. This will eventually change the role of the family physician into one of more participation in clinical research and more history taking oriented toward risk factors for cancer. This, in turn, will lead to individual health-risk appraisals with recommendations for constructive changes on the part of the patient.

The two major arms of cancer prevention are the identification of the contributors to the causes of cancer, usually practiced by epidemiologists and astute clinicians, and the action taken in response to this knowledge, usually enacted by legislative control or preferably by voluntary actions taken on the part of concerned individuals. It is a sobering fact that we could possibly know the cause of every neoplasm and, at the same time, not be able to prevent a single case of cancer. Persons who continue to consume cigarettes, for example, epitomize this potentially tragic situation.

There are several important messages in this volume that come through clearly. First, cancer prevention is a series of several positive actions; taken together, these actions are greater than the sum of their individual components. Second, cancer prevention has not one but two natural constituencies: the primary care physician, whose responsibility is now to keep people well, and those people who have more financial resources and leisure time to devote to staying well. Working together, this combination can create an enormous positive force. Third, everything does not cause cancer, but those things that do should be considered extremely seriously. Substances that might cause cancer (usually reported by the news media from incomplete information) should be carefully considered but should not excite overreaction. They should, instead, be considered with guarded skepticism because our scientific knowledge is woefully incomplete. Fourth, fundamental research is still required and should be supported with enthusiasm by the public both conceptually and financially. Fifth, cancer is not one disease but hundreds of diseases, each with a personality and endurance of its own. However, three kinds of cancer account for 46% of all human cancers: lung, breast, and large bowel cancer. If every person adopted a prudent anticancer life-style, we could begin reducing the toll of cancer among Americans tomorrow, if not today. These include primary prevention by abstinence from tobacco consumption and adherence to proper diet, coupled with a program of secondary prevention for early detection of breast cancer in women and bowel cancer in men and women.

In summary, this book is edited by a nationally recognized expert in cancer management for the understanding of cancer prevention by primary care physicians and especially for persons who want to be a part of the movement toward helping themselves minimize their risks of getting cancer. Cancer is not an inevitable part of aging or of living. Knowledge and its proper application can go a long way toward helping one stay healthy and free from the disease dreaded most by the American public.

Guy R. Newell

Director of Cancer Prevention,
Professor of Epidemiology,
The University of Texas M.D. Anderson Hospital
and Tumor Institute at Houston

Preface

Of the three most feared diseases in the United States—heart disease, cancer, and stroke—cancer is the most dreaded. According to public opinion polls, Americans fear cancer more than they do war. For over a century scientists have probed for the cause of cancer in hopes of defeating this disease or at least improving the number of cancers that can be cured. The search for a miracle cure, a magic bullet, or a preventive vaccine is by now legend, but so far nothing miraculous has come of it. The cure rate has improved, but cancer is still rampant, striking one in every four Americans. Meanwhile, researchers, philanthropic organizations, private societies, and various government agencies continue the quest.

One of the facts about cancer after more than 30 years of research is that several different factors probably interact to cause cancer: the environment, nutrition and diet, genetics, exposure to viruses, and life-style choices. As more and more information is gathered, it is also clear that many cancers—probably up to 60% to 80%—are preventable. This book addresses the issue of cancer and cancer prevention. My own work with people after they have developed cancer has been the motivating force for helping others to avoid this disease, which often is an unnecessary killer. Many cancers *can* be prevented, primarily through life-style changes and appropriate screening techniques.

We have summarized the latest information available on the various factors known or believed to cause cancer: smoking, diet, and alcohol, environment, genetics, and life-style, which includes sexuality and stress (or the effect of the mind on cancer). Chapter One discusses what cancer is, how it develops, and its probable causes. The succeeding chapters are on each of the cancer-related components, explaining the cancer risk factors and making specific recommendations with health guidelines for prevention.

The sources for this information have been the latest research findings on cancer reported in medical journals and at medical conferences as well as recommendations from the Committee on Diet, Nutrition and Cancer (National Life-Sciences Council), the U.S. Senate Committee on Nutrition and Human Needs, the McGovern Committee, and the yearly United States Surgeon General's report on smoking, especially *The Health Consequences of Smoking for Women* and *The Health Consequences of Smoking: Cancer*.

Analysis of the vast amount of data gathered so far pinpoints two factors that probably contribute to over 50% of the cancers today—smoking and diet. Other known contributing factors appear to be immoderate use of alcohol, overexposure to sunlight, and exposure to other environmental factors, including chemicals, industrial wastes, and radiation, in our occupations and in our homes.

On the whole, it appears that our affluence — our "good" way of life — is the major contributor to the high death rates we have from cancer, as well as heart disease, stroke, emphysema, and obesity. The enemy, it seems, is us. The "miracle cure" for cancer available to all of us turns out to be *prevention* — our own ability to make the right choices in our nutrition, our smoking and drinking habits, and our other life-style behaviors.

The public is bombarded daily with stories and articles, amounting to a fear campaign, that state we live in a sea of carcinogens. People inundated by this media campaign question whether it is really worthwhile to change some of their daily habits of drinking, eating, and smoking to save their lives when they are surrounded by cancer-causing agents they cannot control. Many people say it's just not worth the effort. Therefore, it is important that we be not only convincing but factual as well. Unfortunately, all the facts on cancer causation are not yet in. There has to be some meeting ground between the two opposing sides: the one that says everything causes cancer so why try, and the other that believes there are preventive measures against cancer that work. We take the second side and believe preventive measures do exist. This book presents a sequence of data to help the person who wishes to make some changes to reduce his or her cancer risk factors and thus avoid illness and possible death from a disease that may largely be preventable. The topic is highly emotional, inflamed on all sides by those who participate in this "game of life."

Until we unlock some of the secrets of why one of two similar people gets cancer and the other does not and until we can understand the genetic patterns better, we are going to have to use general guidelines involving avoidance of certain substances, products, or chemicals, as well as recommend efforts to reduce the risks and alter our life-styles. It will not be as simple as John Snow turning off the Broad Street pump valve in 1849 in London, thus stopping sewage-contaminated water from infecting that part of the city with cholera. Snow had found the exact cause of the cholera epidemic, and by removing the offending agent, he cut off the source of further infection.

Solving the riddle of cancer has certainly not been easy, since there are hundreds of different forms of cancer. Just as is the case with cancer, cholera did not occur in everyone who drank water from the Broad Street pump because some people had a certain "internal resistance" to cholera. There is also a genetic resistance in many people against cancer, which we do not yet understand.

Sometimes, epidemiologists* can broadly determine what substances or exposures cause cancer by analyzing populations exposed to certain agents and comparing them to others. An association between certain viruses and specific types of cancer has been found, but whether the virus itself causes the cancer is still unknown. Looking at the data of the American Cancer Society, we note *there is an increase in the general cancer rate, but this is primarily a result of smoking.* If one examines age-adjusted death rates and removes smoking and the subsequent increase in lung cancer, one can see a general improvement in the cure rates for cancer. In other words, there has been no recent epidemic of cancer.

Since each chapter is a unit unto itself, there is some necessary overlap of information. However, the purpose of this book is to clear up as much confusion about cancer as possible, to dispel fear, and to provide a practical approach to help prevent cancer.

---

*Those whose job is to search and analyze the association and causes of cancer — the "cancer detectives."

Ernest H. Rosenbaum

The list of terms below are included to help the reader understand some common cancer concepts; other terms can be found in the glossary at the end of the book.

benign	A tumor that is not malignant.
cancer	The proliferation of malignant cells that have the capability for tissue or organ invasion.
carcinogen	A cancer-producing agent or substance.
carcinoma	A cancer that begins in tissue lining, an organ, or duct.
cocarcinogen	An agent that increases the effect of carcinogens.
epidemiology	The study of a disease and its relationship to other diseases through such factors as cause, rate or occurrence, and distribution in a human community.
malignant	Having the potentiality of being lethal if not successfully treated; all cancers are malignant by definition.
metastases	The spread of cancer from one part of the body to another; cells in the new cancer are like those in the original tumor.
mutagen	A factor that can make a normal cell transform into a malignant cell.

Acknowledgments

We wish to give special credit and recognition to our Chief Editor, Jay Stewart, for her endurance, creativity, devotion, and skillful editing that helped to bring this book to completion. Her creative talents helped us project and integrate a strong neutral direction in a very cloudy field so that we could achieve concise, clear, and readable concepts.

We wish also to thank Ruth Gladstone for the initial editing and data compilation that helped form and develop this book. We also extend our thanks and appreciation to Mary Cassanego for collecting and arranging data for the initial draft of Chapter 5; to Joan Borysenko, Ph.D., Sandra Levy, Ph.D., and Bernard Fox, Ph.D., for ideas and inspiration for Chapter 9; and to Isadora R. Rosenbaum, Mary Anne Stewart, and Mary Spletter for constructive critique, advice, editing, and support. Special creative editing by Jack Tucker made Chapter 8 appear alive and informative.

We would like to acknowledge Peter Tucker for his efforts in developing the graphics; David Pearlman, Science Editor of *The San Francisco Chronicle,* for thought-provoking commentaries; Lawrence Mintz, M.D., Lawrence Drew, M.D., Anthony Cosentino, M.D., Thomas Addison, M.D., Howard Brody, M.D., Lawrence Margolis, M.D., T. Stanley Meyler, M.D., Richard Krieg, M.D., Bruce Ames, Ph.D., Philip Kivitz, M.D., Bernard Gordon, M.D., Clifford Grobstein, M.D., George Herzog, M.D., and Alan Glassberg, M.D., for constructive criticism and advice; and Carmel Finigan for managing the "project" and making each obstacle surmountable.

We wish to acknowledge and thank Stanton A. Glantz, Ph.D., Virginia L. Ernster, Ph.D., James L. Repace, Warren Winkelstein, M.D., John H. Holbrook, M.D., Susan Chapman, and Jack O'Brien for sharing their expertise and for providing guidance and source materials on smoking and health.

We wish to thank and credit Diane McElhiney for typing the major part of this manuscript, along with Elizabeth Oliver, Eleanor Iida, Janice Ladnier, Kaye G. McKenzie, Ann Zapponi, Mary H. Barber, and Karen Call for assistance in preparation of the manuscript. Further gratitude is extended to Jeanne A. Dean, Mt. Zion Hospital; to Mt. Zion librarians Angela Wesling and Gloria Won; to Cathy Beecher; and to Kathryn Tester, Carolyn Amberry, and Edythe Newman for typing and supportive assistance.

Contents

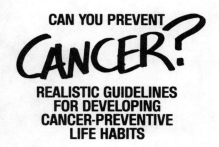

CAN YOU PREVENT

CANCER?

**REALISTIC GUIDELINES
FOR DEVELOPING
CANCER-PREVENTIVE
LIFE HABITS**

CHAPTER 1

An Overview of
Cancer and Cancer Prevention

Prevention is so much better than healing because it saves the labor of being sick.

THOMAS ADAMS
17th-century physician

ERNEST H. ROSENBAUM

When the disease is cancer, prevention is particularly desirable—you can avoid a disease that alters your life and is debilitating, potentially painful, costly to treat, and fatal in 50% of cases. Most people believe that either avoiding or getting cancer is something outside of their personal control. Cancer is often viewed as a thunderbolt of fate, striking at random with no cure or cause. This is *not* true. Many effective ways of treating cancer now exist, and more are being researched all the time. We also know more about the causes of cancer and that certain substances or life-style habits greatly increase the risk of cancer or actually cause cancer. Thus individuals can take specific steps to reduce their risk of cancer.

Oddly enough, there is a growing body of scientific information that has in itself led to confusion and even despair on the part of many people. "Why bother?" asked a young male friend. "Every day you read about something else that causes cancer. It's too much, so I don't even think or worry about it any more." Many people have come to share this attitude: if it isn't the saccharin *in* the coffee, it's the coffee; if it's not the nitrates in hot dogs, it's the nitro-

samines in beer. These are all substances about which the media have warned, and it is no wonder that the average person feels confused and helpless.

The other side of the coin is that current American Cancer Society data already state that we can improve the cure rate this year by approximately 10%—more than 100,000 lives can be saved by using some of the already known and accepted prevention principles (see Table 1-1).

In this book experts in cancer treatment and prevention discuss various aspects of cancer so that you can learn what scientists currently know about cancer, including the possible causes and means of prevention. The basic belief of these experts is that you can make choices that will help protect you from cancer. Simply put, the risk of cancer can be significantly reduced by taking practical, straightforward steps. But before discussing how to protect yourself against cancer, we need to look more closely at the sources of the confusion that most people have about what does and does not cause cancer.

Sometime during the 1970s the World Health Organization announced that medical science had conquered smallpox—a deadly disease that

1

TABLE 1-1   Estimate of preventable cancers (1980)

Association	Site	Incidence	Preventable
Cigarette smoking plus alcohol	Lung and larynx	90,000	80,000
	Head and neck and esophagus	13,500	8500
Industrial exposure	Bladder	9000	5000
Diet	Breast	30,000	10,000
	Colon	30,000	10,000
Sex	Cervix	7500	7500
Sunlight	Melanoma and other skin	5000	1500
Total		185,000	122,500

Modified by Guy Newell and based on National Cancer Institute data (Schneiderman).

had killed and disfigured people all over the world for generations. This worldwide major medical triumph was briefly mentioned in a half-column notice in a major New York paper; other papers gave the good news about the same notice. However, in March 1981 the *New England Journal of Medicine* carried an article by several researchers that indicated an *association* between coffee consumption and pancreatic cancer. These scientific findings were presented with *due restraint,* which was not true of the media coverage that followed. The original tentative findings were reported on the covers of major magazines, the front pages of newspapers, and on television news programs. Any caution about the research results was deleted, and coffee was directly linked as a cause of pancreatic cancer. This relationship has thus far *not* been verified or confirmed.

The finding of some association between coffee drinking and pancreatic cancer certainly deserves *follow-up research* to prove or disprove any actual relationship. In the meantime the general public thinks that coffee causes cancer because of the overblown media coverage on a preliminary research report. The same hype has occurred with other substances. Calum S. Muir, a noted epidemiologist, sums up this media perversity: "Good news is no news, and bad news is good news." In this case the good

news that was no news was the conquest of smallpox. The bad news that became such "good" news was the *association* between pancreatic cancer and a popular American drink, coffee.

This astute Scottish physician goes on to describe the entire process:

A new risk is discovered. There is a scientific paper which appears after peer review and it is full of the normal caveats and cautions, needs to be repeated, etc. Then increasingly frequently there is a press or television conference in which these entirely proper warnings about the findings are thrown to the winds. There is public alarm, and then after a while, the public begins to think, 'You know, these people keep telling us that this is dangerous, that's dangerous, and then I just don't believe it.'

Muir's analysis was borne out by a study reported in the July 1982 *New England Journal of Medicine.* More than 500 randomly selected subjects were questioned about their coffee-drinking habits. Of the 70% who were coffee drinkers, only one person had specifically reduced coffee consumption because of the findings linking coffee to pancreatic cancer, although 50% had heard about the reputed findings.

The unfortunate result of these overblown false alarms is that they take away from the truth of what is, in fact, known about cancer. For example, although it is now a scientific fact that smoking is linked directly to lung cancer, some people still reject this as speculative theory or a mere alarmist approach. They disregard this fact that may have life-or-death consequences for them.

To be able to make intelligent life-style choices, people must first have good information. They have to be able to sort out the latest media hype from basic sound knowledge. This is not always easy because new findings are turning up every day, and some are tentative and some certain. Yet the truth is that cancer remains in many ways a mystery even to those deeply involved in studying it. Despite any mysteries of cancer that remain, we currently know enough about cancer to establish workable guidelines for risk reduction. We know that certain habits or exposures either cause or encourage the risk of cancer. We also have many working theories about what cancer is and how it operates.

WHAT IS CANCER?

To discuss what cancer is, we first need to understand the term. When they hear the word "cancer," most people think of a single disease, such as measles or whooping cough. In fact, the term "cancer" is used to refer to more than 200 diseases that can originate in any cell or organ in the body. But all cancers do have something in common: they always involve the production of abnormal cells that are capable of irregular, independent growth and that invade healthy body tissue.

It is this malignant, uncontrolled, and invasive growth of normal, healthy cells that make cancer what it is, no matter where it occurs. Cancers that arise in different parts of the body are given different names, such as lung cancer and breast cancer. But there can be different types of cancer with different characteristics in one location, such as several kinds of breast cancer or lung cancer.

Cancer appears as tumors in the body, but not all tumors are malignant or cancerous. Tumors are abnormal masses of tissue, and they can appear anywhere in the body. Benign tumors, however, do not invade or destroy surrounding structures or tissues; they remain local. Malignant or cancerous tumors do invade the surrounding tissues, the lymphatic system, or the bloodstream and thus may spread to distant areas of the body.

Specific cancers are named for the body tissues in which they originate. Three general categories are:

1. **Sarcomas,** which arise from bone and soft or fibrous tissues such as muscles, or blood vessels
2. **Carcinomas,** which arise from the epithelium—the cells that make up the skin and lining of the body organs—including lung, breast, ovarian, colon, pancreatic, and cervical cancers
3. **Leukemias** and **lymphomas,** which arise from the blood cells of the bone marrow or lymph node cells

Treatment of cancer can start as soon as a malignant tumor is discovered, the extent evaluated (staged), and the type properly defined. However, a tumor has to be roughly the size of a pea—approximately 1 centimeter (⅜ inch) in diameter—for it to show up on an x-ray film or in a careful physical examination. By the time a cancer has become this size, it has been around for some time; this is what creates many of the problems. The indirect cause of these problems is the delay between the time when a tumor starts and the time it finally becomes noticeable, using current techniques. Cancer starts with one abnormal cell that divides, becoming two cancerous cells. These two cells divide, becoming four; the four become eight, the eight sixteen, and so on. It may take from 1 to 5 years for this duplication process to take place 20 times to the point where the tumor contains 1 million cells. By this time, after being in the body for up to 5 years, the cancerous tumor is still only the size of a pinpoint and weighs only 1/100 of a gram (35/100,000 ounce).

A tumor this size is still too small to be detectable, but not too small to spread the disease. While it has been growing, the tumor may have been releasing cancer cells. Hundreds of thousands of these cancerous cells may spread to other parts of the body, or *metastasize*. Fortunately, many of these metastasized cells die. Because they do not implant—like a seed that does not grow—they do not actually become cancers when they reach another part of the body. Some may become implanted, however, and grow; this means cancer has started developing in another location in the body.

It is only by the time that the original cell has divided 30 times that the tumor has reached pea size and so may be detected by an x-ray film or a good physical examination. Cancers that start in the abdomen or chest cavity have to grow even larger, to a size that will cause both interference with organ function and some symptoms before they are suspected. This is why cancers in these locations are usually detected late and are more difficult to treat successfully. *Successful treatment is linked to early detection.*

Since cancer always involves the production of *abnormal* cells, the essential question is what makes that first cell become cancerous and start duplicating itself. In other words, what causes cancerous growth to begin from a normal cell? Despite several differing theories about what causes this, the experts agree on some points. For a cell to become cancerous, some basic change has to take place in its genetic code (DNA—deoxyribonucleic acid). The genetic change is then transmitted to the newborn cells. A limited analogy might be that of a pattern used for stamping out cookies. Once the pattern is changed, all subsequent cookies are changed. The DNA of a cell holds the cell's genetic code or pattern. DNA is a protein that makes up the chromosomes, tiny threads in a cell nucleus that contain genes. The genes are where the genetic pattern or information of a cell is located, and it is here that a change takes place. About 15 readily identified genes are

known to cause cancer. These are *transforming genes* or *cancer (onco-) genes*, since they can transform laboratory tissue cells into a cancerous state as compared to normal cells. Recent research thus suggests that we all have normal cells in our body containing *oncogenes*, which are inactive. Following certain cellular assaults, stimuli or chemical agents may "turn on" a genetic "light switch" that will activate these genes and thus transform a normal cell into a cancerous cell.

For example, the MYC gene, found in cancers of chickens, has been identified in the chromosomes of a patient with Burkitt's lymphoma (the cancer of the lymphatic system common in equatorial regions of Africa). This may represent an important step in identifying gene/chromosome changes that make a normal cell turn into cancer. Thus a gene known to be involved in cancer of birds has been linked to human cancer.

The change from a normal cell to a malignancy is thought to be a two-step process. First, the DNA is somehow initially changed. Then a second, more decisive change takes place in the DNA that transforms the now receptive cell into an actual tumor cell. This explains the diagnostic value of the Pap smear for cervical cancer. The smear can reveal abnormal cells (dysplasia) before they have become cancerous. These suspicious cells serve as an early warning sign of cancer potential, which indicates a need for more frequent medical checkups.

But what causes these changes in the cellular DNA in the first place? Cancers may develop from perfectly normal cells, and until recently scientists believed that a normal cell became cancerous after receiving multiple injuries over a period of years. These assaults, known as *hits* or *insults*, were thought to work like the proverbial straws on a camel's back; they accumulate over the years until the final straw—the one that breaks the camel's back—hits the cell and causes a transition to a malignant cell. The cell then abandons its original genetic pattern and grows independently and irregularly, invading surrounding healthy tissue.

Dr. Takeo Kakunaga reported at the Thirteenth International Cancer Conference in Seattle in September 1982 that chemicals could transform a normal cell into cancer by a genetic DNA mutation. He observed more than 20 different proteins in the induced cancerous cells of laboratory mice, which are believed to result from gene (chromosomal) alterations. Thus a genetic, *molecular event at the gene level* occurred, with progression into a cancer cell. This suggests that events changing a normal cell into cancer may be caused by a series of chemical mutations.

Traditionally, cancers are believed to take long periods to develop, from 1, 10 to 30, or more years. Thus there may be a time lag between the accumulating hits or exposures and the changeover to actual malignant growth. This makes it difficult to pinpoint the agents that cause the cancer to occur. In addition to the multiple-hit theory, cancers have been caused in animals by exposure to certain viruses. This suggests that viruses may also play a role in human cancer, but only one virus so far has been shown to have a direct causal relationship to cancer in humans, the *Epstein-Barr virus.* However, other viruses have been associated with certain cancers in humans. Five DNA viruses are now being linked to human malignancy, including the hepatitis B virus, cytomegalovirus, herpesvirus (both I and II), and the papilloma virus. Current evidence involving viruses is discussed in Chapter 10.

Recently, there has also been some evidence that a single assault on a cell can cause cancerous change. According to this view, it may be possible that a "single carcinogenic bullet" hitting a cell in the appropriate spot can change the cell so that it is genetically susceptible to cancer or becomes cancerous.

These three theories—the multiple hit, the viral cause, and the single hit—all differ, yet it is possible that they are all correct. There are also many other mechanisms and theories currently being evaluated by research. It is highly unlikely that research will ever unearth a single cause or cure because there are so many types of cancer. This does not mean, however, that most cancers cannot be effectively prevented, treated, and cured. Proof of this is that the cure rate for cancer has been improving steadily since 1930, when it was 20%. The current cure rate is now at 50%.

To dwell on what is unknown about cancer is to open the door for speculation about the causes and cures for cancer, with wilder claims such as cancer being contagious or being caused by use of aluminum cookware, neither of which is true. The advance in the cure rate has been matched by an increase in reliable knowledge about substances and exposures that can lead to increased risk of cancer and specific substances that are *carcinogens*, or cancer-causing agents. Some understanding of how scientists track down a definite relationship between a particular agent and cancer can help you develop confidence in the results of scientific findings.

HOW WE KNOW WHAT WE KNOW

In 1775 a physician named Percival Pott studied the abnormally high incidence of scrotal cancer among London chimney sweeps. He described these young men and boys "thrust up narrow and sometimes hot chimneys, where they are bruised, burned and almost suffocated; and when they get to puberty, become particularly liable to a noisome, painful, and fatal disease," scrotal cancer. The sweeps often worked naked, rarely bathed, and were full of soot, especially in their groin areas. Pott concluded that the soot was the cause of their scrotal cancer.

In 1915, 140 years after Pott published his observations, Drs. Katsu Saburo Yamagiwa and Koichi Ichikawa at the Imperial University of Tokyo tested the effects of coal tar on the ears of rabbits. Cancer developed on the tar-painted area just as cancer had developed on the soot-covered scrotums of the London chimney sweeps.

Two methods were used in this case to arrive at the conclusion that soot causes cancer: (1) observation of specific populations (the sweeps with their high incidence of cancer) and (2) laboratory experimentation. The first is called *epidemiology*—the observation and study of how diseases affect different populations. Epidemiology has revealed a lot of what we know today about cancer. For example, it has been well established that as specific populations, such as Japanese people, move from one country to another they acquire the cancer rates of their new countries for some cancers. This observation has helped scientists understand that changes in life-style habits such as diet play an important part in many cancers, since the inherited genetic susceptibility to cancer would remain the same in these migrating populations.

Epidemiologists study the frequency of cancer occurrence according to characteristics such as age, sex, ethnic background, occupation, social class, and life-style habits, including diet, smoking, and drinking.

The original discovery of a link between smoking and lung cancer was made by epidemiologic studies showing that a high proportion of lung cancer victims were also smokers. Once a certain population is found to have an unusual incidence of a specific disease, then researchers can start to look for patterns unique to that group, such as a particular diet, occupational exposure, or life-style. After a particular risk factor that seems to have a strong association with a specific disease has been isolated, researchers can design further population studies and/or laboratory experiments to establish whether or not there is a causal relationship or just a strong positive association between the substances in question and cancer. Research techniques are becoming more sophisticated and advanced methods of statistical analysis using computers more available, so that we are increasingly more certain that some substances do cause cancer.

We know, for example, that we can receive injuries to our cells from a variety of known external sources as well as substances we take into our bodies and that may have a relationship with cancer: sunlight, radiation, drugs, tobacco smoke, excess fats, chemicals, hormones, industrial pollutants, and polluted water. In addition, our life-style choices have been found to influence cancer susceptibility: how much alcohol we drink, the viral diseases we are exposed to, and the amount of stress in our lives. Finally, the development of cancer may also depend on an individual's genetic predisposition. One can inherit a genetic susceptibility to cancer, although a strong susceptibility has been found to be rare, so that in the total analysis, environment and life-style probably are major contributors of up to 80% or more of human cancers. This means that we can take measures to improve our life-styles and so reduce the risk of cancer.

CANCER-CAUSING AGENTS OR EXPOSURES

Getting to specifics, it is estimated that 32% of all cancers—not just lung cancer—are caused by smoking tobacco. Another 4% of cancers are thought to result from excessive alcohol use. It is well known that an increased consumption of alcohol is associated with cancers of the head and neck as well as cancer of the liver. Alcohol also acts together, or synergistically, with cigarette smoke to further increase the risk of cancers of the mouth, larynx, respiratory tract, and esophagus. Excessive beer drinkers have been found to have an increased risk of rectal and colorectal cancers.

Stomach cancer has decreased in this country but still has a high incidence in Japan, where the people consume many highly salted and pickled foods, which are thought to be the contributing factors. Skin cancers and malignant melanomas are, not surprisingly, highest in areas with the most intense sun. They primarily affect people who spend considerable time outdoors, such as farmers and ranchers; fair-skinned, freckled and red-haired people are particularly susceptible.

Our affluent life-style and specific dietary abuses, such as increased ingestion of fats and calories, obesity, consumption of meats, and a decrease of grains in our diets, have a relationship to breast cancer, colon cancer, and uterine cancer. The relationship between breast cancer and diet is well established in several respects. For example, during World War II in England when there was a shortage of sugar, dairy products, and meat, people substituted cereals and vegetables. A sharp decrease in the incidence of breast cancer ensued. The dietary and cancer trends were both reversed after 1948, when the English returned to their prewar eating patterns. In a study done in Japan, women from the higher socioeconomic levels of society who eat meat daily had eight and a half times the risk of breast cancer than did poorer women who did not eat meat daily. Obese women have shown a higher incidence of breast and uterine cancer in several studies.

People want to know whether they can completely avoid cancer if they avoid these exposures and risks. This question is impossible to answer with certainty. A complex sequence of events leads to the development of a carcinoma or cancer. The process involves stimulation by various carcinogens and/or *promotors* (factors that act in combination with carcinogens to initiate cancer). Another factor in the process is the timing and frequency of exposure to a carcinogen or cocarcinogen, which affect the cellular DNA and may eventually cause irreparable damage, leading to cancer initiation. The effect of carcinogens and promotors is not unique or singular; it occurs in relation to other factors, including a person's resistance to cancer, the strength of the individual's immune system, a dietary deficiency or excess, exposure to radia-

tion and sunlight, genetic susceptibility, and any previous damage to an organ by a virus. Thus cocarcinogens and promotors may act in conjunction with environmental factors to effect a change in the health of the tissue at the cellular level.

The answer to the question of how best to avoid cancer is, however, currently available to us. Certain elements have been linked to cancer, and there is some evidence of the cancer-inhibiting qualities of other substances.

CANCER PREVENTION

The average life expectancy in 1900 was 52 years; since then it has reached 74. This remarkable change, which adds 22 years to the average life, resulted from advances in public hygiene, vaccinations, medical technology and drugs, and our growing understanding of disease and how to treat it. People, however, often fail to reach this life expectancy of 74. Two diseases in particular keep us from living to our full potential and beyond—heart disease and cancer, the most common causes of death in the United States today.

Recent data show that there has been a decline in cancer deaths (except for lung cancer in females), as reported in March 1983 by the American Cancer Society. Early diagnosis, improved therapy, and life-style changes have led to the results listed in the boxed material shown on p. 8.

As in the past, when threatened with a health problem or illness, people turn to the medical profession for an answer, a cure. In the case of cancer medical scientists continue to look for a cure, and new discoveries are hoped for daily. The desperation of some people has even led them to grasping at untested, unproved methods or worse—drugs or healing approaches that have no known effectiveness. Sometimes these sidetracks in search of a supposed "miracle cure" keep people from conventional therapies that have proved successful.

Decline in cancer deaths — percentage change from 1968 to 1979

Breast cancer (female)

Ages 20-34   Down 17%
Ages 35-49   Down 15%

Lung cancer (male)

Ages 20-44   Down 18%

Lung cancer (female)

Ages 20-44   Up 16%

Cervical cancer

Ages 20-44   Down 48%

Testicular cancer

Ages 20-44   Down 43%

Stomach cancer
    (male and female)

Ages 20-44   Down 33%

Bone cancer
    (male and female)

Ages 20-44   Down 19%

Hodgkin's disease
    (male and female)

Ages 20-44   Down 16%

Non-Hodgkin's lymphomas
    (male and female)

Ages 20-44   Down 29%

Data from National Cancer Institute, Biometry Branch.

cancer, even conquered, is physically debilitating, sometimes painful, and costly to treat. More important than any of these facts is that *many cancers can be prevented,* and the means of prevention are not expensive, exotic, or time-consuming. The most important fact of all is that protecting you from cancer is not something that anyone from the medical world can do. There is currently no available cancer vaccine or general cancer antibody. The only one who can take steps to prevent cancer is the person you confront in the mirror every day. That is the sum of it — the good news and the bad.

If you have been a heavy smoker for 20 to 30 years, drink a moderately large amount of alcohol, and have a family history of cancer, the news could be bad, although it is *never too late* to make changes that can have beneficial results. If you stop smoking and reduce your drinking today, your cancer risk will gradually return to normal for lung, head, and neck cancer.

Several experts have stated that we have control over 70% to 80% of the causes of cancers. Not all experts agree. Cecil Fox, in a letter to *Science* (October 8, 1982), stated, "All evidence now available indicates that cancer *is* inevitable in most people and that cancer *is* a part of the human estate." He believes that the common epithelial cancers (lung, breast, prostate, colon) are precocious and occur earlier in life than normally expected. These cancers may develop between the ages of 30 and 60 instead of 90 and 100 and in part are related to our life-style via exposures to cigarettes, alcohol, and asbestos, as well as to genetic insults such as electromagnetic radiation or alkylating chemotherapy drugs. He states that the longer one lives, the greater chance one has to develop cancer. Therefore, elderly people may develop small amounts of epithelial cancer if they live long enough (90 to 100 years plus), but they usually *die of other causes — not from cancer.*

Fox believes that there are *no* guarantees against cancer, nor will there ever be a cancer-

The fact is, as stated earlier, that because of the complexity of cancer, no one cure or cause will probably ever be found. This leaves us with a serious disease that strikes 1:4 Americans and 2:3 families in some form. Several means of treating cancer exist, some completely successful in bringing about a cure, others less so. But

free society. One can use one's intelligence to help prevent or delay cancer by living an appropriate life-style. Fox stated in a personal communication that "cancer can be postponed if one lives a sensible Hippocratic life, among other things." He gives an example of a life of moderation with proper rest, diet, not smoking or using excess alcohol, and from an occupational standpoint, not working in an asbestos mine.

Many pathologists believe that "80% to 90% of men who live long enough develop cancer of the prostate." These cancers may never grow large enough to be detectable or to cause symptoms. They may be unavoidable, but most cancers are preventable; they are not inevitable.

The main actors in the drama to prevent cancer are ourselves. The annoyance of changing our life-style—one we like and are used to—from steak to soybeans, from too much to just enough, from a high-fat to a low-fat diet, can be considerable. Yet millions of people with heart disease have done it. They have taken the responsibility for their own health maintenance. The advantages of choosing to live as healthy a life as possible are many, including increased energy and interest, more opportunities for physical enjoyment, and reaching a ripe old age, as well as fewer medical bills and hospital stays.

The first step to take toward preventing cancer is to gather the necessary information, which is what this book provides. The next step is to analyze your current life-style in terms of the new information that you have gathered. Then, you can make plans and begin the lifestyle changes needed for a turn toward better health and away from the risk of cancer. The following list of questions should help you*:

What do I really want out of life?
What is really important to me?

*Adapted from Rosenbaum, E.H., and Rosenbaum, I.R.: A comprehensive guide for cancer patients and their families, Palo Alto, Calif., 1980, Bull Publishing Co.

What are my priorities, and where have my own health and happiness been on the list?
What habits do I have that could lead to cancer? Are they worth dying for?
What realistic steps can I take to change my lifestyle?

The life-style choices that endanger us often do not seem like dangers or even choices at all but rather the fruits of our labors, the very rewards for which we all work. Don't we all want plenty to eat and as much ease as possible, surrounded by gadgets that make our lives more pleasurable? This is what many of us strive for, yet we are finding that the very advantages of the "good life" are killing us. We have air and water pollution from too many machines and too many poisonous substances used to make items for our daily use. In terms of our personal life choices, "*six of the ten* leading causes of death in the United States have been linked to our diet," according to the McGovern report.

First on the list of dangerous life-style choices is smoking, related to 32% of all cancers (see Fig. 1-1). Next is poor dietary habits, also influencing approximately 32% of cancers, according to many investigators. Changes in our diet since the early 1900s have been followed and recorded by the Department of Agriculture. Overall, there has been an increased consumption of fats; sugars; salt; and salted or pickled, barbecued, and smoked foods. Increased consumption of these categories of food is correlated with an increased incidence of cancer occurrence. In contrast, a high-fiber, low-fat diet that includes abundant fresh fruits and vegetables is correlated with a decreased incidence of colon cancer. No one knows precisely how this works or what causes these relationships, but we do know they exist.

In the early 1900s 40% of the average person's diet came from fruits, vegetables, and grains. The only canned food was home canned, and most people lived on farms or close enough to them to get farm food, which was simple, unaltered, unadulterated, and nonprocessed—

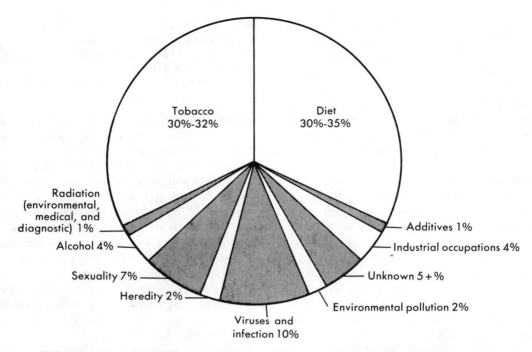

FIG. 1-1 Cancer risk factors—approximate percentages in relation to influence on all cancers (statistical averages, male and female combined). (Modified from Doll, R., and Peto, R.: The causes of cancer, Oxford University Press; and Higginson, J.: Cancer and environment: Higginson speaks out, Science **205:**1363, 1979.)

meat, fruits, vegetables, dairy products, grains, legumes, and so on. Since then, our consumption of primary fruits, vegetables and grains (rather than secondary products made from them) has dropped from 40% of our diets to 20%. Use of fresh potatoes, for example, is more than two-thirds lower now than it was 100 years ago, and the use of processed potatoes has increased by 44% over the last 30 years.

In addition, research studies indicate that in 1976 every man, woman, and child in this country consumed 125 pounds of fat and 100 pounds of sugar a year. Compared with 1910, fat consumption increased 31% (from 32% to 42% of our calories), and sugar consumption increased 50% (from 12% to 18%). For example, the average per capita consumption of 12-ounce cans of soft drinks per year is 295! And that's

an average; many people do not drink *any* soft drinks at all.

These dietary changes accompanied what seemed like natural, unquestioned "improvements" in our life-style. Foods came to be commercially canned or frozen, and a whole new range of processed food products became available. These changes have meant a host of new and different chemical food additives in our diets. For example, the per person intake of food coloring additives has increased 10 times from 1940 to 1977.

Today, eating has become more than a pleasure; it is a kind of recreation—seeking out new food forms or exotic taste treats. Food-as-recreation is, of course, a profitable industry, and we are barraged with advertisements for sugary snacks, high-fat foods, "fast foods," and soft drinks. In every setting, even schools and hospitals, the "American marketplace provides easy access to sweet soft drinks, high-sugar cereals, candies, cakes, and high-fat beef," according to Dr. Beverly Winekoff from the Rockefeller Foundation, speaking before a Select Committee of the U.S. Senate on Nutrition and Human Needs. Access to foods likely to improve our nutritional health is often more difficult. It is almost always easier to buy a piece of cake or a soft drink than an apple at most cafeterias and restaurants, although the situation is beginning to change.

Almost all Americans have a relatively affluent life-style, surrounded by constant temptations, and so there has been a dramatic increase in what could be called the life-style diseases—cancer and heart disease. In the case of cancer, there is no doubt that prevention is the best cure, and we need to look at the means of preventing cancer or reducing our risk of cancer. To begin with, cancer prevention has two levels. The first, called "primary prevention," is prevention of the cancer itself, and this involves life-style choices that are discussed shortly. The second and equally important level of cancer prevention, termed "secondary prevention," consists of ways of preventing the consequences of the disease once it has started. This means early detection and intervention through screening for cancer.

Screening can be a very effective means of reducing cancer risk, as shown by the 70% decline in the cervical cancer death rate over the last 40 years. This impressive decline is exclusively a result of early detection through the use of the Pap smear. Two factors influenced the effectiveness of this screening technique: (1) development of an effective diagnostic technique for early detection, in this case, the Pap test; and (2) public education so that everyone potentially susceptible can make use of the screening technique available.

The chest x-ray film for lung cancer is another screening test, although unfortunately, by the time a tumor shows up on an x-ray film, it has already been around for a year or two, making it more difficult to cure successfully. In other words, some screening techniques are more effective than others because they detect cancers earlier, which leads to more chance of a successful cure. New screening techniques are constantly being researched, and some tests are inexpensive and readily available; others are not. Specific screening techniques are covered in detail in Chapter 4, which includes recommended tests.

Screening is important, especially after a lifetime of exposures, but keeping yourself from getting cancer in the first place is the most effective form of prevention. When people think of cancer prevention, they often tend to focus on avoiding the known or suspected causes of cancer; they should extend their prevention approach to more general and positive-oriented health guidelines. For one thing, although we know many substances that cause or promote cancer, thousands more are not yet known and may never be discovered. Also, other factors that are almost impossible to assess affect cancer initiation, such as the timing and frequency of exposure to carcinogens or promotors. The effect of such exposures is neither unique or singular. Rather, it occurs in relation to many other factors, including, as already mentioned, a person's resistance to cancer, the strength of the individual's immune system, dietary factors, exposure to sunlight and other radiation, and previous damage to an organ by a virus or vitamin deficiency.

In short, the situation that causes cancer to begin is complex. Some things are known about the cause-and-effect relationship between certain life-style practices and cancer rates; a lot more is theorized about, intimated, and analyzed without precise conclusions—and much remains unknown and open to speculation. In many cases, because we can point to certain clear associations between life-style and disease or specific cancer rates, general guidelines for health practices are possible. But because specific cause-and-effect relationships have not yet been clearly established in many cases, we should avoid the small worries and a panic approach to changing our life-style.

For example, for many years people have been adopting different life-style patterns in hopes of preventing disease. They may improve their diets, start an exercise program, take vitamins, reduce calories—all to the good. But some specific dietary changes can be either insignificant or harmful. A good instance of this is substituting brown sugar for white when both sugars are chemically the same. The appropriate approach to take in assessing health risks is probably best expressed in a Burl Ives song called, "Watch the Donut, Not the Hole." The donut, in this case, is the general health guidelines offered here.

HEALTH GUIDELINES

Of the substances and practices to avoid, the two most important are smoking and excessive use of alcohol, especially hard liquor (three to four drinks each day). Additionally, high doses of hormone supplements for menopausal women and diethylstilbestrol (DES) have been linked to cancer, as have numerous artificial flavorings, colorings, and other food additives and burnt foods such as barbecued meats.

We know that diet affects cancer, although we do not have a precise formula for "minimizing the incidence of cancer." A diet high in consumption of animal fat and red meat and low in fiber (from grains, fruits, and vegetables) correlates with increased risk for cancer. Thus you should reduce your dietary intake of red meat and animal fat, if it is currently high.

You should also increase consumption of fiber from leafy vegetables, fresh fruits, bran, grains, and whole grain cereals. Dr. John Higginson, founding director of the World Health Organization's International Agency for Research on Cancer (IARC), says this about fiber: "There are lots of hypotheses regarding the ac-

tion of fiber besides regularity. I am sufficiently convinced of the possibility that I now take All Bran at breakfast, which I didn't do before. That is the sum total of the dietary changes that I have made, apart from not overeating, in the past thirty years."

Certain vitamins and minerals are also thought to have an effect in cancer prevention. These include *vitamin C,* found in citrus fruits, red tomatoes, and bell peppers, and *vitamin A,* which comes from dark green and yellow vegetables, and some fruits, such as spinach, chard, carrots, squash, and apricots. In recent studies people who consume vitamin A foods regularly develop the least amount of lung and other cancers. Vitamin E, from fresh whole cereals, nuts, seeds, grains, and vegetable oils, is thought to hinder production of carcinogenic nitrosamines in the stomach and intestines. Two minerals are also associated with cancer prevention—*zinc* and *selenium.* Zinc is found in whole cereals, grains, and gran; selenium in seafoods and organ meats.

People are beginning to make healthy life-style choices, especially individuals who see the beneficial effects. A survey of 595 physicians done for the *Harvard Medical School Health Letter* found that most physicians had made health-promoting life-style choices: only 8% smoked, down from 38%. Sixty-nine percent use margarine; 44% restrict their consumption of red meat; 79% eat three eggs or less per week; and 71% say they are within 10 pounds of their ideal weight. The physicians are "careful about indiscriminate pill-taking," and 93% say they have two or less alcoholic drinks a day.

Populations of people who already follow special dietary habits for religious reasons, such as the Seventh Day Adventists, who are vegetarians, often show a significantly lower incidence of both cancer and heart disease. The Mormons in Utah have a rate of cancer incidence that is one-third lower than non-Mormons in the same geographic area. Utah residents as a whole have a cancer rate 16% lower than the national average. Mormons traditionally abstain from smoking, alcohol, and extra-marital sex.

The relationship between cancer and sexual activity is covered in Chapters 9 and 10. These two areas are difficult to generalize about because so much remains unknown, and in the case of sexuality the subject is emotionally clouded. Tentative findings so far indicate an association between cancer of the cervix in women and an exposure to sexually transmitted herpes simplex II virus.

Among homosexuals who make a life-style choice that involves many sexual partners, there has been a tremendous outbreak of a skin cancer called Kaposi's sarcoma, as well as rectal carcinoma and Burkitt's lymphoma. These cancers are also associated with viral or multiple viral infections.

Because the evidence is limited, it is difficult to make specific recommendations, although simple common sense dictates that a person try to avoid exposure to genital herpes, and homosexuals might consider restricting the number of their partners or else restricting transmission directly by using a condom. Condoms may also be effective as a means of protecting against herpes among heterosexuals and homosexuals.

Stress, or the influence of the mind on cancer causation and cure, is just beginning to be scientifically investigated. It is a difficult arena for research because it is almost impossible to devise experiments that illustrate how the mind acts on the body. Meanwhile, speculation is wide open, with almost too much room for wild theories.

Some things are known, however, and it seems best to stick with these facts. Stress, tension, emotional upsets, anxiety, and worry can cause chemical and hormonal changes in the body. On the level of personal experience, during a stressful time or situation, you can feel muscular tension, including tightening of the neck, shoulders, leg and possibly back muscles. Your heart may beat faster, and breathing often becomes shallow and faster. These felt re-

sponses are matched by biochemical changes that could influence and weaken the effectiveness of your immune system. It is commonly accepted knowledge that you are more liable to illness when you are "run-down." This weakness in your immune system could have some influence on your susceptiblity to cancer (see Chapter 9), as well as to colds and flu. Until more is known, definite conclusions are not possible. However, it certainly cannot hurt to develop and practice enjoyable techniques for managing or reducing stress. These will undoubtedly have some overall health benefits. Stress can lead to overindulgence in drink, cigarettes, rich food, and so on. Even if stress is not a direct cause of cancer, there are good reasons for learning stress reduction techniques.

With respect to environmental exposures and cancer-causing agents, you have complete control over some things and no control over others. You can, for example, restrict your excessive exposure to sunlight, which is a cause of skin cancer. This is most important for fair-skinned people who have less natural protection from the sun and thus are more susceptible to skin cancers.

Radiation, water pollution, and air pollution are other indirect environmental causes of cancer and are difficult to avoid. Some naturally occurring radiation is impossible to avoid and is probably harmful, but we can reduce unnecessary exposure to x-rays. As workers and consumers, we can educate ourselves about the possible carcinogenic effects of the substances we use (see Chapter 8) and thus act to reduce our exposure to these substances or protect ourselves if we have to be exposed. As citizens, we can act to clean up air pollution and water pollution and to control radioactive contamination by enacting laws that establish standards of safety. In times of such technologic complexity, fair and broadly accepted standards of safety are essential to our well-being as individuals and as a society.

Many factors may lead to the development of cancer—some known, some poorly understood.

Chapter 2 reviews many changes in various populations on different continents, through migrations or racial variations. Another example of a change has become apparent recently in the American black population.

THE RISE IN CANCER RATES IN BLACKS VERSUS WHITES

In general, a comparison of cancer rates from 1957 to 1971 has shown a doubling in the cancer rate for black males, whereas the rate remains fairly constant for black females. The rate of esophageal cancer in black males has increased three times. The lung cancer rate increased four times in males and three times in females; the colon and pancreas cancer rate increased in both sexes; prostate and bladder cancer increased in men; and breast cancer increased in women. (See also Appendix A.)

The exact reason for this is not known, but it has been suspected that differing carcinogenic effects may be playing a role in the black population and the white population and that lifestyle habits may differ as well.

A 1982 study by Drs. William J. Miller and Richard Cooper in the *Journal of the National Medical Association* discussed a comparison of results from 1950 to 1977, with the age-adjusted cancer rate for nonwhite men in the United States rising an astonishing 68.2%, whereas the rate for white men rose only 22%. Rates fell slightly for women of both races. The bulk of this rise was primarily related to the increased incidence of lung cancer and in part to the relative importance of occupation. For example, coke oven workers who were involved in coal carbonization had a greater susceptibility to lung cancer, and more blacks in Pittsburgh, for example, were employed in this occupation than whites. There was also an increased risk in those who worked in shipyards and were exposed to asbestos during World War II, as well as a known synergistic relationship between shipyard workers and cigarette smoking.

For social and economic reasons a larger percentage of blacks have had to accept more dangerous and lower paying jobs. A disproportionate number of blacks work at unskilled and blue collar jobs and are more exposed to industrial carcinogens. Bricklayers, for example, have been found to be at increased risk for leukemia, as well as esophageal and stomach cancers and nose, lung, and both kidney and bladder cancers. Blue collar workers, as well as service workers and office workers, also smoked more. In addition, many of their jobs included exposure to chemical dust, fumes, and other toxic airborne particles involved in industrial development.

Malignant melanoma is a common disease, involving approximately 1% of all cancers. Its occurrence in blacks is only approximately 5% of the total number of cases. It appears to be more aggressive in blacks. It occurs more prominently in the feet when first seen and has a poorer prognosis in blacks, with a 5-year survival rate of 23%, compared to 70% for the general population. The reason why is unknown. Thomas Paul wrote in 1931 that "the pigment of the skin stands as a sentinel guarding the underlying tissues from the baneful effect of the sunlight."

One of the paradoxes in breast cancer has been the difference in the incidence between blacks and whites. Dr. La Salle D. Leffall, Jr. noted in 1982 that black women tend to have breast cancer less frequently than white women, but that blacks had a consistently lower survival rate at each stage of disease. An analysis was done of their estrogen receptor and progesterone receptor activity. An association was made with receptors and tumor differentiation, and in 146 black women whose breast cancer was monitored at Howard University over 3 years, a relatively low incidence of ER-positive* tumors was

*ER—estrogen receptors. A test that measures the degree of hormonal sensitivity of breast cancer cells; a predictor of the response to hormonal therapy.

noted in the black patient population, as well as a higher incidence of poorly differentiated tumors and a lower incidence of well differentiated tumors, both risk factors for more aggressive disease. This in part *could explain the survival difference;* this could also be an ethnic difference. In Japan there is also a different distribution of estrogen and progesterone receptors in postmenopausal women when compared to Western women. The data are still preliminary and merit a much more extensive and comprehensive review.

It is worthwhile to recognize that several studies are in progress to help to explain the differences that exist between cancers in blacks and whites so that more specific measures can be taken. Until this is done, and in view of the increased cancer incidence among the black population, these additional recommendations are provided:

1. Give up or reduce smoking. A smaller proportion of blacks are quitting than whites at present. The use of filtered cigarettes should be emphasized for those who cannot quit, as past studies have shown that blacks use more nonfiltered cigarettes. Effective preventive programs to reduce the incidence of smoking should become a community effort.
2. Attempt to reduce the rate of cervical cancer (in blacks twice that of whites) through sexual hygiene, including regular Pap smears and pelvic examinations, which has proved to be effective in past studies.
3. Lighter-skinned blacks should use a sunscreen such as PABA and guard against excessive sun using appropriate protection.
4. Follow general guidelines (boxed material in the following summary).

SUMMARY

If you smoke, drink a lot, eat beef and other red meats seven or more times a week, are 20 to 25 pounds overweight, and work in a stressful environment or in an industry that exposes you to known carcinogens, you have considerable room for improvement. You can cut your smoking, drinking, and red meat consumption in half just for starters. This is already a significant change and a major step toward a healthier life-style.

**General guidelines
for reducing your cancer risks**

Diet

1. Reduce consumption of red meat and animal fats.
2. Avoid obesity; keep trim and fit.
3. Increase consumption of foods with vitamins A (beta-carotene), C, and E and the minerals zinc and selenium.
4. Increase proportion of basic whole foods in your diet, such as grains, fresh fruits, and vegetables. Increase intake of fiber.

Life-style

1. Do not smoke.
2. Limit alcohol use to less than 2 to 3 ounces per day; limit wine and beer intake.
3. Do not drink and smoke together.
4. Reduce stress or practice stress management.
5. Protect yourself from sexually transmitted viruses.
6. Use care in taking medications and hormones.

Environment

1. Avoid excessive exposure to sunlight or use a sunscreen.
2. Reduce or control exposure to known chemical carcinogens and industrial asbestos with protective techniques.
3. Avoid using dangerous or carcinogenic chemicals whenever possible.
4. Help enact legislation to establish clean air and water standards.

Even without knowing specifics, you can make some simple, practical life-style choices that will benefit you for the rest of your life. The earlier you make these changes in your life, the more beneficial the results will be. But it is important to make the changes, no matter how old you are; your children and grandchildren are still young, and you can help them develop healthy life patterns from the start. You can give them the immensely valuable legacy of good health and the knowledge of how to live a long, vigorous, and healthy life.

The general guidelines listed in the boxed material are the place to start. (It is interesting to note that these are the same recommendations for reducing your risk for heart disease.) You can gain more specific information from the individual chapters, which cover the current and more detailed information now available concerning cancer prevention. Our hope is that you make full use of the information and enjoy the results — a longer, healthier life.

CHAPTER 2

Cancer Epidemiology

It is not necessary to know the precise mechanism in disease pathology before preventive measures are taken.

ERNST WYNDER

NICHOLAS L. PETRAKIS

Epidemiology is the study of the patterns of disease among people, and it has been a part of medicine since the time of Hippocrates, the father of medicine, who lived more than 2000 years ago. During the past 100 years the methods of epidemiology have been used to study the causes and prevention of infectious diseases such as diphtheria, smallpox, and in recent years cancer and other chronic diseases.

Epidemiology studies the complicated interplay of cancer-causing chemicals, radiation, viruses, and so on in the environment with the hereditary and nutritional factors of individuals and their behavior or life-style and then theorizes how these factors interact to produce cancer in some people and not in others. The epidemiologist describes how often a specific cancer occurs in people of differing ages, sex, racial background, socioeconomic level, life-styles, habits, and so forth. Finding that a certain type of cancer is noticeably more common in a particular group of people leads the epidemiologist to develop ideas or hypotheses as to what might have caused the cancer. These early ideas and

hypotheses are then tested by further research studies.

Two types of special studies can be done to test hypotheses. In *case-control* studies a suspected cancer-causing factor that occurs commonly among people who have a specific type of cancer is also studied in persons who do not have cancer. The latter is called the control group. If the suspected factor is more statistically frequent among the people with cancer than among the control group, an *association* between the suspect factor and the cancer is said to be present.

Proving that the suspected factor is an actual "cause" of cancer requires *cohort* or *prospective* studies. In this type of research, two large groups of people are studied: the first group, those who are exposed to or have the suspect factor in their lives, and the second group, those who do not have the factor. After 5 to 10 years the number of cancers that have developed among the first group with the suspect factor is compared to the number of cancers that have developed among the unexposed group.

This type of study provides information on the *risk* factors for a given type of cancer. The results of case-control studies can tell us about the association of suspect factors and a specific type of cancer, but proof of such a *cause* using cohort studies is costly and requires an extended period.

Although laboratory and animal experiments have provided a great deal of knowledge on the nature of cancer, the known causes of human cancer have come largely from epidemiologic studies that focused on human populations. It should be stressed that whereas some causes of cancer in humans have been shown to be direct and simple (for example, cigarette smoking and lung cancer), most cancers are probably the result of a complex interplay of many factors, and no simple direct cause or substance has been found.

This chapter covers what is known of the epidemiologic features of the major sites of cancer in adults. Each cancer site is briefly presented in the form of descriptive and risk factors.

MOUTH AND THROAT CANCER

Cancers of the mouth and throat tend to occur in older persons and make up 6% of all male and 2% of female cancers. The ratio of male to female rates is about 2:1. Like most cancers, those in the mouth and throat occur more frequently with advancing age and may involve the lips, tongue, gums, and inner surface of the cheek and floor of the mouth. Identified risk factors include tobacco smoking or chewing. Cancer of the lip is commonly found in persons extensively and chronically exposed to sunshine, such as farmers and sailors.

It is also known that heavy drinking of alcohol, more than five or six drinks of hard liquor per day, is a causal factor. In addition, alcohol and tobacco appear to interact with each other to produce higher risks of mouth cancer than are caused by either tobacco or alcohol alone. A common precancerous change associated with these factors is a whitish patch (*leukoplakia*) on the mucous membranes of the mouth. Any chronic nonhealing ulcer or leukoplakia noticed in the mouth or on the lips should be brought to the attention of a physician, as cancer of the mouth is curable in its early stages.

LUNG CANCER (BRONCHOGENIC CARCINOMA)

Cancer of the lung accounts for 34% of deaths in males and 16% in females. The highest rates of lung cancer are found in Western countries; the lowest rates are found in Asia and Africa. The risk of bronchogenic cancer increases with age. The rate is rapidly increasing in women; by 1984 it will surpass cancer of the breast as the leading cancer among women.

The key risk factor identified as causing lung cancer is cigarette smoking, and the risk to an individual increases progressively with the number of cigarettes smoked per day. Other factors that relate to industrial occupational exposures have also been identified, including exposure to asbestos fiber, uranium ore dusts, nickel refining, and smelter working. The combination of smoking with asbestos exposure or uranium mining increases the effect over the use of either alone up to 90 times, according to some reports. There may be a hereditary factor that increases susceptibility to lung cancer, and more recently some evidence suggests that patients with lung cancer have low levels of vitamin A, a vitamin important for maintenance of the lung cells of the bronchial tree and other organs.

Prevention of lung cancer can be achieved by discontinuing smoking and avoiding specific industrial exposures. It is also prudent to increase the dietary intake of vitamin A by including dark green leafy and yellow vegetables such as spinach, chard, carrots, and yellow squashes.

A major educational effort must be made to discourage smoking in young people to prevent lung cancer as well as to reduce the risks of cancer of the bladder, mouth, esophagus, and cervix—not to mention coronary heart disease and emphysema. Unfortunately, the cigarette industry has targeted advertising for young people, especially young women. This campaign is directed toward addicting young people to cigarettes as a way to guarantee the future earnings of the tobacco industry. Dr. Virginia Ernster of the Department of Epidemiology and International Health at the University of California, San Francisco, has found that at least 10 to 15 cigarette ads are placed in every issue of all major women's magazines. These ads emphasize the desirability and sexual attractiveness of women who smoke. More than $1 billion a year is spent on the promotion of cigarette smoking by the tobacco industry, whereas the National Cancer Institute, the American Cancer Society, and other voluntary health agencies together spend only about $10 million per year to counter tobacco advertising. Efforts in Congress to strengthen the warning printed on cigarette packs of the health risks of smoking were defeated once again in 1982 by the efforts of the tobacco lobby.

STOMACH CANCER

Cancer of the stomach was formerly one of the major cancers of men and women. For unknown reasons this cancer has declined progressively since 1930. However, it still accounts for 3.5% of male and 2.8% of female deaths and is among the nine most common cancers in both sexes. In Japan, Iceland, and Colombia stomach cancer is still the leading cancer. It is more common in American blacks than whites. In general this cancer is twice as common in men as in women, and risk of occurrence progressively increases with age.

Stomach cancer appears to be caused by an environmental factor. This is suggested by the experience of immigrants to the United States, who show a striking decrease in stomach cancer rates in America after they left countries with high rates of stomach cancer. For example, cancer of the stomach is the most common cancer in Japan. Yet among second-generation Japanese-Americans the stomach cancer rate has fallen dramatically.

Risk factors for stomach cancer have not been clearly identified, but they seem to be caused in part by dietary factors. The disease is more common in populations with diets that are high in dry, salted fish and pickled vegetables and that use many heated fats. It is hypothesized that these foods contain nitrates, which, in the absence of vitamin C, become converted to carcinogenic substances known as *nitrosamines* that act on the stomach to cause malignant changes. This cancerous change is more likely to occur in persons whose stomach lining is abnormal and does not produce hydrochloric acid (*achlorhydria*).

Other risk factors include cigarette smoking; heavy consumption of alcohol, which can damage the lining of the stomach; and exposures encountered in occupations such as coal mining, possibly related to carcinogenic hydrocarbons in coal. Peculiarly, persons with blood group A have slightly higher rates than those with blood group O. The reason for this is not clear. A recent finding is the identification of a precancerous lesion, *intestinal metaplasia,* in which the stomach epithelium resembles that of the small intestine. The specific cause of this change is unknown, but persons with gastric intestinal metaplasia appear to be prone to develop stomach cancer.

The striking decrease in stomach cancer among migrant ethnic groups previously noted strongly supports an environmental factor, probably diet, in the cause of stomach cancer.

ESOPHAGEAL CANCER

Cancer of the esophagus accounts for about 2% of cancer deaths in the United States and occurs about three times more frequently in males than in females. Although not a common cancer, it is difficult to treat because of its location and the relatively late onset of symptoms. In the United States blacks have higher rates of this cancer than whites or other ethnic groups. Strikingly high rates have been reported from Iran, Siberian Russia, and China. In Iran an extremely high rate of esophageal cancer is found among inhabitants of the area at the southern end of the Caspian Sea. Similarly high rates are present in northern central China.

Recent research in China suggests that a factor in the diet may be a cause of esophageal cancer. This is suggested by the observation among Chinese peasants, in whom a high rate of cancer of the esophagus occurs, that food scraps fed to their chickens produced cancer of the esophagus in the chickens. Studies suggest that a type of mold found on certain foods that produces a cancer-producing substance, called an *aflatoxin*, may be a causal factor. Nitrosamines in food may be an additional cause. Other areas of the world with high rates of esophageal cancer are Japan and the Transkei region of South Africa.

Two etiologic (causal) factors have been identified in Western countries: tobacco smoking and heavy alcohol consumption. The relative risk of esophageal cancer is increased almost five times in heavy smokers, and 10 times in heavy alcohol drinkers compared to nonsmokers and nondrinkers of alcohol. A significant interaction, or synergy, has been reported between alcohol and tobacco in the cause of esophageal cancer in which the relative risk is increased up to 155 times over nonsmokers/nondrinkers.

Other reported risk factors are a plant known as bracken fern in Japan, which is part of the diet; exposure to asbestos; and possibly the late aftereffect in some persons who accidentally ingested lye as children. The actual chemical carcinogenic factors are not clear. Recent studies in China in which both humans and chickens develop esophageal cancer suggest the possibility of such dietary carcinogens as aflatoxins or nitrosamines as the causative factors.

COLON AND RECTUM CANCERS

Cancers of the colon and rectum account for about 15% of cancers of men and women in the United States, and as usual incidence rises with advancing age. The highest rates are among whites, next highest in blacks, and lowest in Asian and American Indian populations. This appears to be correlated with socioeconomic status, with the highest incidence among the more affluent. Very low rates are found among Asian, African, and eastern and southern European populations.

Migrants to the United States from countries with low rates of cancer of the colon, such as Japan, China, Poland, and Italy, have developed the higher rates of colon cancer similar to native Americans. Again, as in the case of stomach cancer, a change in the diet accompanying immigration has been suggested as a possible cause. This finding strongly suggests that environmental factors related to diet play a role in cancer of the colon and rectum.

Of the etiologic factors studied, present evidence suggests that a diet rich in fat and meat and low vitamin A intake is implicated. A slight increase in rates is found among asbestos, shoe, and machinist workers. Persons with ulcerative colitis have an increased risk of developing cancer of the colon, probably because of prior damage to the intestine from this disease. Cigarette smoking has not been found to be associated with this cancer site.

Currently, most epidemiologists believe that diet plays an important role in the etiology of colon cancer. The type of diet consumed has an effect on the time it takes for ingested food to pass through the gastrointestinal tract and can influence the type of bacteria present in the large bowel. The large intestine contains a large variety of bacterial types that actively metabolize the fecal contents. Western people who consume foods rich in fat and meat tend to have a prolonged period of time (called transit time) for food to move through the gastrointestinal tract and are more inclined to have constipated stools. In addition, certain types of bacteria in the colon found to be associated with high-fat, high-meat diets have been shown to produce mutagenic and potentially cancer-causing chemical substances. In contrast, populations subsisting on diets rich in the complex carbohydrates present in the largely vegetarian diets common in the Third World countries have rapid gastrointestinal transit times, and bulky stools. The bacteria of the bowel among people with this type of diet are believed to produce much fewer mutagenic or carcinogenic substances.

It is now believed that dietary differences acting through effects on the intestinal tract may account for the differing rates of cancer of the large intestine and rectum between the Western and less well-developed countries. As noted earlier, this view is further supported by evidence in migrant populations to the United States from countries with low colon cancer incidence. Within one generation these migrants have acquired the high colon cancer rates of the native white American population. Most cancer epidemiologists believe that this is best explained on a dietary basis. However, the actual dietary factors are yet to be identified.

UTERINE CANCER

Approximately 10,500 women die annually from cancer of the uterus. The uterus is divided into two segments, each of which can be affected by cancer. The fundus, or body of the uterus, is the seat of cancer of the lining (endometrium) of the uterine cavity. The cervix, or mouth, of the uterus is affected by cervical cancer. Cancers of the endometrium and cervix account for about 13% of cancers of women and rank third below breast and colon cancer in women. Cervical cancer is about two and a half times more frequent than endometrial cancer.

Cervical cancer

Cervical cancer rates begin to increase at about age 25, leveling off around age 50. In the United States significantly higher rates are found among black and Spanish-American than among white women. High rates of cervical cancer are found in Asian and Latin American countries; the lowest rates occur in Japan and Israel. Cervical cancer is most commonly found in women of lower socioeconomic status. A progressive decline has occurred in cervical cancer rates in the United States that is attributed in part to better vaginal hygiene and to widespread use of the Pap smear. In addition, the detection of cervical cancer and precancer now occurs at a much earlier and more curable stage than in past years. The periodic use of the Pap test can practically guarantee cure of a developing cervical cancer at a very early stage.

Factors that increase risk of cervical cancer include a history of previous venereal disease, particularly of herpesvirus, type II infection; onset of sexual activity in early adolescence; and many sexual partners. Recently, several epidemiologic studies have also linked cigarette smoking to increased risk of cervical cancer. The practice of circumcision of Jewish males was formerly believed to explain the lower incidence of this cancer in Jewish women. However, this view is no longer held, particularly as cervical cancer rates have been increasing slightly among young women in Israel in recent years.

Endometrial cancer

Cancer of the body of the uterus, in contrast to that of the cervix, occurs more frequently in white women and is significantly less frequent in Spanish-American and black women in the United States. Very low rates are reported in Nigeria, India, and Japan. The incidence of this cancer increases with age and is strongly associated with increasing socioeconomic status: the more affluent, the higher the risk.

During recent years a striking increase was

reported because of the widespread use of meno-pausal estrogens. In general, more affluent women are more likely than poorer women to receive treatment with estrogen for menopausal complaints. With the public dissemination that menopausal estrogen was an etiologic factor, lower doses of estrogen have been prescribed by physicians, resulting in the decrease of endome-trial cancer rates. These findings show how sociocultural and environmental factors can in-teract with biologic factors to cause cancer.

Other risk factors identified in endometrial cancer are obesity and polycystic ovarian dis-ease. Excess circulating estrogen is present in women with these conditions and, similar to menopausal estrogen use, is believed to be part of the cause. It is known that in obese post-menopausal women excess body fat can convert the adrenal hormone, androstenedione, into es-trogen. Similarly, the disease of polycystic ovaries is associated with excessive estrogen production. It is strongly recommended that the use of menopausal estrogens be used at the lowest dose that will control the symptoms of menopause. If possible, they should be discon-tinued or used sparingly after the menopausal years.

BREAST CANCER

Breast cancer is currently the leading cancer of women in the United States. More than 100,000 new cases occur each year, and about 30,000 deaths result from this cancer. The high-est rates of breast cancer occur in Western countries, the lowest in Asian countries such as Japan and China and in Africa. Cancer of the male breast is about 100 times less frequent than in the female. Breast cancer rates are di-rectly correlated with socioeconomic status, with highest rates occurring among the more af-fluent. Breast cancer rates begin to rise at about age 30 and in American white and black women continue to increase with age. In Japan, Asia, Africa, Latin America, and countries in East-ern Europe there appears to be an increase in rates of breast cancer up to the menopausal years, and then a leveling off or even a decline. Rates in countries around the Pacific Basin in-dicate highest rates in white American and Hawaiian-Polynesian women, lower rates in San Francisco and Hawaiian-Chinese and Japa-nese, and lowest rates in Japan, China, and the Philippines. These differences suggest that both environmental and genetic factors are impor-tant in the causes of breast cancer.

A number of risk factors have been identified for breast cancer. It is not surprising that a strong association between breast cancer and reproductive factors has been found, since the breast glands respond to the reproductive fe-male hormones. Women with breast cancer compared to those without breast cancer have been found on the average to have had earlier age at onset of menstruation; are more likely not to have had children, but if they have had children, to have been older at the time of their first pregnancy; to have had fewer children; and to have had menopause at an older age. Women whose ovaries have been removed be-fore age 40 have a lower risk of breast cancer than those who retain their ovaries.

Dietary factors have been implicated as a possible cause of breast cancer through the demonstration that geographic differences in cancer rates appear to be related to dietary dif-ferences in fat and meat consumption among countries. High fat and protein intakes corre-late with high breast cancer rates; conversely, low intakes correlate with low rates. However, case-control studies on individual patients compared to control women do not support a strong relationship to diet. Because of evi-dence of genetic factors in susceptibility to breast cancer, it seems likely that breast can-cer risk results from the effects of several fac-tors, such as hormone, genetic, and environ-mental (including dietary) interactions. Ciga-rette smoking has not been found to be a risk factor for breast cancer.

SUMMARY

This has been a highly selective and somewhat cursory review of the highlights of what we know about the epidemiology of selected major cancer sites. Based on this information, let us reiterate and expand on the "General guidelines for reducing your cancer risk" in Chapter 1.

Recommendations based on cancer epidemiology

1. Stop or do not start smoking cigarettes, cigars, or pipes, and do not use snuff or chewing tobacco. Tobacco products contain cancer-causing chemicals when burned or chewed.
2. Limit alcohol intake to not more than two to three ounces per day.
3. Keep weight at levels ideal for your height according to Department of Health and Human Services standards.
4. Avoid too much fat and saturated fat in your diet by choosing lean meat, fish, poultry, dry beans, and peas as protein sources. Limit eggs to two or three per week. Limit intake of butter, cream, hydrogenated margarines, lard, shortening, and foods made from these products. Trim excess fat off meats.
5. Eat more complex carbohydrates daily by substituting starches such as grains for fats and sugars.
6. Increase intake of foods containing fiber and starch, such as whole grain breads and bran cereals, fruits, and vegetables.
7. Avoid or minimize occupational exposures to known carcinogenic substances in industry.

CHAPTER 3

Families and Cancer: the Role of Inheritance

In general, only rare diseases are inherited in a simple manner; in common diseases there is usually no simple pattern of inheritance.

A.E.H. EMERY

PATRICIA T. KELLY

Each day more individuals are realizing that life-style and exposure to environmental substances can affect their susceptibility to cancer. People are becoming interested in diet, pollution control, and the examination of commonly used substances to determine if they are carcinogens. At the same time many individuals want to know if the reduction or elimination of environmental carcinogens can substantially reduce their cancer risk. They wonder if cancer susceptibility might in large part be a result of an individual's genetic makeup and therefore beyond the influence of environmental factors.

The purpose of this chapter is to present a summary of the current scientific thinking about the role played by genetics, or inherited susceptibilities, in the promotion of cancer, particularly common cancers of the breast, colon, and lung. In recent years new information about the occurrence of the common cancers in families has become available, making it possible to give individuals with a family history of cancer more accurate information about their personal risks. A summary of some of this new information follows a brief discussion of some relevant genetic principles.

BASIC PRINCIPLES

When most people think about an inherited or genetic susceptibility to disease, they do not usually think of cancer. They think of such diseases as Tay-Sachs, sickle cell anemia, or Huntington's. Both Tay-Sachs disease and sickle cell anemia are inherited as single-gene recessive traits. A disease that is inherited in this recessive fashion only shows up when an individual has two copies of the gene for that disease. An explanation of basic genetics shows how this works.

You have an estimated 30,000 structural genes and 23 pairs of chromosomes. Each gene can be thought of as occupying a given place on a chromosome, for example, the place for gene A on chromosome 1. However, there may be several or even many different types of A genes that could occupy the A place. These different

This work was supported in part by the Research Support Program of Mount Zion Hospital and Medical Center, the E.H. Rosenbaum Cancer Research Fund, and the Stanton and Corinne Sobel Research Fund.

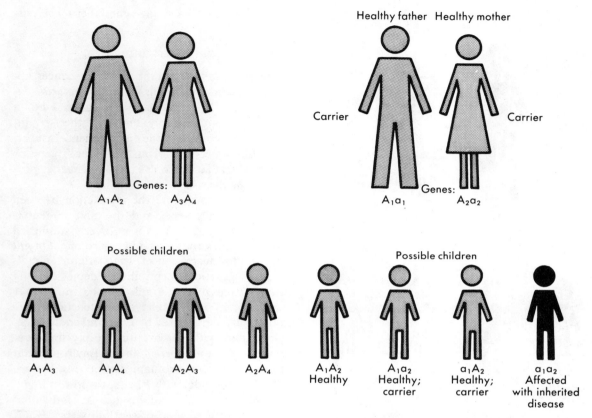

FIG. 3-1 Inheritance of genes from parents.

FIG. 3-2 Recessive inheritance.

types of a given gene are called *alleles*. You have two copies of each gene; one copy comes from your mother and one from your father. For example, as shown in Fig. 3-1, the father transmits either A_1 or A_2, and the mother transmits either A_3 or A_4.

Dominant and recessive inheritance

Sometimes a mutation or change occurs in a gene. When this change results in a gene that will be inherited as a recessive, the changed gene is written as a lowercase letter. An individual who has one copy of a recessive gene with a mutation is healthy (for example, Aa). However, if two people who carry a recessive gene have children, some of their offspring may have the recessive disease (for example, aa), as shown in Fig. 3-2.

It has been estimated that most of us carry at least five genes for recessively inherited diseases. Fortunately, most of the time we marry individuals who carry genes for a different set of diseases; therefore recessively inherited diseases are rare.

Some single-gene disorders such as Huntington's disease are inherited as dominant traits. An individual who has even one copy of a dominant gene (for example, Hh) will have the disease, as shown in Fig. 3-3. About one half of an affected individual's children will also be affected. Note that a dominantly inherited gene is written as an uppercase letter.

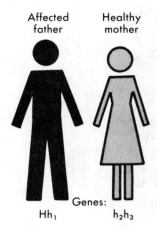

Affected father   Healthy mother

Genes:
Hh_1 h_2h_3

Possible children

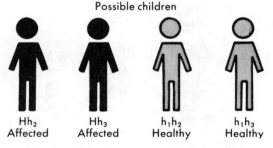

| Hh_2 | Hh_3 | h_1h_2 | h_1h_3 |
| Affected | Affected | Healthy | Healthy |

FIG. 3-3 Dominant inheritance.

Tay-Sachs disease, sickle cell anemia, and Huntington's disease are inherited in what is called simple, single-gene fashion. The presence of even one copy of a dominantly inherited gene can produce the disease. A recessively inherited disease results from the presence of two copies of a gene. Individuals with only one copy are not affected, although they can pass the gene on to the next generation.

When most people think of genetics and cancer, they tend to think that if a person is unfortunate enough to have a gene or genes that predisposes to cancer, that person will eventually have cancer regardless of lifestyle or environmental influences. Scientists have found that usually the situation is far more complex. In most families cancers are *not* the result of a single-gene inheritance pattern.

Multifactorial inheritance

In most cases the propensity for cancer appears to be the result of *multifactorial inheritance*. In multifactorial inheritance a disease is not entirely due to either an individual's genes or to the environment. Instead, it is the *interaction* of an individual's gene or genes with that person's environment that produces the disease.

One way to picture the interaction between an individual's genes and the environment is shown in Fig. 3-4. This is an overly simplified model of how the genes and environment *might* interact to cause a cancer. In this figure an individual's genetic susceptibility is depicted along the bottom of the graph by the numbers 1 through 5. Those who have little genetic susceptibility are represented by the numbers 1 and 2, while those with a great susceptibility are represented by the numbers 4 and 5. Environmental factors that can promote cancer (*insults*) are listed on the side, with 1 being the lowest and 5 the highest number of insults. An individual who has little genetic susceptibility (for example, 2 units) can withstand more environmental insults without developing cancer than can someone with a greater genetic susceptibility (for example, 5 units).

Of course, this figure is a model, not an accurate diagram of what actually happens. We do not know exactly how the genes and environment interact. For example, some individuals with 5 genetic susceptibility units may be far more susceptible to environmental agents of a given type, for example, radiation or a high-fat diet, than those with 4 units. We also do not know how many or which genes make an individual susceptible or even what many of the environmental insults are.

We have learned a great deal from changes in disease incidence over time as well as in migrating populations. Stomach cancer offers a good example of how a changing environment

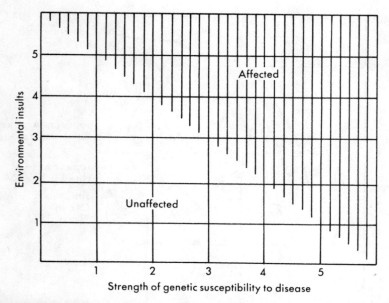

FIG. 3-4 Multifactorial inheritance—possible interaction of genes and environment on cancer susceptibility.

can result in a change in the incidence of a cancer. There has been a marked decrease in the incidence of stomach cancer in both men and women in the United States from 1935 to the present. It is thought that this decrease is largely a result of a change in diet. As food preservation techniques improved, individuals ate fewer highly salted and pickled foods, both of which are believed to increase the risks of stomach cancer. The genetic propensity of the population has probably stayed the same (for example, 3). However, the environmental insults decreased (for example, from 4 to 2) because of better food preservation methods, resulting in fewer stomach cancers in recent years.

SUSCEPTIBILITY TO COMMON CANCERS

Breast cancer

Breast cancer is the disease American women worry most about today. The American Cancer Society estimated that in 1983 114,000 cases of breast cancer occurred in American women.

The average women's lifetime risk of breast cancer is about 9%. To many people, this may seem an uncomfortably high risk; however, the 9% refers to the average woman's risk from birth to age 110. The average woman's risk to age 70 is about 6%; up to age 50 the risk is about 1.5%.

Age. Most people do not realize that the greatest risk factor for breast cancer is age (see Fig. 3-5). In the United States, as women get older, their risk of breast cancer increases. Women in a country such as Norway have a breast cancer incidence that also increases with age; however, the overall incidence of breast cancer in Norway is lower than that of the United States. Japan, on the other hand, has a lower incidence as well as a different pattern of occurrence; the incidence of breast cancer does not continue to rise with age.

Diet appears to play a part in the lower incidence of breast cancer in Japan. When Japanese women move to Hawaii and the continental

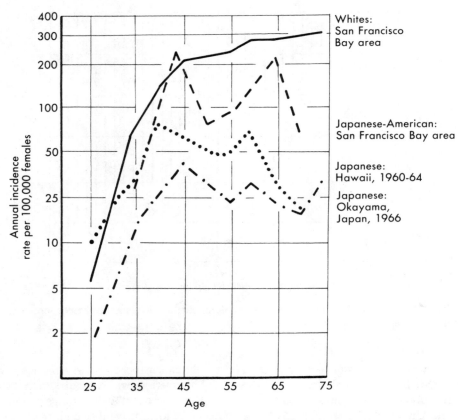

FIG. 3-5   Incidence of breast cancer in Japanese living in Japan, Hawaii, and the San Francisco Bay area. (Modified from Buell, P.: Changing incidence of breast cancer in Japanese-American women, JMCI **51**: 1479, 1973.)

United States, the incidence of breast cancer increases (Fig. 3-5). It is thought that as these people move, they give up their traditional eating patterns and change to a more Westernized diet that is higher in fat. Several studies have found that groups of people who eat a diet high in fat have a greater incidence of breast cancer than people whose diets are more lean. Rats and mice on high-fat diets also develop more mammary cancer than animals whose diets are low in fat.

Family history. For many years studies showed that women who had a mother or sister with breast cancer were two to three times more likely to have breast cancer than women who had no affected mother or sisters. More recently, the studies of D.E. Anderson have shown that all women who have a mother or sister with breast cancer are not necessarily at the same risk. In fact, two women who seem to have similar family histories can have very different risks.

In general, a woman's risk from family history is influenced by the ages at which her relatives were affected, if they had cancer in one or both breasts, and by the pattern of occurrence in the family. For example, in those few families where a woman's mother and grandmother had breast cancer before menopause and in both breasts, a woman's lifetime risk may be as high as 50%. The same woman's risk to age 50 would be much lower—about 10%. If a woman's mother and grandmother had breast cancer after menopause and each in only one breast, the lifetime risk is generally lower—about 16%.

Of course, other factors such as age, benign breast disease, age at birth of first child, age at menopause, and diet also influence a woman's risk of breast cancer. These two brief examples on family history only illustrate that the risks can be quite different in families that appear to have similar histories.

Colon cancer

Cancer of the colon and rectum is the second most common cancer in the United States. The American Cancer Society estimated that in 1983 there were about 89,100 new cases of this disease. The average risk of colon cancer to age 85 is about 3% for males and 4% for females.

There are several different types of colon cancer. One very rare type is associated with polyps (nodular growths of tissue) in the colon and is inherited as a dominant disease. If a parent has this type of colon cancer, the children have a 50% chance of also being affected. Fortunately, less than 1% of all colon cancers are of this type. Several other types of colon cancer are not associated with polyps but are also inherited as dominant traits. The dominantly inherited types of colon cancer tend to occur early—by about age 50. This contrasts with the later onset of colon cancer found in the general population—about age 70.

Colon cancer rates differ in different geographic areas. This suggests that environmental factors are important in promoting this type of cancer. When groups migrate from one area to another, they tend to take on the colon cancer incidence of the new area. Populations that move to an area of higher colon cancer incidence acquire a higher incidence themselves.

Populations that move to an area of lower incidence soon show a decrease in colon cancer rates.

Diet is thought to be one of the most important environmental factors affecting the incidence of colon cancer. Studies have shown that populations of people who eat more fiber and less fat have a lower incidence of colon cancer than do those who eat less fiber and more fat. Diets that are high in green leafy vegetables such as cabbage, broccoli, and brussels sprouts are also associated with decreased colon cancer rates.

However, an estimated one quarter of the colon cancers not associated with polyps are thought to have an appreciable genetic as well as environmental input. In most families this inheritance is thought to be of the multifactorial type, in which a gene or genes interact with the environment. These are termed "familial" colon cancers to distinguish them from the more rare and dominantly inherited colon cancers discussed earlier.

Interestingly, the familial colon cancers seem to arise in different parts of the colon than do those that occur sporadically and that are thought to be largely environmental in origin. Patients with a family history of colon cancer are far more likely to have cancer in the transverse or right side of the colon. Patients with no family history of colon cancer are more likely to have cancer in the left side of the colon. In groups that migrate from an area of low colon cancer incidence to an area of higher incidence, most of the increased incidence of colon cancer appears in the left, or nonfamilial, part of the colon.

Individuals who have a family history of colon cancer are often concerned about their risk and want to know what type of ongoing medical checkups they should have. An appropriate health plan can be devised based on the type of cancer their relatives had, the location in the colon, the ages of onset, and the pattern of occurrence in the family. If their risk is found to be increased, individuals will want to be followed regularly by a physician who specializes in diseases of the colon (an internist or proctologist). Because familial colon cancers occur more frequently in the right part of the colon, care must be taken to include this part of the colon in examinations.

Lung cancer

Lung cancer is the most common cancer in males and the most rapidly increasing cancer in females. The American Cancer Society estimated that in 1983 lung cancer constituted 22% of all cancers in men and 9% of those in women. (In contrast, colon and rectum cancers constituted an estimated 14% in men and 15% in women; breast cancer accounted for 26% of the cancer incidence in women.) From 1952 to 1978 the death rates from lung cancer increased 172% for men and 256% for women.

Lung cancer is a disease that most people as-

sociate with smoking and pollution, not family history. Yet studies show that genetics as well as environmental exposure play a role in susceptibility to lung cancer. One study compared the incidence of lung cancer in smokers and nonsmokers, some of whom had close relatives with lung cancer and some of whom did not. In this study nonsmokers with a family history of lung cancer were four times more likely to have lung cancer than were nonsmokers with no family history.

As might be expected, smokers had a higher incidence of lung cancer than nonsmokers. Smokers with no family history had a fivefold increase in risk. Smokers with a family history had a risk about 14 times greater than nonsmokers with no family history.

These differences in risk are shown in Fig. 3-6. If genetics played no role in lung cancer susceptibility, we would expect to find no difference in the risk of lung cancer in smokers

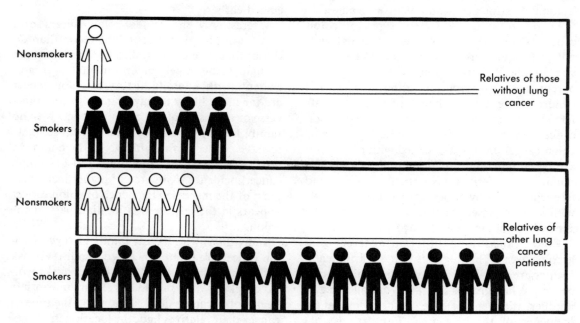

FIG. 3-6   Incidence of lung cancer in smokers and nonsmokers who do and do not have family history of lung cancer.

and nonsmokers, regardless of their family history. Instead, a difference was found, suggesting that both family history and smoking influence an individual's risk of lung cancer.

FAMILIAL AND NONFAMILIAL CANCERS

Can you tell whether the cancers in your family are caused more by genetic or more by environmental factors? No precise answer to this question is possible without a careful analysis by a medical geneticist. However, in general, cancers that are the result of an appreciable genetic component have the following characteristics:

1. Three or more close relatives in one family are affected with one or more types of cancer.
2. At least two generations are affected.
3. Cancer occurs at younger ages than in the general population.
4. Cancer develops anew in several parts of the body (not a spread from a single cancer).

Of course, a family could meet several of these criteria and still not have a strong genetic propensity. For example, if one is fortunate enough to have long-lived relatives, it is *quite* likely that several will have cancer. Usually, individuals who have older relatives with some of the more common cancers are not at significantly increased risk of cancer themselves.

Some rare families have a genetic propensity not just for breast cancer or colon cancer but for several different types of cancer in different family members. For example, in some families there is an increased susceptibility to breast and ovarian cancers or to breast and various types of gastrointestinal cancers. In such a family a sister might have breast cancer and her brother a gastrointestinal cancer. Although these families are rare, their detection is important because the genetic susceptibility to cancer can act as a dominant. Remember that in dominant inheritance the risk to a child of an affected person is about 50%.

Individuals with cancer in their family history may worry a great deal about their own or their relatives' cancer risks. In some cases they may feel doomed and without hope. It is important for these individuals to talk to a medical geneticist about their concern so they can learn what their risks really are. The unknown is usually far more frightening than the known.

Several centers that specialize in cancer risk analysis now exist in the United States. One of the first of these was instituted in 1981 at Mount Zion Hospital and Medical Center in San Francisco. Individuals come to the Stanton and Corinne Sobel Cancer Risk Analysis Service at Mount Zion Hospital to learn what their own risks are, to receive help in evaluating the significance of their risks, and to begin thinking about the type of health care program they would like to follow to ensure early detection of cancer.

An important part of the Cancer Risk Analysis Service is the concern for each individual's personal experiences, thoughts, and feelings about the cancer in his or her family. Individuals find that when they face their fears, when they are given the most up-to-date information, and when they realize that there is hope, they can set up an appropriate surveillance program with their physician and go on with the rest of their lives in a more content and productive manner.

TWO-HIT THEORY

Why are individuals from a family with a strong genetic propensity likely to have cancer at younger ages and in multiple locations? The two-hit theory of A.G. Knudson, Jr., proposes that two mutations or changes in the genes of a cell are needed for a cell to become malignant or cancerous. According to this theory, all cancers arise from two changes or hits to the genes in a cell. Sporadic or nonfamilial cancers are thought to result from two hits from the environment, both of which occur after birth (Fig. 3-7). Because time is required for two hits or

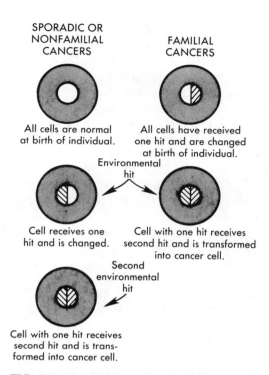

SPORADIC OR NONFAMILIAL CANCERS

FAMILIAL CANCERS

All cells are normal at birth of individual.

All cells have received one hit and are changed at birth of individual.

Environmental hit

Cell receives one hit and is changed.

Cell with one hit receives second hit and is transformed into cancer cell.

Second environmental hit

Cell with one hit receives second hit and is transformed into cancer cell.

FIG. 3-7 Knudson's two-hit theory.

changes to malignancy to occur, most nonfamilial cancers occur in older people.

According to the two-hit theory, familial cancers are also the result of two changes in the genes of a cell. However, in the familial cases the first change or hit occurs at or before conception so the individual is born with one cancer-predisposing change in every cell. Therefore, it takes only one more hit from the environment to produce the second change. Familial cancers occur earlier than nonfamilial cancers because

only one change after birth is needed for a malignancy to occur. This theory also explains why familial cancers are more likely to be multifocal, or to occur in several locations. Every cell of an individual from a cancer-prone family has received one hit before birth so only one more hit is needed from the environment to produce a second new cancer in any location in the body.

The two-hit theory provides us with one way of thinking about how genes and the environment might interact to produce both familial and nonfamilial cancers.

SUMMARY

Genetic susceptibility for some of the common cancers does exist. In rare families the genetic propensity is of the strong single-gene type. In such families a propensity to cancer is inherited as either a dominant or a recessive trait.

Fortunately, families with a strong genetic propensity to cancer are quite rare. In most families, the cancer is brought about by a complex interaction between an individual's genes and the environment.

New services are becoming available to give individuals more precise information about their cancer risk resulting from genetic and environmental factors. Based on the information they receive, individuals at risk can plan health care that will give them the security of knowing that if they should have a cancer, it will be detected in its early stages when treatments are most effective.

CHAPTER 4

Cancer Screening—
a Commonsense Approach

An ounce of prevention is worth a pound of cure.

MARY E. WHEAT
ERNEST H. ROSENBAUM

This book focuses on *primary prevention* of cancer—eliminating or avoiding the causes of cancer. It is primary prevention that is referred to in the still-valid saying quoted above. Cancer in particular is best totally prevented because it can involve many, many pounds of cure in terms of expense and physical discomfort. Cancers can be difficult to treat; some are not treatable; others respond successfully to treatment, but it may be costly and result in other negative side effects. Primary prevention of cancer is always the best choice *when it is still a choice.*

For some people primary prevention and lifestyle changes may start too late. Fortunately, there is a second line of defense against cancer—early detection. Cancer that is discovered early is more curable because it has had less time to spread (metastasize) to other parts of the body or to become enlarged in its original site, affecting nearby organs and body systems. Early detection or screening for cancer, called *secondary prevention,* is an effective means of preventing the consequences of cancer if the screening is appropriate. With early detection practices now used, cancer is one of the most

curable of the chronic diseases; more than half of all people who get cancer live more than 5 years—a better survival rate than patients with cirrhosis of the liver or severe heart disease.

This chapter deals with secondary prevention; it covers the general requirements for valid cancer screening methods and then discusses the specific cancers and tests appropriate for each. We will make screening recommendations for the general public as well as outline some specific recommendations for people at particular risk for individual cancers, such as heavy smokers for lung cancer.

Everyone should be concerned with cancer screening because cancer will eventually affect almost everyone in some way. According to present cancer rates, one in every four persons will eventually have cancer. Those statistical odds mean that someone close to you will have cancer even if you do not. Cancer also kills more children in the age group from 3 to 14 than any other disease. On the average more than 440,000 people die of cancer in the United States each year. Of these, the American Cancer Society estimates that 139,000, or 32% could be saved by "earlier diagnosis and prompt

---

Cancer's seven warning signals

Change in bowel or bladder habits
A sore that does not heal
Unusual bleeding or discharge
Thickening or lump in breast or elsewhere
Indigestion or difficulty in swallowing
Obvious change in wart or mole
Nagging cough or hoarseness

---

treatment." Knowledge of screening techniques can become the key to prolonged survival.

Cancer treatments are becoming more effective and the overall cancer cure rates are continuing to improve. A key factor in this success has been early detection, which often depends on individuals acting to ensure that they are screened for cancers according to the broadly accepted medical guidelines listed under each disease and summarized at the end of the chapter. We discuss screening by site of cancer because cancers in different body sites behave differently. However, certain principles, such as the value of early detection and treatment, apply to all cancers. The American Cancer Society warning signals summarize important changes that may be early signs of cancer (see boxed material).

SCREENING CRITERIA

Because early cancer detection leads to better chances for a successful cure, medical researchers try to develop tests and screening programs that will reveal cancer in people who do not yet have any physical symptoms. However, since resources are limited, choices must be made. We cannot screen everyone for everything. For this reason certain criteria must be set for a screening test or method to be considered useful. One of the most important criteria is incidence—the frequency of the cancer being sought. The disease may occur only in about 6500 out of approximately 300 million persons annually, as is the case with gallbladder cancer. Compare this with colon cancer, which is the second most common cause of cancer death in men and women and is found in 126,000 people each year. If you were asked to decide which disease should receive funds for developing a possible screening test, the choice would be simple—colon cancer.

Then a second set of criteria comes into play. A screening test must be sensitive, that is, accurate with few or no falsely normal results. It must also be specific—when a test is positive, it means that cancer is present and not some other disease process. These effective tests, once devised, must also be easy to use and available at a reasonable cost, or people will not make use of them.

An excellent example is occult blood testing of the stool for colon cancer. This costs less than $1 for the materials involved, is painless, and can be collected at home. Compare it to a colonoscopy, the visual examination of the entire large bowel using a flexible tube. This costs roughly $400 per person, requires 1 to 2 hours, involves some discomfort, and must be performed in a hospital or outpatient surgery setting. Colonoscopy would not be a good choice for mass cancer screening of asymptomatic people, whereas occult blood testing of the stool is.

Another factor to consider is whether or not early detection makes any difference. Does treatment started before the symptoms appear lead to an improved cure rate? If not, it is best to wait until the symptoms indicate the disease, since early detection and treatment offer no advantage. The decisive element in this decision is the growth rate of the cancer. Some cancers are slow growing and some grow very rapidly. A certain lung cancer, small cell cancer, can double in size in 20 days; with this kind of rapid growth, even very frequent and intensive screening in high-risk populations has failed to show any benefit of early diagnosis to patients. This particular cancer cannot yet be detected soon enough to improve survival, so intensive screening offers no advantage. However, with cervical cancer discovery of early lesions called *carcinoma in situ* (on the spot, not yet spread) can lead to a cure rate of more than 99%. Research has shown that cervical cancer progresses very slowly, remaining at the in situ stage for many years, which is why the Pap smear for the detection of cervical cancer has been so effective in reducing death rates from this cancer. Clearly cervical cancer is worth screening for *before* symptoms develop.

A final factor in designing or discovering a screening technique is that it be focused on the population at risk. This, too, is an economic consideration. For example, breast cancer is currently the most common cause of cancer death in American women—obviously a disease well worth screening for if the other conditions of effective testing can be met. Breast cancer also occurs in men, although rarely—about 1% of all cases. It would not make any sense to direct a screening program for breast cancer toward men. Another example is colon cancer, which is the second most common cause of cancer death in both men and women. However, colon cancer is rare in young people; almost all cases occur after age 40. In this case *age* is what determines the population at risk, and screening should be directed toward the appropriate age groups.

Specific risk factors can also be associated with a particular cancer, such as smoking with lung cancer or exposure to asbestos with lung cancer. People in high-risk groups for specific cancers need to be watched more closely if cancers are to be found early. High-risk factors are listed in this chapter under each individual cancer site.

A final consideration for screening is that the detection process be risk-free or of such low risk that it is balanced by the diagnostic value of the test. For example, use of mammography 15 years ago for detecting breast cancer involved an exposure of 7 rads (radiation absorbed dose) per x-ray evaluation, which had a potentially significant risk; the test itself might have increased the incidence of breast cancer. The technology of mammography has been greatly improved so that screening can now be done at under 0.5 rads and sometimes less than 0.1 rads. This is less than 10% of the former exposure and means that more than 10 mammographic examinations can now be done at the same risk as only one of the old-style evaluations.

Because cancer is actually a complex collection of many diseases, each with particular characteristics and growth patterns, and because of the many criteria that must be met for an effective screening program, the screening systems we have evolved so far all have some limitations. The ideal cancer detection test would be 100% sensitive for diagnosis with few false positives, would have no psychologic or physical trauma, would cost very little, and would test for a fatal or serious disease that could be successfully treated when detected early.

The closest example of this ideal test is the Pap smear for cervical cancer. This cancer is frequently fatal if not diagnosed in a localized stage but is almost completely curable with early detection. The Pap smear meets most criteria for a good screening test: it is readily available, relatively inexpensive, and easy to perform and interpret. It also offers a high level of consistently accurate results, and false positives are not common. Falsely normal results because of inadequate sampling can, however, be a problem. It also meets the test of improved survival. Since Pap testing has been widely used, death rates from cervical cancer have fallen by more than 50%. Before this there had been a steady increase.

OBSTACLES TO
EFFECTIVE CANCER SCREENING

Three factors contribute to the difficulty of obtaining good screening results: (1) no tests have yet been developed for detecting some cancers, (2) people do not always use available screening, and (3) the effectiveness of early detection is sometimes hard to establish. The first factor relates to cancers deep in the body tissue, which at present are only discovered when they have grown large enough to cause symptoms to appear, that is, the individual notices something different. By that time the cancer may have spread and become implanted in other areas as well. Examples are pancreatic cancer and ovarian cancer, for which there are at this time no effective early detection techniques.

When an inexpensive and sound test exists and is readily available but still not used, then screening is still ineffective. Thus noncompliance may invalidate the most effective screening tests medical science can devise. People have to use appropriate screening techniques for them to work. Sometimes this means conducting an education program to promote the value of a screening technique, such as the stool test for occult blood in finding early colon cancer, the Pap smear for detecting early cervical cancer, or the breast self-examination for finding abnormal breast changes.

Finally, it is sometimes difficult to tell whether or not early detection of a particular cancer does make a difference in the cure rate. For example, a short-term test of a screening device may indicate that those screened lived 2 years beyond diagnosis, whereas those not screened who turned out to have the same cancer only lived 1 year. The question is, did the early detection make a difference because of treatment or did it just identify the patients a year earlier and thus make it appear they had lived longer? This second explanation is called *lead-time bias,* and to avoid making judgments on the basis of this, cancer detection and treatment studies must last a long time. That is why cancer statistics are usually reported in terms of 5-year disease-free survival periods. By 5 years the effect from lead-time bias will usually have evened out.

Another essential factor in assessing the effectiveness of early detection programs is a comparison group—people similar to the group screened who were not screened. This comparability of groups can be established by first selecting a given population and then randomly assigning individuals from this population to the screening group or the control group.

Even though one out of four Americans will be diagnosed with cancer sometime in his or her lifetime, any given cancer occurs in a relatively small proportion of the population, and even fewer people die of it. This means that thousands of people have to be studied and followed for many years to demonstrate the effectiveness of any screening program. Research such as this is very expensive in terms of both time and labor. For this reason we do not always have as much data as we would like to determine the best detection policy for a particular cancer. Given those limits, we must choose the most reasonable and cost-effective policy for a given cancer based on the information we do have. This is not to say that research has stopped in this area. Many highly qualified individuals continue to work toward better cancer-screening techniques all the time. Furthermore, changes in screening recommendations are made toward greater cost-effectiveness whenever the safety level can be maintained (see "Cervical cancer" later in this chapter). The bottom line, however, is that primary prevention—avoiding known causes of cancer entirely—is still the most effective approach to cancer prevention. Preventive techniques, such as no-smoking programs and patient education regarding known risk factors, should be included in every cancer-screening program.

COLON CANCER

When men and women are considered together, colon cancer is the major cause of cancer mortality in the United States; in 1983 an estimated 126,000 new cases were diagnosed and 57,100 individuals died of this disease. Only lung cancer in men and breast cancer in women cause a greater number of cancer deaths. However, colon cancer, like breast cancer, shows significant improvement in cure if diagnosed early. This makes screening for colon cancer important. (See Fig. 4-1.)

Risk factors

As with many cancers, the incidence of colon cancer increases with age: 95% of all cases occur in people over 45. Dietary habits also appear to be important, based on worldwide studies of colon cancer incidence. In Africa, where people eat a very high-fiber diet of fruits, vegetables, and grains with relatively little meat protein and fat, there is a much lower incidence of colon cancer. One of the factors may be the stool *transit time*—the time it takes for waste products from food to pass through the bowel. Another factor is bulk. Africans have much greater stool bulk and faster transit times—three times shorter than the average Westerner. The normal 3-day transit time in the United States means that any carcinogens present in the food we eat, either as additives or toxic substances (bile salts) produced by the body during digestion, are in contact with the bowel for a longer time, possibly encouraging the development of cancer. Lower bulk means that these carcinogens are in closer contact with the bowel wall as well.

In spite of the association of colon cancer with diet, recommendations for specific foods are not yet available. Thus far it seems wise to avoid a high-fat, high–red meat diet and to follow instead one that includes lots of fiber from fruits, vegetables, and grains.

Certain diseases are also associated with an increased incidence of colon cancer, such as *ulcerative colitis* (when present for more than 10 years), the hereditary disease *Gardner's syndrome,* and familial *polyposis,* in which hundreds of *polyps* (stalklike protrusions of bowel tissue into the center of the intestine) are present throughout the colon. Individuals with these conditions require special and frequent evaluation by their physicians because they are at higher risk of developing colon cancer. An annual sigmoidoscopic examination of the colon with a flexible tube may be required. Occult blood testing may be less helpful in this subset of the population because the underlying condition itself means that blood is often present.

Warning signs

Unfortunately, symptoms from colon cancer are often not noticeable until the disease has spread beyond the limits of the bowel wall. If this happens and the cancer has spread to nearby lymph nodes, the survival rate at 5 years is reduced to about 25%; if distant organs such as the liver or lung are involved, the rate is only 5%. Conversely, the survival rate is nearly 100% if the cancer is localized to the bowel wall lining (mucosa) when discovered.

Symptoms to consult your physician include:

Abdominal pain that lasts more than 1 or 2 weeks
Difficulty in passing stools or a change in bowel
   habits or stool size
Blood in the stool or very dark (black) stools
A mass or lump in the abdomen

These symptoms do not mean you have colon cancer; for example, an individual can have blood in the stool because of hemorrhoids. However, if these signs appear, consult your physician for follow-up. Early cancers may only bleed intermittently; therefore, if you ever notice blood in your stool, even if it disappears, you should see your physician.

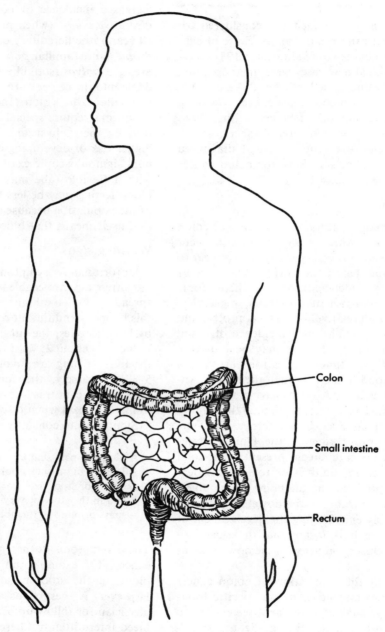

FIG. 4-1 Anatomy of colon and rectum. (Redrawn from What you need to know, U.S. Department of Health and Human Services, Public Health Service/National Institute of Health.)

Screening

Fortunately, colon cancers are slow-growing; there is usually a significant period during which they can be detected by screening techniques *before* actual symptoms appear. Three tests are available to detect colon cancer before it becomes symptomatic. The first is the digital rectal examination by a physician or nurse practitioner. The second is testing the stool for occult (microscopic) blood. The third is sigmoidoscopy, which involves using a specially designed flexible instrument (hollow tube) to view the interior of the bowel and remove polyps if any are found.

In the *digital rectal examination* a gloved finger is used to examine the rectum (the last 5 or 6 inches [12.5 or 15 centimeters] of the colon) for any lumps or masses; the prostate gland in men can be examined at the same time. Testing for occult blood can be done at this time, but this test should also be done at home after the individual has followed a preparatory diet. The examiner's finger can potentially cause some microtrauma that shows blood, or something the patient has eaten can cause a false-positive test result. In addition, a single specimen of stool is not an adequate sample, since blood in the stool from a very early cancer or polyp may be only intermittent.

The *occult blood test* done at home requires the patient to use wooden sampling sticks and to smear a small amount of stool on special filter cards. These are stored in a cardboard container in a cool, dry place until brought to the physician or screening center within 5 days. The American Cancer Society currently recommends that two stool samples be collected each day over 3 days. Some authorities say that three stool samples total will yield virtually the same benefit at a much lower total cost of screening.

Occult blood screening appears to meet most of the necessary criteria for effective screening. It is readily available and inexpensive; materials for six tests cost about $1, and patients are generally charged between $2 and $10 for processing. The incidence of false positives, with no abnormality found on follow-up evaluation, is only about 2% when the appropriate diet has been followed before the test. Certain foods may cause the same changes in the filter paper as occult blood does, giving a false-positive result. For this reason, it is necessary to follow a restricted diet for 3 days before the test and while you are sampling your stools.

The specific diet requirements are no meat, no vitamin C, and a high-fiber diet that includes cooked rather than raw vegetables. High-fiber foods are primary foods such as fruits, vegetables, whole grains, cereals, and bran. Vitamin C has been shown to cause occasional false-negative tests, and meat protein and the peroxidases in large amounts of raw vegetables can cause the occult blood test to be falsely positive. It is important to avoid these foods while you are testing.

Many large-scale studies have proved the benefit of occult blood testing in detecting colon cancer. In one study 48,000 people between the ages of 50 and 80 have used occult blood screening every year or every two years. Of the cancers found thus far in the screened group, 63% have been localized, compared to only 15% among the control group not screened. In a cancer that is almost totally curable in the localized stage, a screening device this effective should be used as widely as possible.

Recently, however, several large-scale trials of stool occult blood *mass screening* have been the subject of much controversy. Questions of the efficiency of the test under these conditions, which did not include personal physician contact, have been raised by the American Cancer Society, The National Cancer Institute, and other professional bodies. It is important to realize, however, that this controversy centers around *compliance* and *use* of the occult blood test, not its technical effectiveness. When used as we have recommended, it has been shown to be effective.*

*For further information on occult blood mass screening, contact the San Francisco Regional Cancer Foundation, Building 1805, San Francisco, CA 94129.

The final screening test is *sigmoidoscopy,* and it may be performed along with an x-ray examination (barium enema) if there is reason to suspect a malignancy. Sigmoidoscopy involves looking at the bowel through a tube with a light and a magnified viewing system that is much like a telescope. The newest flexible sigmoidoscopes can reach 24 inches (55 to 60 centimeters) into the colon with less discomfort to the patient than earlier rigid instruments that only reached up to 10 inches (25 centimeters). With the new instruments, a biopsy can also be performed, or a small polyp can be removed entirely without any additional surgery. Performed by an experienced person, it usually takes 5 to 10 minutes for the actual examination and can be done in an office setting. Because the bowel must be clean to be clearly visible, the patient uses any laxatives and enemas before the test as instructed by the physician. There is very little risk involved when the test is performed by an experienced examiner — only a one-in-several-thousand chance of perforating the bowel wall.

The improved reach of the flexible sigmoidoscope (24 as compared to 10 inches) is also important because currently more polyps and cancers are found in the higher portions of the bowel. Forty years ago 75% of all masses were located in the lower 10 inches of the colon; now that figure is only 50%.

Sigmoidoscopy is recommended for independent screening as well as for follow-up on a positive test for occult blood. In a large 25-year study of 18,000 patients over age 45 who received repeated sigmoidoscopic examinations, including removal of any polyps that were found, only 13 colon cancers were found in the group. This represented 15% of the 87 cancers that would normally have been expected using average colon cancer statistics. Although this was not a controlled study, such a dramatic decline in cancer incidence indicates a clear benefit of sigmoidoscopy. Furthermore, many scientists believe it suggests that colon polyps may

evolve into cancer, although this remains somewhat controversial. In any event, sigmoidoscopy dramatically decreased the incidence of cancer in this large study, and it is considered a beneficial test in colon cancer screening. It should also be performed in any patient who has a positive occult blood test, as should a colon x-ray examination *(barium enema).* In large studies when sigmoidoscopy was performed on people who have never had it before, polyps or cancer were found in 1 in 630 examinations. When the test was repeated in people who had had it done previously, no matter how long before, the incidence dropped to 1 in 4400 examinations.

If a polyp is found on sigmoidoscopy, a good radiographic examination (barium enema) is an essential follow-up. If one lesion is found anywhere in the colon or rectum, the chance of another mass or polyp being present increases from two to five times. Any polyp or mass means the entire colon is at an increased risk. Pathologists have also recognized that the larger a polyp, the more likely it is to contain cancer. Those less than 0.5 centimeter (about $\frac{1}{5}$ inch) carry a cancer incidence of less than 1%; those larger than 3.5 centimeters (about $1\frac{3}{8}$ inches) have a cancer incidence of 29%. *Adenomas* are also risk factors; these are growth changes in the glandular mucosal lining of the bowel that are considered premalignant.

When a barium enema is used for radiographic examination, it should be a *double-contrast (air-contrast) enema,* in which both the dye substance and air are used to outline the surface of the bowel. A number of studies have shown that the chance of missing a small polyp or mass declined from about 25% to 5% when the double-contrast procedure was used.

When no cancer or polyp is found after sigmoidoscopy and a good barium enema examination, one can be virtually certain that no large polyp or cancer is present. A small polyp may have been missed, however, particularly in the right side of the colon, although, as we have said, there is less than a 1% chance that a polyp this size will contain cancer. A colonoscope can be used to see the right side of the colon, but the test is expensive and carries a somewhat higher risk of complications (1:1000), although it is still a very safe procedure. Also, colonoscopy may require admission to the hospital, depending on local community practice. This procedure would probably be used only on patients with a history of colon cancer, polyps, adenomas, or a family history of colon cancer. It should also be used in patients with long-standing ulcerative colitis or other major risk factors. You should discuss with your physician whether colonoscopy would be indicated for you in the follow-up of a positive stool occult blood test.

Summary and recommendations

Cancer of the colon is a common disease; screening should be done on a regular basis before any symptoms occur. Controlled studies have shown that reduced mortality occurs when screening procedures such as the digital rectal examination and sigmoidoscopy are used. Other research has shown that periodic occult blood testing detects colon cancer at an earlier and hence more curable stage. The combination of these three available screening techniques should significantly improve the cure rate for this most common cancer.

Current American Cancer Society recommendations suggest two sigmoidoscopic examinations 1 year apart after age 40, followed by examinations every 3 years after that. Many authorities point out that this will not be acceptable to patients because of expense and discomfort and would cost several billion dollars to implement if done for all Americans over 40. Because of the difference in yield between initial and repeat sigmoidoscopy (1/630 compared to 1/4400), it is thought that with the additional screening potential of occult blood testing, sigmoidoscopy can be done much less frequently. We agree with this second approach, as long as the occult blood testing is negative. Of course,

---

> **Recommendations for colon cancer screening**
>
> ════════════════
>
> 1. Have digital rectal examination annually beginning at age 40 (including prostate checkup for men).
> 2. Begin annual stool occult blood testing (three to six cards, with appropriate diet) at age 50.
> 3. Have sigmoidoscopy with flexible sigmoidoscope at age 55 and every 10 years thereafter.
> 4. If at higher risk (including personal or family history of colon cancer or polyps; Gardner's syndrome, familial polyposis; long-standing ulcerative colitis), begin annual sigmoidoscopic or colonoscopic examinations at an earlier age. Discuss with your physician whether colonoscopy or sigmoidoscopy is indicated for you.

---

individuals at increased risk, such as from ulcerative colitis or familial polyposis, or those with prior history of colon cancer or polyps should have sigmoidoscopy or colonscopy much more frequently (at least annually) and should be followed closely by their physicians. (See boxed material.)

LUNG CANCER

Lung cancer is not only one of the most common cancers in both men and women, it is also one of the deadliest. Only 8% of those diagnosed as having lung cancer survive for 5 years. Lung cancer is the most common cause of cancer death in men and the third most common in women. Unfortunately, its incidence in women is rising, since the effects of increased smoking are beginning to show up in women's lung cancer rates. Scientists estimate that by 1985 it will be *the* most common cause of cancer death in

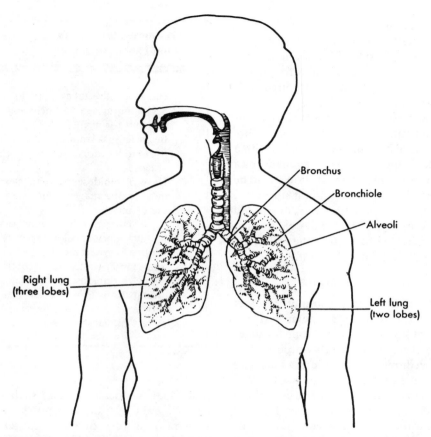

FIG. 4-2   Anatomy of lungs. (Redrawn from What you need to know, U.S. Department of Health and Human Services, Public Health Service/National Institute of Health.)

women. In 1983 an estimated 135,000 new cases were diagnosed and 117,000 people died of lung cancer. One of the main reasons lung cancer is so deadly is that only 20% of lung cancers are diagnosed while they are still in the localized stage when they could possibly be treated more successfully. (See Fig. 4-2.)

Risk factors

Perhaps 90% of all lung cancers result from environmental carcinogens—things we inhale from the air into our lungs. The most common exposure is tobacco, specifically cigarettes. The danger of lung cancer increases with exposure; the more you smoke, the greater your risk.

Other environmental carcinogens play a role in lung cancer, but a far smaller portion of the population is exposed to them so that the impact of these elements, some of which are as deadly as tobacco, is far less. The lungs are particularly vulnerable to airborne carcinogens because with each breath we take, more than 60 square yards (48 square meters) of lung surface are exposed to potential pollutants.

A number of substances found in industrialized and urban areas have been linked to lung cancer, including coal and tar fumes, petroleum oil mists, lead products, copper and zinc smelting by-products, asbestos dust, uranium dust, and arsenic. Many of the cars and industries that generate these poisons are concentrated in urban areas, making urban dwellers slightly more at risk. However, researchers estimate that only a small percentage (about 1% to 2%) of lung cancer cases can be attributed to urban air pollution. Moving to the countryside may not provide any additional protection, since current agricultural practices make extensive use of insecticides that also include a number of known carcinogens.

An additional risk factor with lung cancer is the possible additive or interactive effects of various exposures. Nonsmoking asbestos workers, for example, have a sevenfold increase in the rate of lung cancer over nonsmokers in general. If they smoke as well, their relative risk increases up to 40 to 90 times.

It is often hard to assess the cancer risk of a particular substance or to determine if it is linked to cancer because there can be a long time between exposure and the subsequent development of cancer. The most famous example is people who were exposed to asbestos when they worked in shipyards during World War II. Increased lung cancer rates first turned up for these people 20 years later. If a large population has not been exposed, as in the shipyards case, it may be very difficult to trace back to a particular occupation or environmental exposure that took place years before (see Chapter 8).

The final risk factor for lung cancer, age, is also related to the lag time between exposure and development of the disease. Lung cancer is not a disease of young people. It occurs primarily in people between ages 40 and 80, with the decade between age 50 and 59 having the greatest number of cases. However, the most striking increase in cases is occurring in the 60 to 80 age-group.

Individuals at risk for lung cancer are those over age 40 who smoke and/or have a history of occupational exposure to carcinogens, such as uranium miners or asbestos or petrochemical workers. During the past decade OSHA (Occupational Safety and Health Act) has worked to establish threshold limits for known carcinogens in the workplace. Physicians trained specifically in occupational medicine will be increasingly valuable in identifying people at risk so we can work to make job sites safer by reducing environmental exposure (primary prevention) as well as by instituting more intensive and well directed follow-up (secondary prevention).

Warning signs

The following symptoms do *not* mean you have lung cancer; they mean you should contact your doctor for a discussion and evaluation of the symptom(s):

Persistent cough
Chest pain with breathing or coughing
Sputum or phlegm streaked with blood
Recurring bronchitis, pneumonia, or other respiratory illness
Persistent hoarseness

Screening

Two tests are currently available to screen for lung cancer—the chest x-ray film and sputum cytology examination. Unfortunately, neither has proved particularly effective in helping us find lung cancer early enough to make much difference in the survival rate. The survival rate of lung cancer does depend on the stage at diagnosis; when an individual is discovered to have an isolated malignant lung nodule with no evidence of disease spread outside the lung, surgery is performed and there is a 5-year survival rate of 40%. Overall, however, the survival rate for lung cancer is only 8% after 5 years, in part because only 20% of cases are diagnosed in a localized stage.

The kind of cancer is relevant to the survival rate as well. Lung cancers include epidermoid or squamous cell cancer, small cell cancer, adenocarcinoma, and large cell cancer. Each of these behaves in different ways. Squamous cell cancer is most strongly associated with smoking and represents 30% to 40% of the cancers in high-risk individuals. These cancers usually grow in the large bronchi or breathing tubes near the trachea. They can be very difficult to detect on an x-ray film until some spread has occurred. However, because many do occur centrally, abnormal cells may be shed that can be found in sputum cytology tests (lung Pap tests).

Small cell cancer is an aggressive tumor, growing rapidly and spreading early. Only about 10% of individuals who have this cancer live for 5 years. No screening test yet works to find small cell cancer early enough for surgery to be effective. Treatment has improved, however, and it is possible that increasingly effective chemotherapy will help control small cell cancer until better screening techniques are available.

Adenocarcinoma typically arises in the periphery of the lung, where it can be detected at a relatively early stage by chest x-ray film. It is not associated with smoking, although it may be associated with scars in the lung from earlier infection or previous surgery. Sputum cytology rarely detects this type of lung cancer. Large cell cancer of the lung also occurs in the peripheral areas and can more easily be detected by x-ray film than by sputum cytology. Peripheral

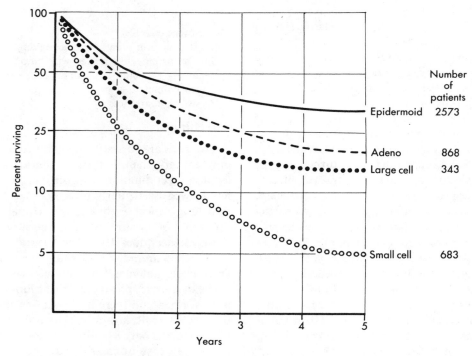

FIG. 4-3 Postsurgical survival in relation to cell types in patients with lung cancer. (Modified from Selawry, O.S., and Hansen, H.H.: Lung cancer. In Holland, J.F., and Frei, E., III: Cancer medicine, ed. 2, Philadelphia, 1982, Lea & Febiger.)

cancers are difficult to detect by cytology because the abnormal cells must travel a greater distance to reach the sputum.

Survival for these different kinds of lung cancer varies considerably, as can be seen from Fig. 4-3.

As you can tell from this discussion, neither of the tests for lung cancer detects all the possible types, so that the two tests may be best used in a complementary way. The x-ray film can distinguish peripheral lesions more easily than central ones because the central shadows of the heart and blood vessels can mask small lung cancers. Sputum cytology, however, may be more effective for centrally located cancers, usually squamous cell cancers, because abnormal cells can reach the sputum more easily.

To perform the *sputum cytology examination,* sputum is collected over a 3-day period and then examined under the microscope for abnormal cells. Even if the test shows cancer, it does not indicate where the cancer is located. If the chest x-ray film does not indicate a lesion, the entire lung has to be examined by means of fiberoptic bronchoscopy. This involves using a flexible, telescopic tube to view the interior of the lungs. If abnormalities are found, cell samples can be taken by both brushings and washings. In the case of a definite mass or ulceration, a biopsy can be done. If no abnormalities are seen in the bronchi, washings and brushings are taken from different areas of the lungs to determine where the cancer cells originated. These procedures can be lengthy and costly, sometimes involving a stay of several days in the hospital.

Summary and recommendations

Over the past several decades, eight major studies have assessed the effectiveness of lung cancer screening, and so far no screening program has been shown to reduce lung cancer deaths. Large programs have been run at the Mayo Clinic, Johns Hopkins University, and the Sloan-Kettering Clinic. At the Mayo Clinic intensive evaluation, using chest x-ray films and sputum cytologies every 4 months, has been done since 1971 for heavy smokers over age 45. Even though there has been an increase in the number of cancers detected in a localized stage (from 20% in the control group to 50% in the screened group), there has been no improvement in the survival rate.

In addition to not prolonging survival, mass screening of all smokers over 45 done according to the Mayo Clinic procedures would cost in excess of several billion dollars annually. In other words, mass screening for lung cancer at present is not worth the cost and effort, as it has had no demonstrable positive effects. Individuals who are at risk, however, such as heavy smokers and people with occupational exposure, may decide through consultation with their physicians that individual screening is appropriate. If recommended, only the 4-month screening interval has increased the number of cancers found in a localized stage.

The best approach to controlling lung cancer is not to smoke or to quit smoking, since quitting does make a health difference if maintained. Lung cancer rates slowly return to just above normal if an individual quits smoking for 15 years. Lung cancer cannot be effectively detected or treated at present; we must rely on prevention. (See boxed material.)

**Recommendations for
lung cancer prevention and screening**

1. Do not smoke.
2. Be aware of occupational risks.
3. If at risk (over age 45 and a smoker or a worker with occupational exposure), discuss possible screening with your physician.

BREAST CANCER

Breast cancer is the foremost cause of cancer deaths in women, according to the National Cancer Institute survey. Yet, breast cancer is a disease that lends itself to earlier diagnosis and therefore more successful treatment. In 1983 an estimated 114,900 new cases of breast cancer were diagnosed and 37,500 women died from this disease. It is estimated that 1 in 11 American women will have breast cancer sometime in her lifetime. Unlike lung cancer, however, the survival rate for breast cancer can be very high *if* it is detected early when the disease is localized without lymph node involvement. Currently, of those who have breast cancer, 50% will be cured through surgery and/or radiotherapy. Using early detection methods, this cure rate can be raised to as high as 80% to 90%.

Women particularly at risk are those who have already had breast cancer or those who have a sister or mother who has had breast cancer, especially if the relative's cancer occurred before menopause and in both breasts. Breast cancer also appears to be a hormone related cancer. Its incidence is increased in women who first have children after age 30 (this means they have had more continuous stimulation with the female hormone estrogen), or who have never had children, and slightly increased in those who start menstruating early (before age 11) or who enter menopause late (after age 55). Early menstruation and late menopause also reflect the estrogen influence. There has not, however, been an increased incidence of breast cancer noted in users of oral contraceptives.

Recently, there has been an association between breast cancer and obesity and high-fat diets. This does not mean that obesity or a high-fat diet cause cancer, only that there is an association between the two.

In summary, risk factors for breast cancer include:

1. Prior history of breast cancer
2. Family history of breast cancer (mother or sisters)
3. First child conceived after age 30 or no children
4. Early menstruation (before age 11) or late menopause (after age 55)
5. High-fat diet or obesity (?)

Warning signs

Since 1 of 11 women will probably have breast cancer, it is important that every woman know the signs. These symptoms do not mean that you have breast cancer, but they do suggest that you should consult your physician:

Any lump or thickening of the breast
Any swelling, dimpling, or skin irritation
Change in the shape of the breast
Discharge from the nipple
Any retraction or scaliness of the nipple
Any change or tenderness that lasts beyond that normally associated with the menstrual period

It is important to realize that of every 10 lumps found in breast tissue, eight are not malignant, that is, are not cancer. But they are your early warning system and should be reported promptly.

When a new lump is found, mammography (a soft tissue x-ray film of the breast) is done and a biopsy may be performed. This will determine whether the tissue is cancerous or benign; 4 of 5 biopsies are benign. A pathologist examines, interprets, and diagnoses tissue samples. If the tumor is benign, no treatment is necessary and only observation is required. If it is malignant, then the individual consults with her physician in a decision-making process, with the recommended treatment depending on the pathology, the size of the lesion, and whether obvious spread to the lymph nodes under the armpit has occurred. The form of treatment has to be decided: surgery, radiation, or possibly chemotherapy. The smaller the cancer, the more treatment options that exist. For small (less than 1 inch, or 2.5 centimeters) cancers that have not obviously spread to the lymph nodes, both less extensive surgery—*lumpectomy,* or segmental resection *(tylectomy)*—and radiation therapy have been shown to be as effective as the more extensive surgical procedures previously used.

In any case, the lymph nodes should be sampled because this gives important information about additional treatment that may be required, and about the prognosis. Even if the entire breast needs to be removed, with modern techniques the surgeon can already plan for reconstructive plastic surgery. Breast cancer does not have to result in the permanent loss of a breast.

Many discussions are held at this point if cancer is diagnosed, and a medical evaluation is indicated, including specific scans, a chest x-ray film, blood chemical tests, and further information on the hormonal status of the tissue that was removed, known as an estrogen receptor assay. The receptor assay can give predictive information regarding both aggressiveness of the tumor and potential success of hormonal therapy.*

The most important thing to remember is that when you find a new lump, you need to have a diagnosis made as soon as possible. You should see your physician promptly. Depending on your physical examination, he or she may re-examine you immediately after your period. If the lump persists, other tests (mammography and biopsy) will generally be done. If the lump is cancer, then a more extensive evaluation is performed and an appropriate decision for therapy in each case is recommended. It is also important to appreciate that cancer may involve both breasts in approximately 10% to 15% of women, and thus the other breast merits more careful observation each year.

Screening

There are three common and effective early detection techniques for breast cancer in women. One is free and you can do it yourself —breast self-examination (BSE). The other two are breast examination by a physician or nurse and mammography.

*In California, state law requires that a woman be informed of the different methods of treating breast cancer whenever the diagnosis is made. See Appendix D for a full statement of these alternatives.

Mammography is the most technical and expensive; it is complementary to physical examination, since it can discover as many as 30% to 40% of nodules not yet detectable by palpation, or touch. Mammographic techniques have improved dramatically in recent years. Older two-view mammography released 5 to 7 rads (a measure of radiation dose), whereas current xeromammography only releases about 0.5 rads. Even more exciting is the new low-dose screen film technique whereby radiologists use a single-purpose x-ray machine developed solely for breast examinations. When gentle pressure is used to compress the breast tissue, only 0.1 rads are released for the two-view examination. Using these newest techniques, between 40 and 60 mammographic examinations can be done for the same radiation exposure as a single examination 15 years ago. The original higher dose of radiation was considered a risk factor and received a lot of negative publicity, but the new low-dose mammograms are much safer. The mammogram can be used for a baseline after a woman presents with suspicious symptoms, or it may be used as a primary screening technique. You should discuss with your physician what kind of mammography is available in your community.

The American Cancer Society recommends a baseline mammographic examination between ages 35 and 40, with mammography every 1 to 2 years beginning at age 40 and annually after age 50 in average-risk women.

There are other less common screening tests for tumors as well. *Ultrasound* is the most important of these. It uses sound waves in a radar-like technique to examine the sound waves in the interior of the breast and involves no radiation exposure. Its effectiveness is currently being compared to better studied tests such as mammography, and researchers are very hopeful that it will prove helpful in the examination of younger women, whose dense breasts are more difficult to examine with mammography.

Another technique is *thermography,* which involves measurement of heat from various areas of the breast to detect warmer areas that may reflect increased metabolism or tumors. This does not involve radiation exposure but has been much less reliable than mammography or physical examination, with a number of false-positive and false-negative tests. *Diaphanoscopy* involves the use of light for transillumination through tissues to detect nonpalpable breast lumps and to evaluate palpable lumps by the shadows they cast. It is still experimental for detection of nonpalpable tumors, although it can be helpful in differentiating benign from malignant masses. However, it is not as yet a procedure to be used in place of x-ray mammography, which has been and remains the technical keystone for diagnosis of breast cancer. Further evaluation must be done of both diaphanoscopy and thermography to establish their reliability.

Breast self-examination and medical examination are similar procedures, except that self-examination can be done monthly by the individual at home, and a medical examination is done less frequently by a medical practitioner. The technique is described in detail here, but we also recommend that you ask your physician or nurse to teach you the technique on a one-to-one basis, as this has been found to be the most effective approach. There may also be special clinics in your area to teach women this simple, effective technique as well.

Screening for breast cancer works. A large study done by the Health Insurance Plan of Greater New York (HIP) over a 5-year period in the 1960s showed approximately a 30% decrease in mortality for women over age 50 who were screened versus those who were not. The screening process involved both mammography and breast examination by medical personnel. One third of the cancers were found by mammography alone in women over age 50. Since then, mammography has improved even more. Not only is the radiation exposure much less, but the ability to detect small cancers has increased. Beginning in 1973, the American Cancer Society

screened 280,000 women through the 27 centers of the Breast Cancer Demonstration Detection Project (BCDDP). In this study 41% of cancers were found by mammography alone (compared to 33% in the HIP study). The most dramatic increase was noted in women *under* age 50, among whom 85% of all cancers were detected by mammography, compared to 38% in the HIP study. Furthermore, in the BCDDP study the percentage of cancers detected in a localized (without lymph node spread) stage had increased from 70% to 80%. Reports from the BCDDP and other studies also suggest that women who perform regular breast self-examination find their cancers at an earlier (and thus more curable) stage.

The important thing to remember is that physical examination and mammography are complementary. Even though mammography has improved, it is no substitute for physical examination. More cancers have been found earlier when *all* detection methods have been combined than when any one is used in isolation.

Breast self-examination

Breast self-examination (BSE), if used routinely, represents an important opportunity for each woman to protect herself from the possibly devastating effects of breast cancer. The examination is painless, takes little time, and costs nothing. It may save your life. The advantage of doing it regularly (monthly) is that you develop a sense of how your breasts normally feel and thus will be able to tell if there are any changes. Most breast lumps are noted by women themselves, not by their physicians or nurse practitioners. If you find a change, you should consult your physician promptly. Also, as shown in the BCDDP, for women who do develop breast cancer, those who practice BSE often find their cancers at an earlier, more curable stage.

The first step is timing. Examine your breast just after your period has ended, preferably about the same time each month. You will have

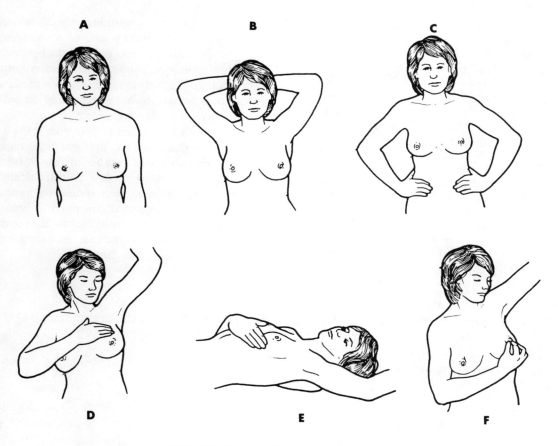

FIG. 4-4 Breast self-examination (BSE).

fewer hormones affecting your breast at this time. If you do not menstruate, choose a specific day of the month. One woman uses the first of the month—she waters her plants, does a self-examination, and pays her bills all the same day. The BSE procedure follows:

1. Examine your breast standing or sitting in front of a mirror for any change in shape or alteration in the skin of the breast (Fig. 4-4, *A*). Clasp your hands behind your head or raise them over your head and look for the same things (Fig. 4-4, *B*). Lean forward a little and look again to see if there is any puckering of the skin or changes in the nipples or in the general

contour. Put your hands on your hips and tighten your arm and chest muscles, again looking for any changes (Fig. 4-4, *C*).

2. Some women do this next part in the shower after soaping themselves, because they can feel the tissue of the breast more clearly. Others do the viewing sitting up and then lie down for the second part; some lie down and do the whole thing. The main focus of this part of the examination is to feel for unusual lumps that were not there before. If this is your first self-examination, keep in mind that some women have naturally lumpy breasts and you may be one of them. Your physician can tell you if all the lumps are the usual kind, and you can also be-

come familiar with your own breasts and their relative lumpiness. Starting with three or four fingers of one hand held flat, examine the opposite breast by pressing the flat part of your fingers over a small part of the breast. Have the arm on the side you are examining up over your head (Fig. 4-4, *D*) and a pillow under your shoulder if you are lying down (Fig. 4-4, *E*). This flattens the breast and makes it easier to examine. Moving in circles this way, go from the outside edge around the breast and slowly in toward the nipple. Do not forget the area between the armpit and the breast and the armpit itself.

3. Gently squeeze the nipple and look for a discharge or any unusual puckering. (Fig. 4-4, *F*).
4. Repeat steps 2 and 3 on your other side, using the opposite hand.

Try all approaches — standing, lying down, or in the shower — to get a sense of which feels most comfortable to you. BSE works best as a screening technique if you do it every month. When you go for a checkup, have your medical practitioner review the breast examination with you to check out your technique.

Gallup polls have shown that only 25% to 33% of American women perform BSE regularly. Sometimes this is because of fear of finding cancer or of losing a breast. Yet, ironically, it is this same *early warning system* we have a tendency to postpone that can make a breast cancer curable. In addition, early diagnosis means more treatment options, including the possibility of saving your breast.

Recommendations for breast cancer screening

Ages 20 to 40

1. Perform breast self-examination (BSE) monthly, shortly after menstrual period.
2. Have examination by physician every 3 years, with review of BSE.
3. Arrange for baseline mammography between ages 35 and 40.

Over age 40

1. Perform BSE monthly shortly after menstrual period or on a set date.
2. Have examination by physician every year.
3. Arrange for mammography every year *after* age 50.*
4. Check with your physician for recommendations for ages 40 to 50.

*There is as yet relatively little data to establish the most appropriate interval for mammographic screening. The HIP study previously cited mentioned an interval of 1 year, and it is primarily on this study that the ACS recommendations are based. However, other screening programs are underway looking at the effectiveness of other screening intervals, such as 2 years. Currently, mammography every *1 or 2 years* after age 40 is a reasonable recommendation for average-risk women and should be discussed with your physician. Women at higher risk or with breasts that are difficult to examine should have annual mammography after age 50 and every 1 or 2 years between ages 40 and 50.

In 1983 the American College of Radiology issued revised guidelines for mammography in hopes of increasing the use of this modality. Two new recommendations are:
1. After age 40 mammography should be used every 1 or 2 years.
2. The recommended radiation should be less than 1 rad to midbreast for both breasts.

This recommendation was supported by a recent Swedish study in which 94,000 women older than 39 were screened. The initial screening evaluation determined that 1020 (62%) of 1649 subjects had no breast abnormalities. The remaining 629 (38%) underwent further diagnostic procedures — needle aspiration biopsy and cytology or galactography (x-ray pictures of breast ducts). In 267 of the 629 cases benign lesions were found. The remaining 362 (58%) underwent biopsies; in 235 (65%) there were malignant lesions. The Swedish study suggests that in the United States 1 in 5 biopsies are positive for cancer, whereas 2 in 3 of their biopsies were positive, thus reducing unnecessary surgery and stress to patients. This preliminary report is important as support for the American College of Radiology guidelines that mammography is currently our best screening test. Only 5% of U.S. women undergo yearly mammography, which could potentially save 7500 yearly breast cancer deaths. (Merz, B.: JAMA **249:**2142-2143, 1983.)

Summary and recommendations

Although it is the number one cause of cancer deaths in women, breast cancer can be detected earlier, resulting in successful treatment and a higher survival rate. Furthermore, one of the most effective screening devices for early detection, breast self-examination, can be done at home routinely at no cost. Women at high risk should follow the specific recommendations of their physicians; the general population should follow the recommendations listed in the boxed material, which are those of the American Cancer Society. Remember, physical examination by patient and physician, as well as mammography, all make important contributions to finding breast cancer early.

Women who have had breast cancer should have mammography every year regardless of age. Other high-risk women (family history of breast cancer in mother or sister; prior breast cancer; first child after age 30; two or more breast biopsies) should discuss with their physicians the advisability of regular mammography after age 40.

UTERINE CANCER

For purposes of cancer description and screening, the uterus (womb) is divided into two sections: the mouth, which is called the cervix; and the body of the uterus, called the corpus. Cancer in the cervix is called cervical cancer, and cancer in the uterus body is called uterine or endometrial cancer, since it almost always begins in the inner lining of the uterus, the endometrium. This is the tissue that is shed monthly during menstruation. These two cancers are different in many respects, including risk factors, and are discussed separately. (See Fig. 4-5.)

Cervical cancer

Each year approximately 16,000 new cases of cervical cancer are diagnosed and about 7000 women die of this disease. As with other cancers, cervical cancer cure rates improve with early detection. Cervical cancer, or invasive cancer of the cervix, is preceded in most cases by *carcinoma in situ,* which means that cancerous changes have already taken place on the

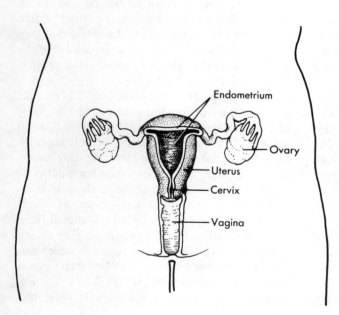

Endometrium

Ovary

Uterus

Cervix

Vagina

FIG. 4-5 Internal anatomy of female genitalia. (Redrawn from What you need to know, U.S. Department of Health and Human Services, Public Health Service/National Institute of Health.)

surface of the cervix; however, the cancer is limited to the cervix alone. Unlike many other cancers, this stage of carcinoma in situ generally lasts a long time, between 8 and 30 years. Also, from 20% to 33% of these localized cancers may disappear spontaneously.

When the changes in cell growth are discovered at any time during this stage, the cure rate is close to 100% because no cells have spread. Furthermore, there are also changes in the local tissue, *dysplasia,* that are not normal but are not yet cancer. Dysplastic changes are premalignant, indicating that the individual needs to be very closely followed. As with carcinoma in situ, a number of these dysplastic changes in cells may disappear spontaneously or may be altered by cryocautery or electrocautery.

Risk factors. The risks are almost the opposite of those for breast cancer, in which risk decreases if you have a child early. With cervical cancer, early sexual intercourse, multiple sexual partners, and history of venereal disease are associated with a higher cancer incidence. Specifically, the herpesvirus is associated with cervical cancer, but we cannot say it causes cervical cancer. It may be another reflection of the association of cervical cancer with expanded sexual activity. Some prostitutes, for example, have a lifetime cervical cancer risk of 8%, much higher than that of the average population. Finally, lower socioeconomic status is also associated with increased rates of cervical cancer.

Warning signs. Symptoms are not common with this cancer, although some women may have spotting between periods or after intercourse or douching. An increased vaginal discharge may be another symptom. These symptoms do not mean that you have cervical cancer, just that you should consult your physician for further examination.

Screening. The specific screening technique for cervical cancer represents the biggest success for cancer screening to date. The Pap test (named after George N. Papanicolaou, who devised it) has been found over the past 30 years to be reliable, inexpensive, and easy for a physician to perform in the office. It is done during a routine pelvic examination; the doctor merely takes a scraping of cells from the inside of the cervix using a small wooden spatula or a Q-tip. The process is brief and painless. The specimen is then preserved and sent to a laboratory where pathologists trained in observing cancer cells evaluate the slide. The changes in shape and structure that take place in cancer cells have been classified into a grading system, and by examining the specimen, the pathologist can tell if any of these cancerous or precancerous changes have taken place. The test does not prove there is cancer, as there can be changes or abnormalities that are not cancerous. However, abnormal cell changes should be closely followed, and your physician might want to perform a further diagnostic test such as a biopsy or colposcopy with biopsy, which involves taking a small section of tissue for microscopic examination.

The Pap test has been successful not only because it is a good test in itself, but also because women have been educated to make use of it. In 1976 almost two thirds of women between the ages of 18 and 34 reported having had a Pap test during the preceding year. Four out of five (82%) said that they had had at least one Pap test in their lives. Compare this with the 25% to 33% who say they perform breast self-examination.

Summary and recommendations. There is no question that the Pap test works. The only medical controversy remaining is how often to have it done. The American Cancer Society recently reviewed all data connected with cervical cancer screening and made new recommendations. These recommendations are generally conservative because they want to prevent as much cancer as possible. They have now altered their recommendation from suggesting a Pap smear every year for women at average risk under age 65 to recommending a series of two Pap smears a year apart, beginning at age 20 or when a woman becomes sexually active. If these are

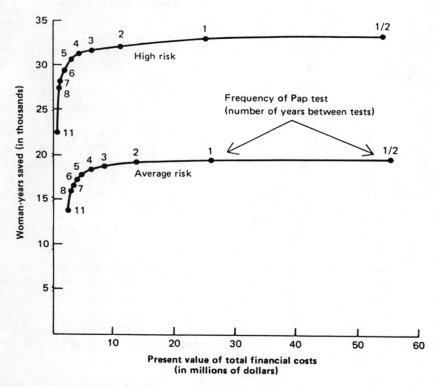

FIG. 4-6 Effect of Pap test frequency on woman-years of life saved and costs for a population of 100,000 average-risk and high-risk women. Main assumptions: (1) testing is begun at age 20; (2) woman will have checkup every 3 years for other malignant diseases from age 20 to age 40 and then annually thereafter. Marginal cost of Pap test is $10; (3) Pap test-detectable carcinoma in situ (CIS) precedes invasive cervical cancer (ICC) by an average of 8 years (range: 0-10 years); (4) 5% of ICC develop very rapidly and do not pass through dysplasia or CIS stage; (5) no cases of dysplasia or CIS regress spontaneously; (6) 5-year relative survival rates from time of detection (lead time adjusted) are: dysplasia and CIS, 98%; local invasive, 78%, and regional invasive, 43%; and (7) high-risk women with multiple sexual partners have 1.7 times risk of controls.

NOTE: If woman must also pay $25 office visit fee for separate visits for Pap test, costs increase to $72.7 million for annual Pap test and $170 million for biannual Pap test.

(From Cancer of the breast, Ca **30**[4]:221, 1980. Reprinted by permission from Ca—A Cancer Journal for Clinicians, © 1980, American Cancer Society, Inc.)

both normal (negative for abnormalities), Pap screening should be repeated every 3 years until age 65. If *all* tests have been totally normal (class I Pap smear) until then, there is very little chance that a woman will develop cervical cancer. Two tests are recommended at the beginning of screening because early dysplastic changes can sometimes be missed by a single Pap test, especially if proper sampling techniques are not used. It is important that cells from the cervical canal be obtained in the sample. You should know, however, that the American College of Obstetrics and Gynecology does not agree with these recommendations and continues to recommend yearly Pap tests.

This change in recommendations was based on the effectiveness of the tests and a cost consideration. Fig. 4-6 summarizes the information, measuring the costs of doing Pap tests against the number of lives saved. Ninety-seven percent of all the cancers that can be found with annual screening can be found with a Pap test every 3 years—but at less than one-half the cost. (This means that 3% of the cancers that would be found will be missed; the estimate applies to *average-risk* women.) The cautious gynecologists, who have seen a Pap smear change in less than 1 year, are concerned about testing less often. This matter should be discussed with your physician. Women who are at higher risk, that is have a history of *any* abnormal Pap test or are sexually active with multiple partners, should be screened more frequently, annually or even more often. You should discuss your individual screening needs and risk factors with your physician.

Part of this controversy arises from medical practitioners who believe that women may not remember to have a test done every 3 years, whereas once a year is easier to remember. Some physicians are afraid that the death rates from this entirely controllable cancer (by means of early screening) may begin to climb again if women neglect to be screened. Our thought is that if you are careful and keep a health diary in

---

Recommendations for cervical cancer screening

1. American Cancer Society recommendation: have two Pap smears 1 year apart. If negative, a routine Pap smear once every 3 years until age 65 or as recommended by your physician.
2. American College of Obstetrics and Gynecology recommendation: have annual Pap smear.
3. Begin yearly pelvic examination after age 40 (see "Endometrial cancer").
4. If sexually active with multiple partners or showing abnormal smears, discuss more frequent screening with your physician.

---

which you record what screenings you have had and when—something like an innoculation record for a child—you should have no problem. In some instances, however, your physician may recommend more frequent screening after assessing individual risk factors. (See boxed material.)

Endometrial cancer

Endometrial cancer is more common than cervical; an estimated 39,000 new cases were diagnosed in 1983, compared to 16,000 for invasive cancer of the cervix. However, deaths from endometrial cancer were estimated at only 3000 in 1983, compared to more than 7000 for cervical cancer. The cure rate for endometrial cancer after 5 years is 75% for all stages and 88% if it is detected early before the uterus has enlarged. This cancer spreads slowly and, like cervical cancer, remains localized for a long period in about 85% of cases, making it an ideal cancer for early detection.

This is a cancer that generally strikes women over age 55, after menopause. Women specifically at risk are those who are obese, have not had children, have a history of infertility or failure to ovulate, have a combination of hypertension and diabetes with their obesity, or are taking estrogen medications such as Premarin. More generally, this is a cancer of affluent populations. Its incidence has increased, whereas cervical cancer has declined because of Pap smears.

Experience has indicated that endometrial cancer is influenced by hormones; specifically, it is more likely to develop in the lining of the uterus when it is exposed to the effects of estrogen for long periods. The constant stimulation of estrogen causes the lining of the uterus to build up; this buildup called *hyperplasia,* may make it more likely that cancer will develop. Hyperplasia can occur when a women is infertile, since if an egg is not released from the ovary, the protective hormone progesterone is not secreted either with regular menstrual cycles or with pregnancy. Progesterone allows the lining of the uterus to shed (as with a menstrual cycle) and thus may prevent the buildup that may precede cancer changes. The risk from obesity is probably caused by fatty tissues converting an adrenal hormone to estrogen. Finally, women may receive estrogen treatments after menopause for symptoms such as hot flashes, depression, painful intercourse (due to thinning of the lining of the vagina), or bone weakness (osteoporosis). All these symptoms are caused by a lack of estrogen. Now that medical practitioners are aware of the possible cancer-inciting side effects of estrogen, they have lowered the dosages prescribed and may also cycle estrogen with progesterone to prevent hyperplasia of the uterine lining. The estrogens are usually given for 3 weeks at a time, using progesterone (Provera) with the last 7 to 10 days of estrogen. (Not all gynecologists use this method, since many women over age 55 object to still having menstrual periods.) This regime allows the uterine lining to remain normal, and cancer incidence is not increased in women treated in this manner.

Warning signs. The earliest symptom of endometrial cancer is bleeding or spotting after menopause. Since menstrual periods are sometimes irregular with the onset of menopause, it may be difficult to tell if the bleeding is the menstrual period resuming or whether it is abnormal bleeding that could indicate endometrial cancer. If there is any question, particularly if the risk factors just mentioned are present, consult your physician regarding endometrial sampling (see following section).

Screening. The Pap test, so successful for detecting cervical cancer, detects only 20% to 40% of the cases of endometrial cancer, so it is not reliable. Cells from inside the uterus must be obtained for an accurate test of endometrial cancer. The most commonly used procedure is *dilation and curettage (D and C).*

This is a surgical procedure usually done under general anesthesia in a hospital, although it may also be done as outpatient surgery. The cervix is dilated or opened, and the inside lining of the uterus is scraped (curetted). The tissue from the endometrium is examined by a pathologist under a microscope to see if cancer is present.

Recently, alternatives to D and C that can be easily and inexpensively performed by a doctor in the office have been developed and tested. Several techniques that use aspiration (or suction) to gather cells from the inside of the uterus appear very promising. These would make screening for endometrial cancer simpler and less costly, and many physicians now do endometrial sampling in their office with local or no anesthesia. If you are at particularly high risk, or aspiration endometrial sampling is inconclusive, your physician may continue to recommend a D and C.

Summary and recommendations. Current recommendations suggest that any woman at increased risk should have an endometrial sampling performed at the time of her menopause. This includes women who are obese, have a history of infertility, or have taken estrogens. A

**Recommendations for
endometrial cancer screening**

═══════════════════════════

1. Have annual pelvic examinations after
   age 40.
2. If at high risk, you should have endometrial sampling done at menopause and
   thereafter as recommended by your physician.
3. Promptly report any postmenopausal
   bleeding and have endometrial sampling.
4. Discuss endometrial sampling with your
   physician before postmenopausal estrogen therapy and annually while receiving
   estrogens.

---

regular pelvic examination may also reveal
masses or changes in the uterus, but this generally indicates a more advanced stage. Nonetheless, endometrial cancer is still highly curable at
this point (65%) because of its slow spread.
Women who require postmenopausal estrogens
should be evaluated by their gynecologist before therapy and should have regular (every 1
or 2 years) endometrial sampling while on therapy. (See boxed material.)

OVARIAN CANCER

The outlook for screening this cancer of the
reproductive system is much more disappoint-
ing than for cervical and endometrial cancer.
Ovarian cancer is the fourth most common
form of cancer in American women but the
most frequent cause of death in cancers of the
female genital tract. Approximately 18,200 new
cases are diagnosed each year, and 11,500
women die of this disease annually. Put in percentage terms, ovarian cancer accounts for 4%
of the cancers in women but 6% of the cancer
deaths. The average survival at 5 years is 37%,
but this is somewhat misleading. If found when
localized, the cure rate is as high as 80%, but

most ovarian cancers are found late in their
development when they have already spread. At
this point the cure rate drops to 20%. New
treatments with aggressive chemotherapy now
appear to be improving these results.

There are no known specific risk factors. The
incidence of ovarian cancer begins to rise after
age 40, with maximum occurrence between ages
55 and 74. However, it may also be seen in
women between the ages of 25 and 50. Current
estimates are that 1 of 100 American women
will die of ovarian cancer. (See Fig. 4-7.)

Warning signs

Abnormal menstrual bleeding occurs in 15%
to 30% of women with ovarian cancer. Other
possible signs may be pain or an increase in abdominal size with vague gastrointestinal complaints. These symptoms do not mean that you
have ovarian cancer, only that if they persist,
you should contact your physician for further
examination.

Screening

Ovarian cancer spreads along a fairly established route. From the ovaries it spreads locally
in the pelvis, then moves throughout the abdomen and, if progressive, may spread to the
lungs, lymph nodes, and other distant areas.
The pattern of spread follows the fluid, or lymphatic drainage of the ovary.

This cancer is very difficult to diagnose early
because it begins deep in the pelvis, where it can
grow to considerable size before it can be detected by physical examination. It is comparable
in this respect to a pregnancy, which would not
be noticed for 2 or 3 months if not for the sign
of missed periods; the early growth of the fetus
is too small to be perceived even by the woman
herself. Regular yearly pelvic examinations
have not usually enabled physicians to find
ovarian cancer at an early stage. By the time the
enlarged ovary is noted during a routine examination or a woman notices abdominal swelling
with other vague discomfort, the disease has

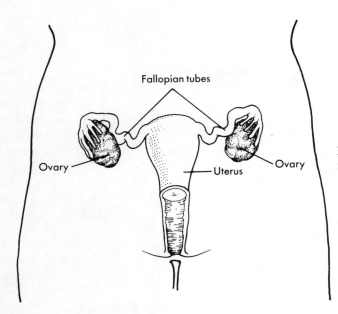

Fallopian tubes

Ovary

Ovary

Uterus

FIG. 4-7   Anatomy of ovary and surrounding organs.

usually spread. Only 1 in 4 ovarian tumors is localized at the time of diagnosis.

No screening test has yet been devised for this cancer. Because the ovaries are deep within the pelvis and not accessible through the vagina, as is the cervix, no test such as the Pap smear can help find abnormal cells to discover the disease at an early stage.

Once a mass has been discovered, evaluation includes examination of the urinary tract, bladder, and kidneys, a bowel examination, and usually a highly sensitive, computed tomography (CT or CAT) scan of the abdomen and pelvis or ultrasound to assess the stage of the spread of the tumor (a diagnostic, not a screening approach) so that treatment can be planned accordingly. Surgery is almost always performed, with additional use of radiation or chemotherapy in selected cases.

Summary and recommendations

This cancer is not currently responsive to early screening techniques. Because it is often not localized when diagnosed, it tends to have a

> ### Recommendations for ovarian cancer screening
>
> 1. Have a yearly pelvic examination after age 40. (A Pap smear and/or endometrial sampling for cervical or endometrial cancer screening will be done as indicated by your physician.)
> 2. Report any unusual symptoms to your physician: vaginal bleeding between periods, abdominal swelling, or vague abdominal discomfort or pain.

higher mortality rate than the other cancers of the female reproductive system. (See boxed material.)

PROSTATIC CANCER

Cancer of the prostate is the third most common cancer among men, accounting for 75,000

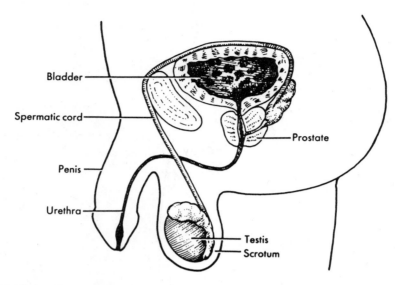

FIG. 4-8   Internal anatomy of male genitalia. (Redrawn from *What you need to know*, U.S. Department of Health and Human Services, Public Health Service/National Institute of Health.)

new cases each year. It follows lung and colorectal cancer. In 1983 an estimated 24,100 deaths occurred from prostatic cancer. (See Fig. 4-8.)

Risk factors and warning signs

The major risk factor is age, since the incidence of prostatic cancer continually increases with age. An association with a high-fat diet has been shown, but this has not been demonstrated to be an actual cause of prostatic cancer. Autopsy series in older men have also shown that microscopic nests of prostatic cancer cells increase with age but these often never cause symptoms or have clinical significance. It is a more aggressive tumor in younger men.

Symptoms for prostatic cancer are the same as for noncancerous enlargement of the prostate, a very common condition in men over age 40 (probably at least half of men over 40 have some enlargement of the prostate). They include painful urination or ejaculation, trouble starting or stopping urine flow, dribbling or a weak stream, and occasionally blood or pus in

the urine. When symptoms of difficult urination develop quickly, they are somewhat more likely to indicate cancer than when onset is slow and gradual. In any case, because all the symptoms can mean disease of the prostate *other than cancer,* they are not specific. They do not mean that you have prostatic cancer, but they do suggest that further tests should be done and that you should see your physician promptly.

Screening

During a digital examination of the rectum the physician can check for prostatic enlargement to detect any irregular or firm areas that could indicate a tumor. This is the best single test for prostatic cancer. If anything suspicious is found, further tests include urinalysis, x-ray films, blood tests, (especially an acid phosphatase test), and examination by a urologist (a specialist in diseases of the urinary system). Acid phosphatase is an enzyme found in the prostate gland that tends to increase when cancer is present. If after testing the diagnosis is not clear, a biopsy is recommended.

**Recommendations for
prostatic cancer screening**

════════════════════════

1. Have a yearly digital rectal examination of the prostate after age 40.
2. Report symptoms of difficult voiding and painful urination or ejaculation to your physician.

**Recommendations for
testicular cancer screening**

════════════════════════

Perform periodic (4 to 6 times a year) self-examination of testes and scrotum.

Summary and recommendations

The best screening for prostatic cancer, a very common cancer of American males, is a physical examination. (See boxed material.)

TESTICULAR CANCER

Cancer of the testis, or testicle, occurs in approximately 1% of males, usually between the ages of 15 and 35. The most common symptom is a palpable mass, sometimes with pain but usually painless. Men with a history of an undescended testicle are at higher risk.

Diagnosis of cancer depends on a pathologic analysis (biopsy) as well as a blood analysis, including special hormonal assays and chest x-ray films with lung and abdominal CT scans to see if spread has occurred. Treatment has improved tremendously over the past 20 years — with early detection the cure rate is almost 100%; even with advanced metastatic spread to the lung and abdomen the cure rate may be 60%. Screening involves periodic examination of the testes and scrotum for any masses (see boxed material). For self-examination examine each testis gently with both hands after a bath or hot shower. Place the index and middle fingers underneath the scrotum and the thumb on top, then gently roll the testis. A small fullness called the epididymis is normally present on the top of each testis. Compare one testicle with the other. There usually is a difference in size, but if lumps or masses are present, see your physician.

BLADDER CANCER

An estimated 38,500 new cases of bladder cancer, or cancer of the lining of the urinary tract, were diagnosed in 1983 and about 10,700 people died from this disease. As with lung, head, and neck cancer, it is associated with cigarette smoking. The carcinogens in the smoke are absorbed into the body and in some way encourage the development of cancers, even in distant organs (for example, the bladder and pancreas). People who work with certain chemicals such as aniline dyes or hydrocarbons also have an increased incidence of bladder cancer. In Egypt and other parts of Africa, along lakes and rivers, bladder cancer is associated with chronic infection with a parasitic disease, schistosomiasis. Bladder cancer occurs in both men and women, although it is more common in men. It is a tumor that tends to recur; each recurrence is usually more aggressive than the previous one. (See Fig. 4-9.)

The earliest symptom of bladder cancer is usually blood in the urine, a condition called *hematuria*. The urine will probably be faintly pink or smoky in color rather than red, and the hematuria may occur only intermittently.

Screening procedures for bladder cancer other than following up the symptom of blood in the urine do not exist at present. Blood can be detected from a simple urinalysis, and the cells in the urine can be studied for cancer cells (a urine Pap test). *Cystoscopy* (a telescopic view of the inside of the bladder) is also used in the evaluation of hematuria or in the follow-up of individuals with previous bladder cancer (see boxed material). However, in Europe, where

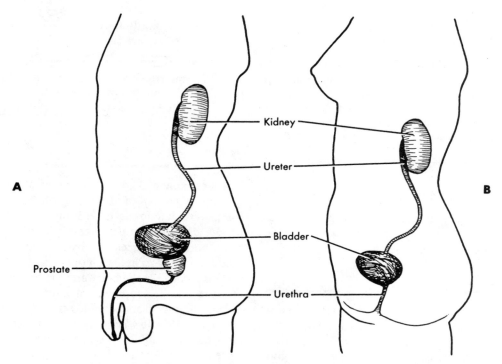

FIG. 4-9   Comparison of bladder and surrounding organs in **A**, male and **B**, female. (Redrawn from What you need to know, U.S. Department of Health and Human Services, Public Health Service/National Institute of Health.)

Recommendations for bladder cancer screening and prevention
1. Have a urinalysis or urine cytology if at high risk only, as recommended by your physician.
2. Avoid tobacco.

they have studied groups of workers at high risk using urine cytologies (examination for cancer cells) and examination for hematuria every 6 months, there has been no improvement in the overall survival nor a shift in the diagnosis to an earlier, more curable stage.

PANCREATIC CANCER

Relatively uncommon in the past, pancreatic cancer is now increasing. It comprises about 3% of all new cancer cases but 5% of deaths from cancer. An estimated 25,000 new cases were diagnosed in 1983 and roughly the same number (22,600) died from the disease. These figures are probably low, since it can be very difficult to detect pancreatic cancer, and it may never be identified as the primary cancer unless an autopsy is performed. The symptoms generally occur when the disease is well established and has metastasized or spread.

Risk factors and warning signs

Although the cause of pancreatic cancer is unknown, certain risk factors are associated with it. Chronic pancreatitis, heavy alcohol use, chronic gallstone disease, diabetes, and smoking have all been associated with increased incidence. Recently, a high-calorie, high-fat, high-protein diet has also been implicated as a possible risk factor. Women have about one and a half times the risk of men, and the incidence may also be slightly higher in blacks. As with many other cancers, it is one that occurs more commonly in older people.

Symptoms include weight loss, abdominal discomfort or pain, and jaundice (yellowish skin color). Depression is sometimes a prominent symptom as well, and occasionally blood clots in the legs may be the first sign. If the cancer originates near the head of the pancreas, which is near where the gallbladder empties into the intestine, it often causes jaundice and liver enlargement. Because of the jaundice, these cancers are more likely to be found early, and surgery is sometimes curative if there has been no spread of the tumor.

Screening and recommendations

There are no useful screening tests for pancreatic cancer before symptoms occur. (See boxed material.) Because the pancreas lies deep in the abdomen, it cannot be felt during physical examination. Once the symptoms occur and pancreatic cancer is suspected, tests to establish the diagnosis include ultrasound, CT scans, *endoscopic retrograde cholangiopancreatography (ERCP)*, and biopsy with either a thin-needle approach or surgery. Unfortunately, once the diagnosis of pancreatic cancer is confirmed, treatment is not much more effective than the screening procedures, and most patients are dead within a year. Of all people diagnosed

---

Recommendations for pancreatic cancer screening and prevention

1. Report jaundice, weight loss, or chronic abdominal pain.
2. Avoid heavy use of tobacco and alcohol.
3. Follow a prudent diet without excessive fat.

---

with pancreatic cancer, about 10% to 25% are candidates for surgery, and 1 in 5 of these die during the operation itself.

STOMACH CANCER

Of all the cancers affecting Americans, stomach cancer is the only one to show a steady decrease in both sexes over the past several decades. During that time, the death rate has declined from 29:100,000 to 8:100,000 in white men and from 22:100,000 to 4:100,000 in white women. In 1983 an estimated 25,000 cases were diagnosed and 14,000 people died, making stomach cancer the seventh most common cancer death. It is unclear why the incidence of stomach cancer has declined so dramatically. Whatever the reason, it has not been a result of early detection, since we have not developed effective stomach cancer screening techniques in this country. Tests that are currently available are relatively complicated and expensive and are usually indicated only in people with symptoms. By the time symptoms occur, the disease has usually spread. (See Fig. 4-10.)

Risk factors and warning signs

Stomach cancer is associated with a diet high in salted, pickled, and preserved foods, for example, the Japanese diet; stomach cancer is much more common in Japan than in the United States. Another risk factor is *pernicious anemia,* a particular form of vitamin B_{12} defi-

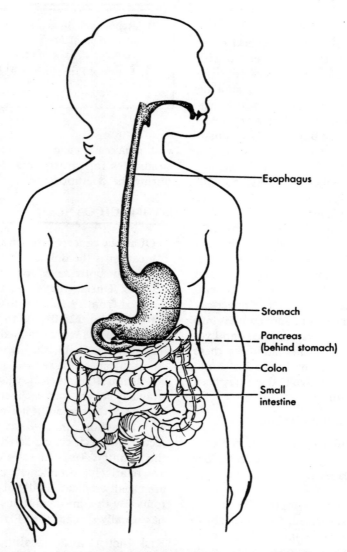

FIG. 4-10 Anatomy of stomach and surrounding organs. (Redrawn from What you need to know, U.S. Department of Health and Human Services, Public Health Service/National Institute of Health.)

ciency associated with absent stomach acid and abnormalities of the stomach lining. This condition predisposes to stomach cancer, with a relative risk as high as 20 times that of the normal population. Pernicious anemia can occur in anyone, but it is most common in blond, blue-eyed people, such as those of Scandinavian, German, or English-Scottish ancestry. If you have pernicious anemia, you should discuss with your physician an appropriate schedule of tests to look for possible stomach problems and detect them early. Also, if you have a gastric ulcer that does not heal completely in 2 to 3 months, this should be biopsied; it may also be an early stomach cancer. Early warning signs of stomach cancer include weight loss, abdominal discomfort, trouble swallowing when eating, heartburn, and diarrhea. These symptoms do not mean that you have stomach cancer, but when they are persistent, they should be checked by your physician.

Screening and recommendations

There is no effective screening technique for asymptomatic people for stomach cancer. (See boxed material.) Once symptoms appear, a variety of diagnostic techniques, such as an upper gastrointestinal series or endoscopy, are used

---

Recommendations for stomach cancer screening and prevention

1. Report any persistent stomach discomfort or weight loss to your physician.
2. Avoid highly salted, preserved foods and food additives.
3. Gastric ulcers that do not heal completely should be biopsied.
4. Discuss periodic testing, such as upper gastrointestinal series or endoscopy, with your physician if you have pernicious anemia.

---

to evaluate whether is is cancer and if it has spread. Because this cancer is very common in Japan, Japanese physicians have developed the most effective combination of detection tests and treatment. Based on early diagnosis and aggressive surgery, their approach has achieved survival rates of more than 50% for stomach cancer. Overall cure rates, however, are about 12%.

HEAD AND NECK CANCERS

Cancers of the head and neck are strongly associated with excessive alcohol and tobacco use. They are usually squamous cell cancers that tend to occur in the oral cavity, the larynx (voice box), pharynx (back area of the throat where the nose joins the throat), and sinuses (see Fig. 4-11). Oral cancers account for about 4% of all cancers, and most of them occur after age 40. They are twice as common in men as in women. This, however, represents a dramatic increase in oral cancers in women, since they were previously four to six times more common in men. As with lung cancer, this increase is probably related to the increased incidence of smoking in women. In 1983 an estimated 38,100 cases of head and neck cancer were diagnosed and about one third of this number—12,850 people—died of the disease.

Risk factors and warning signs

The risk factors, as mentioned, are alcohol and tobacco use, with the risk increasing even more when they are used together. Any form of tobacco, including snuff, chewing tobacco, and pipe smoking, is associated with a higher rate of cancer. Also, the more you smoke and drink and the longer you do this, the greater your risk of a head or neck cancer. It is thought that perhaps 90% of these cancers arise from prolonged exposure to environmental factors (such as alcohol or tobacco) known to be carcinogens or cocarcinogens. Other risk factors may include certain viruses and carcinogens such as betel

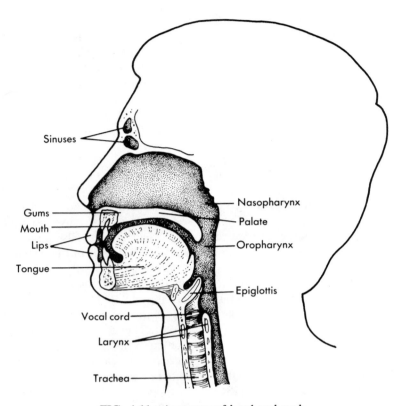

FIG. 4-11 Anatomy of head and neck.

nuts, as well as genetic susceptibility. For example, we know the Chinese have a higher rate of nasopharyngeal (nose and throat) cancer, which is thought to be an inherited vulnerability. Although many oral cancers appear to develop in areas covered by dentures, there is no firm evidence to show that the trauma from ill-fitting dentures or bridges actually *causes* cancer. However, early cancers may look very much like a sore caused by a rough filling or bridge. This means it is important that any persistent sore should be checked by your physician or dentist, and ill-fitting dentures and fillings should be refitted by your dentist.

Not only does tobacco precipitate the development of head and neck cancers, but its use is also associated with a decreased survival rate in individuals who have these cancers. One study of 203 patients with cancers of the head and neck showed a 70% 5-year mortality rate for smokers and a 35% rate for nonsmokers—the chances of survival for a smoker were only half those of a nonsmoker. The 5-year survival rate for these cancers ranges from 22% for pharynx (throat) cancer to 84% for lip cancer. Overall disease-free survival for oral cancer is about 40%, but this is closely related to the time of diagnosis. If an oral cancer or other head and neck cancer is found while it is still small and before spread (metastasis) has occurred, then the disease-free survival is about 70% (and as high as 85% to 90% for a small lip cancer). Once it has spread or enlarged, survival is significantly decreased. This means that it is very

---

Recommendations for screening and prevention of head and neck cancers

1. Eliminate or reduce all tobacco use.*
2. Minimize alcohol intake.*
3. Avoid other known carcinogens, such as betel nut chewing.
4. Have annual dental care and have a good oral and head and neck examination at that time.
5. Report any persistent sores in the mouth, swelling in the neck or under the chin, or repeated bleeding from the mouth or throat.
6. Have ill-fitting dentures or fillings adjusted by your dentist.

*The *combination* of alcohol and tobacco use creates the highest head and neck cancer risk. We suggest you join a support group to stop drinking and/or smoking if this applies to you.

---

important to pay attention to the warning signs.

Warning signs include any mouth sores that do not heal after 2 to 3 weeks. These may be whitish patches (*leukoplakia*), which are precancerous lesions, or red, velvety sores (*erythroplasia*). In addition, any firm swelling in the neck or under the chin, any persistent hoarseness, or any repeated bleeding from the mouth or throat should be promptly evaluated, especially if the individual is over age 40 and has a history of significant use of tobacco or alcohol. Another warning sign may be difficulty in swallowing or in moving the tongue or jaw.

Screening and recommendations

Screening for these cancers should be done by the dentist or physician during annual checkups and whenever any of the warning signs occur. Dentures and bridges should be removed for the oral examination, and tongue blades, mirrors, and good lighting should be used to examine the sides of the tongue as well as underneath the tongue and between the gums and cheek. If hoarseness or bleeding from the throat is a complaint, then mirrors must be used to examine the larynx and pharynx.

The neck should also be checked for any swelling. Other than an annual examination and reporting warning signs promptly, there are no additional screening procedures for head and neck cancer. Remember, if you do notice one of the symptoms described, it does not mean that you do have cancer, but it does mean that you should check with your physician or dentist and have a good head and neck examination.

SKIN CANCER

Skin cancers are the most common form of cancer, accounting for more than 400,000 new lesions each year. Fortunately, the overall cure rate is 90% to 95%. There are several kinds of skin cancer; the most frequent type is a basal cell cancer, which usually appears as a waxy or pearly nodule that may ulcerate. Basal cell cancers usually develop in sun-exposed areas of the body. Squamous cell cancers are the second most common, and they can appear in both sun- and non-sun-exposed areas. They are most frequently associated with precancerous lesions that are called *actinic keratoses*—reddish-brown, rough, scaly areas on the face and hands of elderly people. Other associations are with the white patches of leukoplakia on mucous membranes or the red lesions of erythroplasia in the mouth. These squamous cell cancers generally have a precancerous phase; however, those associated with scars may grow more quickly and aggressively.

Melanoma is a more serious skin cancer that may occur in either dark- or flesh-colored moles. Approximately 17,000 cases develop each year, with 5200 deaths. Melanoma is unpredictable and may be very aggressive. Because it can spread quickly, it has a survival rate of 70% (among whites), compared to the 95%

survival rate of the other skin cancers. It is most common in fair-skinned people and less frequent in dark-skinned people; light-skinned blacks have an intermediate susceptibility. More than 50% of melanoma cancers occur in previously existing moles.

Risk factors

Excessive exposure to the sun is the primary risk factor, but others include radiation and exposure to ultraviolet light. Occupational exposure to creosote, arsenic compounds, radium, coal tar, and pitch also increases the risk. People with fair complexions are at greater risk than those who are heavily pigmented. The dark pigment (melanin) serves as a built-in sunscreen. People who live in areas where there is more sun, such as the Southwest, and those who work outside in the sun, such as farmers or ranchers, are at greater risk. Skin cancers also occur more frequently in older people who have had more exposure to the ultraviolet rays of the sun over their lifetimes. Protective clothing and sunscreens should be used by fair-skinned people and those subject to excessive sun exposure.

How does sun exposure damage the skin? At the base of our protective layer of skin (the epidermis) is a basal layer of growing cells, including the melanocytes, which produce melanin. The amount of melanin in our cells is genetically determined, and its purpose is to scatter the ultraviolet light that hits the skin. Since darker-skinned people genetically produce more melanin, they have more protection from ultraviolet light. It has been shown that this ultraviolet light can damage or delay the repair of DNA in skin cells, thus leading to skin cancer. Obviously, the greater exposure—both in intensity and duration—the greater the damage that can occur. There are several signs of sun-damaged skin. These include roughened, dried skin, the basal cell and squamous cell cancers already described, as well as *Bowen's disease* (a precancerous scaly skin disease), and actinic keratosis.

Sunscreens can help prevent this damage.

They do allow tanning, but they prevent the sun*burn* that occurs with the more damaging frequency of ultraviolet light. The Food and Drug Administration has labeled sunscreens by a numbering system based on an *SPF (sun protection factor)*. An SPF tells you how much longer you could stay in the same sun with the sunscreen on until your skin would redden. For example, an SPF of 6 means you can stay 6 hours in the same sun with the sun screening to acquire the same amount of reddening as 1 hour without the sunscreen. The SPF tells you the time ratio of protection. Tables 4-1 and 4-2 illustrate which sunscreens are appropriate for which skin types.

One cautionary note with sunscreens: if you take thiazides (water pills used for hypertension or edema) or other sulfa-derived medicines, you should avoid para-aminobenzoic acid (PABA)–based sunscreens, as this combination may cause sun-sensitivity. Other protective sunscreen substances, benzophenones, can be used, so read the label carefully. Also, people who are allergic to sulfa drugs or the local anesthetics, procaine or benzocaine, should use benzophenones instead of PABA.

Warning signs

Any unusual skin change that persists, such as pearly nodules or rough scaly reddish brown areas, is a warning sign. A sore that does not heal or any changes in moles, such as growth, bleeding, or color changes, should be checked by a physician promptly. Skin changes may not be cancerous or precancerous, but those that persist should be examined. Skin biopsy may be indicated in any suspicious lesion.

Screening and recommendations

The only screening procedure available to detect any cancer of the skin is physical examination. People themselves can take stock of their skin from time to time, but a physician or nurse practitioner should also check the skin during a physical examination.

TABLE 4-1 Skin types and how they sunburn

Skin type	Sunburn prognosis	Examples
I	Always burns, never tans	Irish, Scots, redheads
II	Always burns, then slightly tans	Blue-eyed, fair-skinned Caucasians
III	Sometimes burns, always tans	Darker Caucasians
IV	Burns minimally, always tans	Caucasians with Mediterranean ancestry
V	Rarely burns, tans well	Spanish, Orientals, Indians
VI	Never burns; deeply pigmented	Black-skinned Negroes

From Hanke, C.W., and Williams, P.A.: To prevent skin cancer: a guide to sunscreens for you and your patients, Your Patient and Cancer, July 1982.

TABLE 4-2 Topical sunscreens—their SPF (sun protection factor) ratings and who should use them

Chemical ingredients	Commercial name	SPF	Recommended for skin type
Absorbers			
Para-aminobenzoic acid (PABA)	Pabanol	15	I, II
in alcohol formulations	PreSun	15	I, II
Broad-spectrum sunscreens	PreSun 15	15	I, II
containing PABA and other agents	Sundown Sunblock 15	15	I, II
	Supershade 15	15	I, II
	Total Eclipse	15	I, II
Esters and derivatives of PABA	Eclipse	10	I, II
	Blockout	6	III, IV
	Pabafilm	6	III, IV
	Sundown	6	III, IV
	Sun Guard	6	III, IV
Non-PABA chemical sunscreens:	Solbar	7	II, III
benzophenones, cinnamates	Piz Buin	6	II, III
	Uval	6	III, IV⁻
Reflectors			
Physical sunscreens:	A-Fil Cream	4-8	I to IV
titanium dioxide, zinc oxide,	Reflecta	4-8	I to IV
and so on	RVPaque	4-8	I to IV
Lip screens			
PABA formulations	Chap Stick	—	—
	Lip Balm	—	—
	PreSun	—	—
	RVPaba	—	—

From Hanke, C.W., and Williams, P.A.: To prevent skin cancer: a guide to sunscreens for you and your patients, Your Patient and Cancer, July 1982.

Recommendations for skin cancer screening and prevention

1. Have skin checked at cancer-related general physical examination — once every 3 years for ages 20 to 40 and every year for ages 40 and over.
2. If at high risk, talk to your physician for specific recommendations.
3. Examine your skin periodically for changes, especially in moles. Have a friend check areas you cannot see or use a mirror.
4. If fair skinned, use a sunscreen or protective clothing and avoid excessive exposure to the sun. (See the list for specific ways to protect yourself from the sun.)

Ten ways to protect yourself from the sun*

1. Avoid outdoor activities, avoid midday sun, (between 10 AM and 2 PM, when rays are strongest), in summer months (therefore, play golf, tennis, swim, and so on in the early morning or late afternoon).
2. If you get minimally sunburned at midday, beware of further exposure. The burn may be made worse by additional ultraviolet exposure late in the afternoon.
3. Remember that burning ultraviolet rays occur on overcast days; they are invisible and *not* screened by clouds. Sand, snow, and concrete can reflect significant amounts of ultraviolet light onto the skin, so protect yourself. Do not depend on beach umbrellas; they offer little protection from sun rays reflected by sand, water, and so on.

---

*Modified from Hanke, C.W., and Williams, P.A.: To prevent skin cancer: a guide to sunscreens for you and your patients, Your Patient and Cancer, July 1982.

4. Some drugs and cosmetics may increase susceptibility to sunburn, such as thiazides (for high blood pressure) or sulfas. Avoid mineral, olive, or baby oil, since oils magnify and increase the sun's burning effect.
5. Wear a hat and long sleeves whenever possible during the summer months.
6. Use a sunscreen on your face at all times when in the sun during the summer, even if you wear a hat. It will protect you from scattered ultraviolet light that is reflected into your face.
7. Use a sunscreen with an SPF recommended for your skin type. For maximum effectiveness, apply it at least 1 hour before exposure. (See Table 4-2.)
8. Always reapply sunscreens after swimming or perspiring.
9. Men should apply sunscreens to the tops of their ears if this area is exposed.
10. Individuals at high risk for skin cancer and degenerative skin changes (outdoor workers, persons who have already had skin cancer) should apply sunscreens daily.

Kaposi's sarcoma

This is a skin cancer that used to be extremely rare and usually occurred in older people of Russian-Jewish extraction. Lately there has been an alarming increase in certain metropolitan areas (San Francisco, Los Angeles, New York City) among certain populations. Called "gay cancer," it is occurring in a very different form among young (ages 20 to 40) male homosexuals in major population centers. This form of Kaposi's sarcoma spreads more quickly and is associated with a generalized abnormality in the immune systems of these young men that makes them subject to unusual viral and protozoan infections (see Chapter 10), as well as certain other rare cancers. Women homosexuals have a much lower incidence of Kaposi's sarcoma, which may be because they make dif-

---

**Recommendations for
Kaposi's sarcoma screening**

1. Have periodic skin examination.
2. Check for enlarged lymph nodes.

---

ferent life-style choices or because of certain different hormonal factors not yet explained. Other groups in whom these cancers and infections have occurred are some drug users, who shoot drugs into their veins, hemophiliacs, and a small group of Haitian refugees, in whom neither drug use nor homosexuality seems to be present. Kaposi's sarcoma and the other immunodeficiency diseases are often associated with a life-style that includes many different sexual partners. Another associated factor is repeated exposure to a venereally passed virus, cytomegalovirus.

At present no one knows if the sarcoma results from constant stimulation of the immune system (for example, from drugs or venereal infections) that ultimately causes it to fail or whether there may be some as yet unidentified infectious agent involved. Since spread seems to occur through sexual contact as well as through blood products and transfusion, recent evidence increasingly suggests that some infectious agent is involved. Research in this area is just beginning.

Warning signs. Kaposi's sarcoma appears as violet or purplish small bumps or nodules, usually on the legs, although these can appear anywhere on the body. It may be associated with fever, feelings of fatigue or enlarged lymph glands, or the individual may feel perfectly fine. If you find any skin changes similar to these nodules, you should consult a physician immediately for a complete and careful examination of the entire skin. This is particularly the case for high-risk individuals—homosexuals who have been sexually active with many

partners. People who notice persistent swellings of any lymph nodes should also consult their physician.

LEUKEMIAS AND LYMPHOMAS

Leukemias and lymphomas are the *hematologic malignancies,* that is, cancers of the various cells found in the blood. When the cancer begins in the bone marrow (where blood is formed) and many abnormal cells are found on a blood smear, then the cancer is called a *leukemia.* Leukemias can involve several different cell types: *myelogenous leukemia* is the abnormal growth of white cells or neutrophils, which normally fight infection; *lymphocytic leukemia* is a cancer of the lymphocytes, cells which produce antibodies that the body uses to protect against infections and foreign substances (for example viruses). Very rarely, erythroleukemia, or cancer of the red cell or erythrocyte, which carries the oxygen in the blood, may occur. The diagnosis of leukemia is established by biopsy of the bone marrow, although it may be suspected when abnormal cells are found on a blood smear.

When a cancer arises in the lymph node system, it is called a lymphoma. This diagnosis is made by biopsy of a lymph node, which is generally enlarged. Together, about 54,600 cases of lymphoma and leukemia occur each year in the United States, and about 30,000 people die of these diseases.

Lymphomas are of two general kinds, Hodgkin's and non-Hodgkin's. In *Hodgkin's lymphoma* a particular kind of giant abnormal cell, the Reed-Sternberg cell, can be found. This differentiation between the different kinds of lymphoma is important because different forms of therapy are most effective, depending on what type of lymphoma is present. The *non-Hodgkin's lymphomas* are further subdivided according to the particular kind of lymphocyte that is abnormal. This subdivision gives physicians important information regarding the most effective treatment as well as the prognosis.

The cure rate for many leukemias and lymphomas has risen dramatically in the past decade, and treatment for most kinds is now much more effective than in past years. In Hodgkin's lymphoma, for example, one of the most curable of these diseases, the cure rate is now 90% to 100% for the more localized stages and 50% to 60% even in more advanced stages. In leukemia, after a bone marrow biopsy is done, no further search for further disease is necessary, but in the lymphomas it is critically important that a complete evaluation (staging) for spread of disease be done. This staging procedure may include blood tests, chest x-ray films, CT scan of chest, abdomen, or both, evaluation of the lymph system (*lymphangiogram,* a dye procedure that outlines the lymph nodes and lymph drainage vessels), bone marrow tests with biopsy, and in some cases laparotomy (abdominal surgery) to check for spread within the abdomen. The laparotomy will include biopsies of the liver and/or spleen. Not all of these procedures are required in every case, but it is very important to determine exactly how far the cancer has spread. Patients are then divided into groups according to where disease has been found in the body and whether or not they have symptoms. The appropriate therapy, radiation or chemotherapy, is then chosen based on this information. Within each group patients without symptoms generally do better than those who do have symptoms.

Risk factors

Radiation exposure (dose-related), certain hereditary conditions (for example, Down's syndrome or mongolism), some drugs (chloramphenicol and many chemotherapy agents), and toxins such as benzol or benzene have all been shown to increase the incidence of leukemia. Radiation may also increase the risk of lymphoma. In addition, abnormalities of the immune system, *immunodeficiency syndromes,* may identify patients at risk for lymphoma.

Certain lymphomas, such as Burkitt's lymphoma, which occurs primarily in Africa, have been associated with specific viruses, in this case the Epstein-Barr virus. Both sexes and all ages are at risk for leukemia and lymphoma.

Warning signs

The early warning signs of lymphoma or leukemia are nonspecific. With lymphoma a persistent, painless swelling of one or more lymph nodes may be all that the patient notices. If you notice a swollen lymph node that does not go away after 3 to 4 weeks, you should consult your physician. Occasionally, swelling may take place deep in the abdomen. Then the patient may be asymptomatic (without symptoms) or may notice abdominal fullness or heaviness, with or without pain. Other symptoms may include sweats at night, fevers, skin rash or bumps, itching, enlarged tonsils, or generalized weakness with loss of appetite or weight loss. It is important to remember that these symptoms are *not* specific. They do not mean that you have cancer, but only that if they persist for longer than about 3 weeks, you should see your physician for a checkup. Many noncancer diseases can cause these same symptoms, for example, hepatitis or infectious mononucleosis.

Certain leukemias may also be present with symptoms of abdominal swelling or discomfort. Other common symptoms include bone pain, paleness, a tendency to bruise or bleed easily, and frequent infections. Fatigue and weight loss are also common with certain types of leukemia. Again, if these symptoms persist over several weeks, they do not mean that you have cancer, but they do mean that you should check with your physician or nurse practitioner.

Screening and recommendations

There are no current screening recommendations for people who do not have symptoms. Watching for the symptoms just discussed and having your cancer-related checkup as we have recommended for other cancers are your best

<table>
<tr><td>

**Recommendations for
leukemia and lymphoma screening**

1. There are no currently recommended screening procedures for lymphomas or leukemias.
2. If at high risk because of radiation exposure or some other factor, discuss an individualized follow-up program with your physician.

</td></tr>
</table>

protection. At the checkup your examiner checks for enlarged lymph nodes and does an abdominal examination; a blood test (CBC, or complete blood count may be done) as well. In general, routine blood counts in asymptomatic people have not enabled us to find lymphoma or leukemia at a more curable stage. Once symptoms do occur, blood tests can be extremely useful in helping identify the cause of the abnormality. If you are a high-risk individual, either because of hereditary factors or perhaps because of some unusual occurrence such as heavy radiation exposure, then you should discuss an individualized follow-up program with your physician.

BLOOD CHEMISTRY TESTS

Thus far no blood chemistry tests have been successful for cancer screening. If a patient has already had cancer, then certain blood tests are important in following that person to check for possible recurrence. Blood tests are also useful in identifying the cause of an abnormality once symptoms have occurred. It is hoped that new organ-specific (breast, stomach, lung, and so on) tests will be developed for early stage cancer detection in the next few years. If such organ-specific blood chemistry profiles become available, then blood screening programs for cancer can be developed.

CONCLUSION

Although cancer screening is a continually developing science, it is already an effective means of preventing the effects of certain cancers when appropriate tests are used. There is generally a significant difference in the approach to screening of those under age 40 compared to those over 40, since most cancers occur more commonly as we get older.

Cancer is a costly disease, not only personally in terms of loss of health and suffering both for the patient and the immediate family, but also economically to society as a whole. Estimates are that U.S. industry could save $800 million yearly if workers would use commonsense rules of screening such as the American Cancer Society prevention and detection recommendations.

The value of a medical examination that is cancer-related cannot be overstressed; it may save your life. A physical examination once every 3 years until age 40 and then once a year after that time is far less costly than finding you have cancer and then initiating treatment—often when it is too late.

In general, it is wise to have these physical examinations, which should include checking for such cancers as testicular and prostatic in males and breast, ovarian and uterine (cervical and endometrial) in females, as well as cancers in the mouth, neck, skin, thyroid, lymph nodes, and colon for both males and females.

Recommendations for specific cancers are given in the sections on each of these cancers and are summarized in Table 4-3 on pp. 72–73.

We urge you to keep a health diary, noting when your next examination is due, and to follow sensible cancer prevention habits such as avoiding smoking and excessive alcohol, following a prudent low-fat, high-fiber diet, and avoiding excessive sun exposure. These simple and relatively inexpensive measures may well save your life.

TABLE 4-3   Timeline for cancer screening checkup*

	Age	20			25			30			35			
Breast	Breast examination, including review self-examination review	X	X		X		X		X		X		X		X
	Mammography†										X BASELINE			
	Breast self-examination			Monthly after age 20										
Cervical and endometrial	Pelvic	X	X		X		X		X		X		X		X
	Pap smear‡	X	X		X		X		X		X		X		X
	Endometrial sampling§													
Colon and prostate	Rectal examination													
	Stool occult blood‖													
	Sigmoidoscopy¶													
Head and neck	Oral and head and neck examination													
Self-reporting and primary prevention	Smoking, diet and alcohol counselling, stress audit	X	X		X		X	⟶	Repeated at every checkup					
	Testicular self-examination			Four to six times a year between ages 20 and 45										
	Report mouth sores and skin lesions	X	X		X		X		X	⟶ Repeated at every checkup				
	Report postmenopausal bleeding													

*These are reasonable recommendations for cancer screening based on the information in this chapter. They should be reviewed *on an individual basis* with your physician.

†Women at high risk should consider annual or biannual mammography after age 40. This should be discussed on an individual basis with your physician. The ACS continues to advise annual mammography over age 50 for all women.

‡Women with a history of abnormal Pap smears, cervical cancer, or sexual activity with different partners should have annual or more frequent screening. Discuss this with your physician. The American College of Obstetrics and Gynecology continues to recommend annual Pap smears.

§Should be considered before postmenopausal estrogen therapy and probably annually while taking estrogens. Discuss this with your physician.

‖Patient should be on appropriate diet.

¶ACS recommendations are more frequent—two annual examinations after age 50 and then every 3 years.

40					45				50				55				60				65				70		

X X X X X X X X ——————→ Repeated annually

X   X   X   X   X   X   X   X   X   X   X   X   X   X   X   X   X   X

X X X X X X ——————————→ Repeated annually after age 40

  X   X   X   X   X   X   X   X

    X   Repeat for postmenopausal bleeding
(At menopause if high risk)

X X X X X X X X X X X X X X X X X X X X X ——————→ Annually

          X X X X X X X X X X ——————→ Annually

    X   X   X
      (Repeat for positive occult blood)

X X X   Repeated annually

X X X ——————→ Repeated annually at checkup

CHAPTER 5

Nutrition and Cancer Prevention

A wise man always eats well.

CHINESE PROVERB

ERICA T. GOODE
ERNEST H. ROSENBAUM

For many years now, the scientific literature has provided increasingly clear statements that connections exist between the foods we eat and the development of cancer in our bodies. Media information is often worrisome and may leave you, the consumer of food, water, alcohol, and some inevitable environmental contaminants, with a sense of fatalistic dismay. This chapter is designed to provide some relief from your fears, since we do have some ideas regarding the helpful aspects of:

1. *Healthy patterns* of eating. These emphasize whole foods, replete with variety and fiber, and are helpful in avoiding cancer and in maintaining overall health.
2. Avoidance, most of the time, of other dietary patterns, such as high-fat, high-calorie, low-nutrient intake.
3. Avoidance of substances that negate healthy food patterns and that may promote cancers in their own right, such as a high-alcohol, high-cigarette, low-nutritional intake pattern.
4. Some general guidelines about food selection, storage, and preparation that should be followed to avoid, as much as possible:
   a. Significant nutrient losses
   b. Increased levels of mutagens in foods introduced, for example, by charbroiling, searing, or browning meats
   c. High levels of food contaminants (such as pesticide residues, diethylstilbestrol [DES] in meats, and vinyl chloride)
   d. Food additives that may be harmful
   e. Naturally occurring carcinogens, which may arise from the foods themselves or through improper storage
5. Information on which cancers (stomach, colon and rectum, breast, endometrium of the uterus, lung) are particularly influenced by diet.

Most of the diet-cancer information, including all these considerations, has recently been summarized in a publication entitled *Diet, Nutrition and Cancer* (Washington, D.C., 1982, Committee on Diet, Nutrition and Cancer, Assembly of Life Sciences, National Research Council, National Academy Press). The Committee, which reviewed the vast array of information, including epidemiologic, animal, and *in vitro* (occurring in laboratory apparatus) studies, also commented on the pitfalls of various methods for collecting data. Remember that many studies provide only *hints* of a connection between food intake and the later development of or protection from certain cancers.

Additional problems in interpretation of diet/cancer association arise because of the following:

1. Some families are more prone to develop cancer than others.
2. "Stress," an almost unmeasurable factor that comes and goes in our lives, may play a role (see Chapter 9).
3. People eat differently at various times in their lives; exposure to harmful and protective dietary substances may change and may be hidden at the time a cancer develops.
4. Levels of *calories* taken in by individuals result in differing degrees of body fat, depending on exercise levels, general lifestyle, and familial factors that affect body metabolism. Being overweight may lead to increased rates of some cancers (especially endometrial cancer and possibly breast cancer) but may occur in women who eat less than their thin counterparts. *Total caloric intake* may lead to increased development of those cancers seen when increased levels of harmful substances are being eaten with these increased calories, but the individual may be lean. Thus, these basic differences must be sorted out, and careful dietary intake studies (which are difficult, especially long-range ones) are the only means of clarifying these points.
5. The aging process leads to increased risks of developing cancer. We know from laboratory rat studies that longevity is doubled by feeding the animals limited calorie, nutritionally adequate diets as "teenagers" and for the rest of their lives. This delayed aging provides protection against tumor development. Should we interpret this to mean that human adolescents should curtail their rapacious appetites?

This chapter attempts to provide a balanced view of some of these issues so that you can decide what your own risks may be and how you want to modify them. We do know that approximately 20% of deaths in the United States are cancer-related and that many of these can be delayed or prevented by changes in life-style. It is thought by most researchers that about 90% of all cancers are environmentally induced and that diet is at least partially responsible for 30% to 40% of cancers in men and 60% in women. The Committee summary of the *Diet, Nutrition and Cancer* report suggests that we understand these associations about as well as the cigarette/lung cancer connections were known when the Surgeon General issued his initial report in 1965. The problem for you, of course, is that you cannot stop eating; thus risks are diminished but never abolished.

WHAT IS A HEALTHY DIET?

When a scientist or researcher is quoted in the media as saying that a dietary substance or nutritional habit *causes cancer*, it is important to ask several questions: Who is this individual? What are his or her qualifications? Is this person's area of work close to the subject on which he or she is commenting?

The next question is the *degree of certainty* that is ascribed to the connection. In general, *very few* substances lead directly to the development of cancer. We all know that many people who smoke heavily for a long time develop lung and other cancers. But we also know people who live long lives *while* smoking and die of some illness other than cancer, emphysema, heart disease, or hypertensive complications—all of which are seen at high levels among smokers. As can be seen in Fig. 5-1, we may fall one, two, or more standard deviations away on the

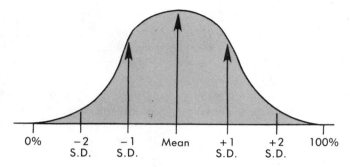

FIG. 5-1 Bell curve showing standard deviation (*S.D.*) and mean chance of developing a particular cancer. Position on bell curve (no chance, 100% chance, or somewhere between) is influenced by such factors as inherent genetic potential, other environmental factors including nutrition, coexisting stresses, and disease. Since the chance for developing cancer is influenced by *many* things, predictions are most difficult. Each individual either "gets cancer" (100%) or does not (0%).

bell curve from the mean chance of developing some type of cancer with some known substance exposure. If we look at one standard deviation in either direction from the mean, we have included 67% of the population. If we look at two standard deviations, plus or minus from the mean, we have included 97% of the population.

The next question is whether the researcher described the *means* of making the connection. Is the diet/cancer relationship based on epidemiologic studies that show a relationship between people's life-style changes, including diet, and subsequent change in disease patterns, including cancer? Or are the statements drawn from mutagenicity studies done *in vitro* (in a "test tube") or from *in vivo* (occurring in a living organism) studies done on animals? If the latter is the case, was more than one animal species used? Was the presumed cancer-promoting substance painted onto the animal? Injected? Used in very high levels that are unattainable in a "normal" diet?

You must raise these and other sensible questions before concluding that food X causes tumor Y. Other chapters in this book explore these topics in greater depth. To help you think

about these topics, you need to know a little about types of studies and levels of certainty about the conclusions drawn from each (see boxed material on p. 77).

The determination of dietary intake is critical to all of these ways of observing people. This is difficult! To prove this, try to recall every item that you ate or drank yesterday. Then try to recall all that you ate last week. Then think of what a typical day's food intake was for you 5 years ago. And finally, recall what you ate at home as a small child. Few of us know the exact amounts, which is the first problem. The second is that different brands of food, their growing location, their transport and storage, and the amounts of substances and the recipes used in their manufacture may introduce considerable variability in terms of additives, nutritional value, calories, fat levels, and other factors that may be important in tumor promotion. These factors may be unknown to you but may be very important to a connection between substance X and tumor Y, simply because none of us is aware of all these things.

Finally, to put some perspective into your approach, consider the following sections on diet and the associations with various cancers.

Type of study	Conclusions (level of certainty)
1. **Description.** These studies characterize one population (or more than one) and a number of factors in the environment, then note and compare the incidence of the disease in that group or groups.	Suggestive
2. **Correlation.** The overall, aggregate exposure of a population to a substance (or substances) is described and related to patterns of disease. The *Dietary Goals* are primarily based on this type of review. Differences in the total percentage of calories derived from carbohydrate, protein, or fat are observed in the population at two different points in time, then related to disease development over that period.	Suggestive only, since *individual* cause and effect is not explored and pitfalls can arise in drawing conclusions from data collected at different times and for purposes other than those of the study.
3. **Case-control.** These studies look at individual behavior and subsequent development of disease. For example, cases and controls are watched for development of tumors; experimental subjects are fed certain substances and control subjects are not. The different length and level of exposure and the statistical evaluation determine the strength of the connection between foods and development of cancer.	Depends on study design—can be effective
4. **Cohort.** These studies look at groups of similar individuals and attempt to watch them over time and to control a number of important variables that might obscure the conclusions. For example, a study might watch two groups of the same sex, similar ages, same residence location, similar occupations and socioeconomic status, then note whether tumor Y occurs less in one group that routinely takes vitamin capsules than in the other, non-vitamin taking group.	Depends on study design—can be effective
5. **Intervention.** These studies provide the most refined results, since these assign closely matched subjects to different groups. The experimental subjects are exposed to various levels of the substance, then watched for an increase or reduction in tumor development. These studies are ideal for establishing causality but are time-consuming and virtually impossible to perform with free-living human subjects. This would be a typical study design for use on laboratory animals.	Best

DIET IN RELATION TO
SPECIFIC CANCERS

Not *every* type of cancer seen in humans is related to dietary intake in any appreciable way that we can recognize. However, epidemiologic studies have observed and recorded relationships between diet and cancer at various body sites, and for a number of these cancers the connection between diet and the tumor involved is clear enough to make an association between the two phenomena. *Diet, Nutrition and Cancer* reviews these cancers and draws conclusions about the degree of dietary causality. For those cancers that are discussed, the connection is clearly present. You should keep these tumors in mind throughout this chapter, since the relationships between dietary substances (fat, protein, carbohydrate, vitamins, minerals, fiber) and nonnutrients (alcohol, food-borne substances such as package and pesticide residues) and tumor development will be better understood in the context of which tumors are most likely to be caused by problems in dietary intake.

Gastrointestinal (digestive) tract cancer

The most obvious connection between diet and tumor development would seem, logically, to occur in the digestive tract, since this area is exposed to the foods we eat on a regular basis. This includes the esophagus, stomach, intestines, colon, and rectum, and a high association between diet and cancer indeed exists for these areas. A relationship for the pancreas, liver, and gallbladder is also present, but it is less strong.

Anatomically, the *esophagus* is the first area under discussion. The mouth could be considered first, except that exposure to foods in the mouth is relatively brief for most of us and in other areas occurs on a much more lingering basis. Cancer of the esophagus is clearly related to the intake of alcohol; a number of studies done in countries around the world have re-

vealed definite alcohol/cancer correlations. Smoking plays its role as well, and in people who drink and smoke the risk of cancer development in the esophagus increases.

Some very interesting studies have been done in specific communities showing that food intake has important effects as well. One such study was done in a small set of communities in China known to have a very high rate of cancer of the esophagus. The people in the villages were selected and followed over time with a special device, similar to a bottle brush, used in the esophagus to collect cells, which were then checked for progressive dysplasia, metaplasia, and finally cancerous change. At the same time epidemiologists were looking at dietary factors that seemed to contribute to the differences between these communities and other areas where the incidence of esophageal cancer was low. After intensive sleuth work they found that these affected people had very low intakes of the trace mineral molybdenum because of soil deficiency. In addition, their intake of fruits and vegetables, animal products and fat, calcium, and riboflavin was quite low. These villagers had a particular way of pickling their vegetables that led to fungus and mold contamination. This was thought to produce nitrosamines, which we know are associated with the development of stomach cancer, particularly when eaten in connection with low dietary vitamin C. This Chinese community was encouraged to make several changes in their ways of producing and preparing foods, and the researchers are currently waiting to see a reversal in the high levels of esophageal cancer in these areas.

In other studies similar kinds of associations have been made. For example, areas of Iran where the people were shown to have low intakes of vitamins A and C due to a low intake of legumes, green vegetables, and fresh fruit, there are similarly high levels of esophageal cancer. The authors believe that a high opium use among these people might contribute. Another epidemiologic review of food patterns in

Africa and Asia showed a diet emphasizing wheat and corn, with relatively low zinc, magnesium, and niacin, was taken by those developing esophageal cancer, while a higher intake of cassara, yamo, peanuts, and millet, containing these nutrients, seems protective.

The conclusion from these studies and others is that a variety of substances may collaborate in the development of the cancer in the esophagus. The Iranian study found that high opium use in subgroups seemed to produce the highest incidence of esophageal cancer, and the Africa, Asia, and other United States studies have demonstrated the contribution made by alcohol and/or smoking and the associated poor dietary habits. Some studies have correlated the temperature of substances ingested with an increased susceptibility to esophageal cancer. However, the connections, as mentioned, are quite clear. If one were to try to prevent the problem, one would eat a diet rich in high-nutrient vegetables and fruits, particularly those with vitamins A and C. One would avoid trace mineral deficiencies, of molybdenum in particular, as well as pickled and moldy foods that might be contaminated with mycotoxins (toxic substances produced by certain fungi) or be rich in nitrosamines.

The next organ we come to in the digestive tract is the *stomach*. Epidemiologists have noted that the incidence of stomach cancer is highest in parts of Asia, particularly Japan, and in South America, and is very low in North America and Europe, where it is actually decreasing over time. The incidence is also high in Iceland; it is thought that the intake of smoked foods in this country, as in Japan, may play a major role in the development of cancer. The problem with smoking of foods is discussed in the section on extrinsic mutagens later in this chapter.

Another factor seems to be the level of nitrate in drinking water or the level of nitrosamines in food. Conflicting reports have occurred among reviewers of this literature concerning various dietary factors and the subsequent development of stomach cancer. However, one interesting study, involving Japanese who lived in Hawaii and still adhered to a Japanese style diet versus those Japanese who had already adopted more Western diet habits, showed that the Japanese use of pickled vegetables and dried salted fish was practiced more regularly by those people who developed cancers of the stomach. Their Westernized counterparts, who began eating fewer of these foods and seemed to be consuming more fresh fruits and vegetables, particularly lettuce and celery, had a lower incidence of stomach cancer. This pattern was studied by a different researcher, who showed that the intake of vegetables and vitamin C–rich foods was inversely related to the development of stomach cancer. A few people have less stomach acidity, which seems to predispose them to cancer of the stomach. However, only a small group of these people have developed this problem. Another study in Japan showed that in people eating a Japanese style diet, those who drank two glasses of milk per day fared better in terms of cancer of the stomach.

To summarize, it seems that although the incidence of cancer of the stomach is quite low in this country, certain people could still be at risk if they eat heavily salted, pickled foods or highly smoked foods and if they have a diet low in vegetables, particularly those containing vitamin C. It is possible that milk intake and perhaps other dairy products may assist in the low level of cancer of the stomach present in the United States and other Westernized countries.

The *small intestine* has not really been studied to any degree in relationship to diet and development of cancer. The association is probably there, but we know that of all people developing cancer of the intestinal tract from the duodenum to the rectum, cancer is progressively greater in areas approaching the rectal end of the tract. This is thought to result from the progressively higher concentrations of toxic substances, waste products, bacteria, and possibly other substances present in the final stool before defecation.

Many studies in the early 1970s attempted to show a clear association between "fiber" in the diet and the incidence of cancer of the *colon* and *rectum*. These studies are extremely complicated since fiber includes a variety of substances, the various subcomponents of which have various effects on cancer develoment, as well as other processes such as nutrient absorption. This subject is discussed later in this chapter; however, the most recent summary of investigations into cancer of the intestinal tract, particularly the colon, shows a much clearer association between "fiber" and these cancers.

One study done in 1979 showed that total dietary cholesterol was strongly correlated with cancer of the colon. It must be remembered, however, that association is not necessarily causation. Other studies have looked at the source of the dietary fat; one study seemed to show that persons who get their fats from red meat have higher rates of cancer than those who obtain their fat primarily from other sources, such as milk; another study was unable to show trends in beef and fat intake as being similar to incidence of cancer of the colon. One study that focused on mutagenic activity of the stool found more mutagenic activity in diets of meat eaters than in vegetarians.

As reviewed by a variety of studies, the consumption of vegetables, which incidentally contain higher vitamin A and crude fiber, seems to be protective against colon cancer. In addition, a series of studies have looked specifically at the cabbage family and found that these are particularly associated with a low incidence of cancer of the colon and rectum. A few studies have shown that beer intake or beer and other liquor intake is higher in people with a higher incidence of colon cancer.

To summarize, cancer of the colon occurs to a greater extent in those who eat a high-fat, probably high-calorie, and possibly high-saturated-fat diet. Dietary fiber has a protective ef-

fect; however, because of methodology and different fiber fractions, many studies are unclear as to which factors within high-fiber foods are useful in reducing colon cancer. And finally, the cruciferous vegetables (from the plant family *Cruciferae*), that is, broccoli, cabbage, cauliflower, and brussels sprouts, may be specifically protective.

Cancer of the *pancreas* is not strongly associated with dietary intake at this time. A few studies have attempted to show how the rate of cancer of the pancreas, which is definitely rising in our population, may relate to various dietary changes in the population. The most notorious study was reported in the media in 1981 and suggested a relationship between coffee intake and cancer of the pancreas. However, the study did not differentiate between decaffeinated or regular, instant or percolated coffees. When this control was used in a different study, it seems that the decaffeinating process may have been partly responsible for the increased cancer rates, since the decaffeinated-coffee drinkers had a higher incidence of cancer of the pancreas than those drinking regular coffee. Another question arises: since most coffee comes from foreign countries, are pesticides or other substances introduced during the growing process culprits for increased cancer? This has not yet been investigated.

In summary, the connections currently existing between diet and pancreatic cancer are questionable. The same holds true for diet and cancer of the *gallbladder*.

Liver cancer, as with that seen in the stomach, is much more prevalent in foreign countries, particularly Africa and Southeast Asia, than in the United States and other Westernized countries. It is thought that a variety of liver carcinogens, which are discussed elsewhere in this chapter and include aflatoxins, safrole, cycasin, and pyrrolidine alkaloids, as well as alcohol, may be inciting agents. Of these substances, only alcohol is found in great supply in diets in the United States. When the incidence of alcoholic cirrhosis is sorted out from other forms of cirrhosis, such as that introduced in conjunction with hepatitis B virus infection, the hepatitis B cirrhosis is much more often linked with eventual hepatoma (liver cancer) than is the cirrhosis seen in alcoholism. It will be interesting to follow individuals in the United States who have hepatitis B antigen positivity and see whether they develop cancer of the liver. It may be that these cancers appear only when two or more factors occur at the same time, such as hepatitis B with concurrent aflatoxin exposure or perhaps with other nutritional factors. At present it is believed that in the United States the risk of diet-induced liver cancer is very limited.

Breast cancer

The relationship of diet to breast cancer has been explored in two major ways: (1) animal experiments and (2) epidemiologic trends in humans. The second includes studying differences in the diets of women who have developed breast cancer and those with fairly long-term dietary habits who are free of cancer.

In one well-controlled animal study, done at Memorial Sloan-Kettering Cancer Center in New York, mice with a genetic predisposition toward cancer were given half the normal number of calories per day, as compared to another group of mice who could eat at will. Those given limited calories developed almost no breast cancer, whereas the controls developed breast cancer at the normal rate. We do know that in some families, women may have a greater risk for development of breast cancer, indicating some genetic predisposition in humans as well as in other animals. Other studies have shown that it may well be the level of total dietary fat that contributes most to the subsequent development of breast cancer.

In terms of epidemiology, it has been known for some time that when people in their native countries, consuming their native diet, move from place to place, their chances for certain kinds of diseases change. For example, one study investigated premenopausal Japanese women who showed a negligible incidence of breast cancer in their native habitat. When they moved to California and adopted the eating habits of the American woman, however, they tended to show a greater susceptibility to breast cancer. It is interesting to note that Oriental women, including the Japanese, have different kinds of earwax (cerumen) and nonlactating breast secretion than Caucasian women. The Japanese and other Oriental women tend to have a dry earwax, and it was thought that their type of breast secretion might be related to this. However, it seems from these migratory studies that this difference in breast secretion confers no special protection in the face of certain dietary changes.

In a third epidemiologic study the diets of women with and without breast cancer are compared. One such study was completed in 1978, with 400 cancer cases compared with 400 neighborhood control women. The overall nutrient intake of both was estimated from dietary histories focusing on six nutrients. In the premenopausal woman the strongest association was found between a high-fat intake in the breast cancer cases and a lower fat intake in the control group. Weaker associations were seen for saturated fat and cholesterol differences. In postmenopausal women the only consistent finding was again an association between total fat consumption and the development of breast cancer. Other studies show constellations of high-fat foods correlated with the onset of breast cancer. In one study the relative risk increased with consumption of beef, other red meat, pork, and sweet desserts. All of these substances are usually high in fat.

Interesting associations have also been observed between a high-vegetable intake and the risk for developing breast cancer. In the migratory Japanese study women in Japan ate a much higher level of vegetables than they did in California. In addition, a study done in England during World War II investigated changes in food consumption at the time of war shortages, during which the incidence of breast cancer fell sharply. When the types of foods eaten were studied, it was noted that the war brought about shortages of sugar, dairy products, and meat and that many more vegetables were consumed at that time. After the war the previous dietary habits returned, and after 1948 the trend in breast cancer was reversed and rose to its previous levels.

Also of interest is a recent study in the *New England Journal of Medicine* comparing 10 vegetarians and 10 nonvegetarians. The fat content of the vegetarian diet was 30% of total calories compared to 40% for the nonvegetarians, and 28 grams of fiber versus 12 grams, respectively. The vegetarians had higher stool weight with increased estrogens (hormones) and lower blood levels of estrogen, whereas the nonvegetarians had the converse. This adds more information to the role of increased dietary fat intake with lower fiber intake and higher blood estrogen levels.

In summary, from all studies including those reviewed in *Diet, Nutrition and Cancer,* it must be concluded that of all dietary factors, the only one definitively linked with the incidence of breast cancer is a high-fat diet.

Uterine cancer

Although numerous studies have not directly linked uterine cancer with any dietary factors, the uterine endometrium is a hormone-sensitive organ and thus responds to changes in the hormonal level in the body. One such change depends on body weight, and in the excessively overweight female it has been shown that cancer of the uterine endometrium does increase. Some studies have attempted to correlate the onset of uterine cancer with the total fat in the diet, as has been done in other types of hormone sensitive tumors. This has not been studied thoroughly enough to make that association.

Lung cancer

Cancer of the lung—bronchogenic (arising in a bronchial tube) carcinoma—which is known to be influenced by an assortment of environmental impacts on the lung, particularly smoking, also has a dietary component to its onset. A variety of studies have studied bronchogenic carcinoma in men, particularly since these are the high-intake smokers and the people at greatest risk for development of this cancer. Several studies have concluded that consumption of dark, green leafy vegetables, rich in beta-carotene (the precursor of preformed vitamin A found in the human and dairy product and animal sources of vitamin A) is lowest in those people who subsequently develop cancer of the lung, when compared with matched smokers who remained healthy.

One extensive study with a 19-year follow-up looked at 1900 men in Chicago, many of whom smoked. There was a very strong inverse association between lung cancer incidence and beta-carotene intake, after adjustment for cigarette smoking. Lung cancer was not significantly influenced by the intake of preformed vitamin A, which is the usual form found in vitamin tablets. Thus it seems important for people to get beta-carotene (the precursor of vitamin A) in dark-green and yellow fruits and vegetables; substitution with a vitamin pill is not sufficient in terms of protection against cancer of the lung, particularly in smokers.

Bladder cancer

One study investigating bladder cancer made conclusions similar to those found in the lung cancer data, in that a low total vitamin A intake correlated with the development of bladder cancers. In this study carrot and milk consumption, both high in vitamin A, were taken into account in the total vitamin A intake assessment. Various other studies have attempted to correlate the development of bladder cancer with intake of artificial sweeteners, coffee, total fats, tea, alcohol, and soft drinks in humans, and fiddlehead greens (related to bracken fern), which cause bladder cancer in cattle. No clear associations have been drawn between any of these substances and human bladder cancer.

To summarize, the only substance in the diet clearly related to bladder cancer is vitamin A, with its protective role. It is not clear whether the beta-carotene form is significantly more helpful than preformed vitamin A.

Other cancer sites

Other cancers, such as cancer of the prostate, may also be related to diet, and these associations may become stronger over time. There is some evidence, as noted in the preceding discussions, that there is an increased risk of certain cancers associated with certain dietary factors, particularly a high-fat, high-protein diet. It is possible that vitamin A or beta-carotene and/or a vegetarian diet prevents cancer of the prostate to some extent. Several studies have tended to support this concept.

Fig. 5-2 should put the relative risks of developing certain nutrition-related cancers into perspective for one group of immigrants to the United States. Most striking in this chart, the risks of liver and stomach cancer were seen to be extremely high in Japanese living in Japan, less but still high in immigrants (Issei), and even less in the sons of immigrants (Nisei). This may reflect, as has been noted, that certain Japanese foods, levels of nitrates relative to vitamins C and E levels of mold (aflatoxins), levels of salted, pickled substances, or other factors of

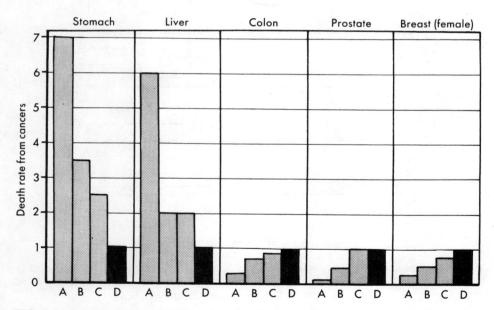

FIG. 5-2 Relative death rates from cancers of Japanese immigrants to United States compared with rate for California whites (averages). *A,* Japanese; *B,* Japanese immigrants to California (Issei); *C,* sons of Japanese immigrants to California (Nisei); *D,* California whites. (Compiled from a variety of sources.)

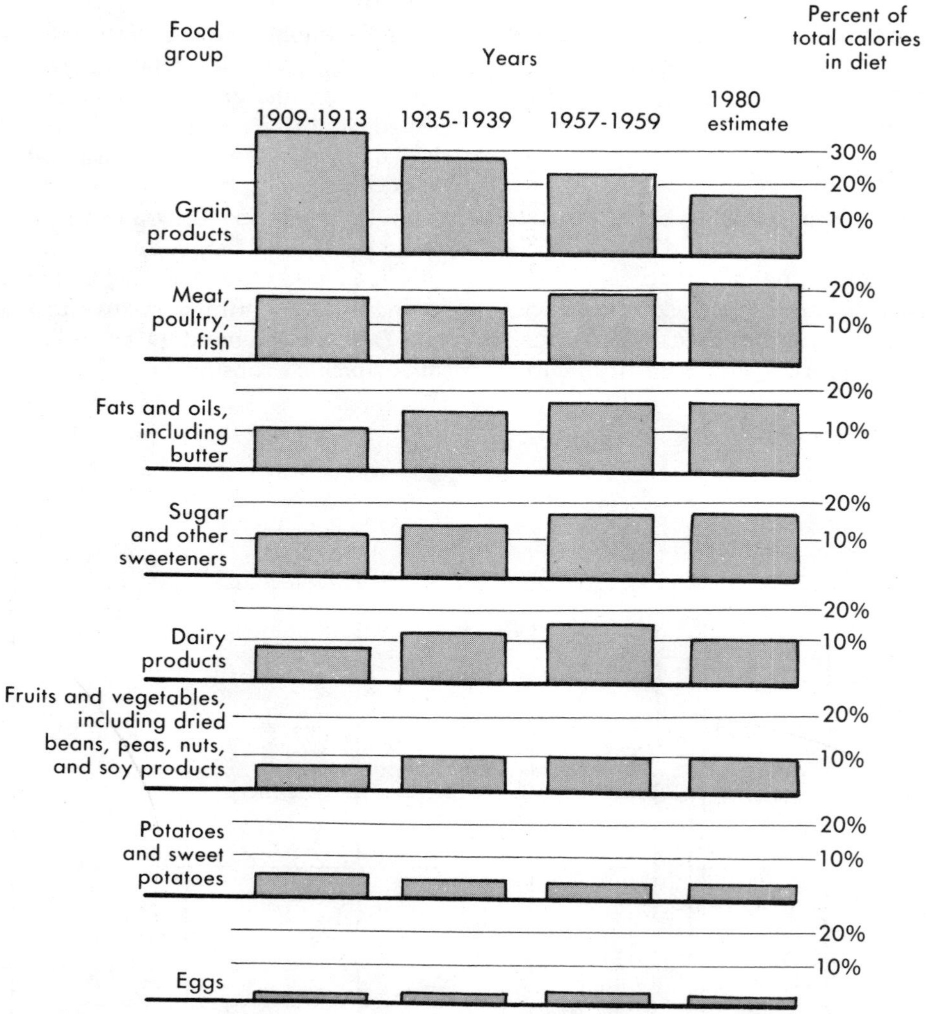

FIG. 5-3 The changing U.S. dietary intake of food groups. (From U.S. Senate Select Committee on Nutrition and Human Needs: Dietary goals for the United States, Washington, D.C., February 1977, U.S. Government Printing Office.)

which we are not aware—whether dietary or environmental—may affect cancer susceptibility.

DIETARY GOALS

The composition of the average person's diet in the United States has changed radically during this century. Early in the twentieth century and before, foods routinely contained complex carbohydrates from grain products and vegetables and "naturally occurring" sugars from fruit, juices, and vegetables. For many Americans these now provide a minor contribution to diet. At the same time the consumption of fats and refined and processed sugars has risen dramatically. These two substances now comprise about 60% of the total caloric intake for the U.S. population, *an increase of 20% since the early 1900s,* as illustrated by Fig. 5-3. It should be noted from the diagram that the meat, poultry, and fish category and the dairy group contribute much of the dietary fat.

In the opinion of expert nutritionists consulted by the Senate Select Committee on Nutrition and Human Needs in the early 1970s, before their reports of 1976 and 1977, these and other food changes are producing overall undesirable effects in terms of both over- and underconsumption of food; these effects may be as profoundly damaging to health in the United States as the widespread contagious diseases of the early part of the century.

The general overconsumption of foods high in fat, especially saturated fat, as well as overconsumption of cholesterol, refined and processed sugars, salt, and alcohol, has been associated with an increase in several of the leading causes of death, including heart disease, some cancers, stroke and hypertension, diabetes, arteriosclerosis, and cirrhosis of the liver. We will not dwell on the multiple purposes of the U.S. Dietary Goals in prevention of disease but will instead focus on those aspects thought to be especially pertinent to the prevention of early cancer development.

The typical overconsumption of food, com-

bined with our more sedentary life-style, has become a major public health problem. In testimony at Senate committee hearings in the early 1970s, Dr. Theodore Cooper, then Assistant Secretary for Health, estimated that about 20% of all adults in the United States "are overweight to a degree that may interfere with optimal health and longevity."

Nutrient density (the nutritional value of a food relative to its calories) is poor in several foods. Fats are relatively low in vitamins and minerals, and refined sugar and most processed sugars have no vitamins and minerals. Reduced-calorie and low-income diets, and often the diets of elderly and disabled individuals, are frequently unbalanced in terms of excess sugars and thus may lead to vitamin and mineral insufficiencies.

Given the wide impact on health arising from such dietary trends, it was thought to be imperative that consumers be provided with certain guidelines for eating. The dietary goals for intake of carbohydrates, fats, and protein listed in Fig. 5-4 have been recommended for citizens of the United States. Each recommended level of intake represents a conclusion based on the opinion of a variety of scientific experts. *Therefore, each specific level should be considered as the center of a range.* The overall recommendation is for a diet that is lower in fat, higher in total and complex carbohydrates, lower in cholesterol, and lower in salt than the diet consumed in 1976. The specific ranges include the following:

Total carbohydrates (55% to 61%)
    Complex carbohydrates and "naturally occurring" sugars (45% to 51%)
Total fat (27% to 33%)
    Polyunsaturated (8% to 12%)
    Monounsaturated (8% to 12%)
    Saturated (8% to 12%)
Protein (10% to 14%)
Cholesterol (250 to 350 milligrams)
Salt (4 to 6 grams)

Changing one's dietary patterns generally requires slow adjustments in food selection; for

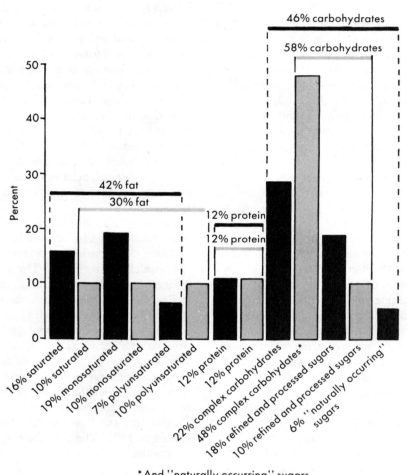

*And "naturally occurring" sugars.

FIG. 5-4 Recommended dietary intake in percentages of fats, protein, and carbohydrates. Dark gray bars represent present (1976) intake; light gray bars show desirable intake. (From U.S. Senate Select Committee on Nutrition and Human Needs: Dietary goals for the United States, Washington, D.C., February 1977, U.S. Government Printing Office.)

example, choosing roast meat instead of fried meat, fresh vegetables instead of macaroni salad, or fresh fruit instead of sweet desserts. The question of whether dietary changes alone can reduce the leading causes of death in the United States remains controversial. Individuals, in exercising freedom of dietary choice, should recognize that these dietary recommendations do not guarantee improved protection from the killer diseases. They do, however, increase the probability of protection.

More specifically, the U.S. Dietary Goals suggest that the individual should make these changes:

1. To avoid being overweight, consume only as much energy (calories) as is expended; if overweight, decrease energy intake and increase energy expenditure.
2. Increase the consumption of complex carbohydrates and "naturally occurring" sugars from about 28% to about 48% of energy intake.
3. Reduce consumption of refined and processed sugars by about 45% to account for about 10% of total energy intake.
4. Reduce overall fat consumption from approximately 40% to about 30% of energy intake.
5. Reduce saturated fat consumption to account for about 10% of total energy intake; balance that with polyunsaturated and monosaturated fats, which should each account for about 10% of energy intake.
6. Reduce cholesterol consumption to about 30 milligrams a day.
7. Limit the intake of sodium by reducing the intake of salt to about 5 grams (2.0 grams of sodium) or less a day.

These goals translate into the following changes in food selection and preparation:

1. Increase consumption of fruits and vegetables and whole grains.
2. Decrease consumption of refined and other processed sugars and foods high in such sugars.
3. Decrease consumption of foods high in total fat, and partially replace saturated fats, whether obtained from animal or vegetable sources, with polyunsaturated fats.

4. Decrease consumption of animal fat and choose meats, poultry, and fish, which will reduce saturated fat intake.
5. Except for young children (under the age of 1 year), substitute low-fat and nonfat milk for whole milk, and low-fat dairy products for high-fat dairy products.
6. Decrease consumption of butterfat, eggs, and other high-cholesterol sources. Some consideration should be given to easing the cholesterol goal for premenopausal women, young children, and the elderly to obtain the nutritional benefits of eggs in the diet.
7. Decrease consumption of salt and eliminate foods high in salt content.

Table 5-1 shows generally how to include a variety of whole, nutritious, low-calorie foods containing limited sodium (salt) as the basis for one's daily diet. Note that highly sweet or fatty foods have been excluded, as have nonnutrient contributors such as coffee, tea, and alcoholic beverages.

An example of a typical day's intake might be as follows:

Breakfast: One-half grapefruit
Bran cereal with low-fat or skim milk
Coffee or tea, black
Lunch: Vegetable borscht (vegetable soup)
Sandwich: whole-wheat bread, low-fat cheese (such as mozzarella, Lorraine, Pre Monde), tomatoes, sprouts
Custard (low-fat milk)
Snack: Peanuts in shells, fresh fruit
Dinner: Stir-fried Chinese dish (chicken, tofu, spinach, Chinese cabbage, onions, green peppers, sesame seeds, with very limited oil and soy sauce)
Brown rice
Cucumber salad with vinegar dressing
Blackberries with yogurt topping
Glass of white wine

Persons with physical ailments who believe that they should not follow these guidelines need to consult with a health professional having expertise in nutrition. Individuals who are limiting calories, have been ill, are pregnant, or are over 65 to 70 years of age may need a different calorie intake and/or a supplemental vitamin that provides the U.S. Recommended Daily Allowances of vitamins and minerals (see following section), since small variations in nutrients occur with daily food differences.

It should be noted that this overall eating pattern runs counter to what one may hear from advertising. In 1975, according to Leading National Advertisers, Inc., about $1.5 billion was spent on food advertising, which represents about 28% of total television advertising spend-ing. A study conducted by Lynne Masover and Dr. Jeremiah Stamler in Chicago analyzed the food advertising on four Chicago television stations during the week of August 4 to 10, 1975, and reported:

A detailed look at this weekly food advertising time—restaurants excluded—found that the group of non-nutritive beverages was, by far, the single most-advertised food group, capturing approximately two-fifths of time, of which nearly one-third was for wine and beer. Sweets took up about 11 percent of the time; non-nutritive beverages

TABLE 5-1 U.S. Dietary Goals chart

Food group	Nutrients supplied	Servings/day*	Examples†	Comments	Salt content
Milk	Calcium, riboflavin, protein, vitamins D and B$_{12}$, pantothenic acid, magnesium, zinc	2‡ 1 serving = 1 cup milk 1 carton yogurt 3 scoops cottage cheese	Low-fat, skim milk Buttermilk, low-fat cheese, low-fat cottage cheese, plain yogurt .... Whole milk, cottage cheese Cheese, fruit flavor yogurt Custards, puddings Ice cream, milkshakes	Less fat and calories More fat and calories	Low salt: Swiss, ricotta, mozzarella, and "unsalted" cheese; dry curd cottage cheese Medium salt: milk, yogurt, ice cream, cheddar, jack and Muenster cheese, salted butter/margarine High salt: buttermilk; parmesan, processed, blue, creamed cottage, and Gouda cheese
Meat and legumes	Protein, iron, niacain, thiamin, vitamins B$_6$ and B$_{12}$, folic acid	2‡ 1 serving = 2-3 oz meat, poultry, or fish 4 tbs peanut butter 2 eggs 1 cup dried peas or beans	Dry beans and peas Poultry, fish Lean beef, lamb, or pork Eggs .... Fatty beef, lamb, or pork Processed meats Nuts, peanut butter	Less fat and calories More fat and calories	Low salt: fresh meat, poultry, fish, eggs, unsalted peanut butter, beans Medium salt: frozen fish, fresh shellfish High salt: all salted, smoked, or pickled products; ham, bacon, cold cuts; canned fish or meat; sardines; TV dinners

*For adults.
†Lower calorie foods are listed first, selections above dotted lines provide the best nutrient density foods.
‡More servings per day for children and adolescents and during pregnancy and lactation.

TABLE 5-1 U.S. Dietary Goals chart—cont'd

Food group	Nutrients supplied	Servings/day*	Examples†	Comments	Salt content
Vegetables and fruit	Vitamins A, C, E and B₆, folic acid, iron, magnesium	4 1 serving = 1 dish vegetable or fruit 1 small glass juice 1 piece whole fruit or vegetable Bowl salad	Cantaloupe, tomatoes, spinach, broccoli, orange, unsweetened fruit juice Apricots, grapefruit, green beans, carrots lettuce, strawberries, peaches, cabbage, pears, potatoes, bananas Corn, apples	Less fat and calories	Low salt: all fresh fruit and vegetables, unless otherwise noted; canned fruit Medium salt: celery canned or frozen vegetables, Swiss chard High salt: tomato juice, vegetable juice, pickles, olives, sauerkraut, relishes, packaged vegetables
			Canned fruits in syrup, canned vegetables Sweetened fruit juice, salted vegetable juice Dried fruit, avocado Canned soup	More fat and calories calories	
Bread and cereal	Iron, niacin, thiamin, vitamin B₆, magnesium, pantothenic acid, zinc	4 1 serving = 1 slice bread ½ bagel or muffin ½ cup hot cereal, potato, rice, or pasta 1 corn tortilla 5 crackers	Whole-grain breads, rolls, cereals Enriched breads, rolls, unsweetened cereals Macaroni, spaghetti, noodles Rice, tortillas Pancakes, muffins, cornbread	Less fat and calories	Low salt: noodles, rice, hot cereal (not instant), low-sodium bread, tortillas, shredded or puffed wheat, unsalted crackers Medium salt: most dry cereals, cornbread, biscuits, muffins, commercial breads, pancakes High salt: foods with baking soda/powder, instant hot cereals, salted crackers or breads, prepared noodle products
			Crackers, presweetened cereals	More fat and calories	

plus sweets — all items low in nutrients, and most of them high in calories — commanded an absolute majority of time. Add to these the oils, fats and margarines, baked goods, snack foods, and relishes, and the proportion of advertising going to low-nutrient, generally high-calorie foods was nearly 70 percent. . . .

Of the restaurants advertised, nearly all were of the limited-menu, fast-food type specializing in foods high in saturated fats and cholesterol.

The study found that only about 25% of the time was devoted to more "nutritious groups," such as bread, cereal, pasta, meat, fish and sea-food, dairy products, fruits and vegetables, soups, and nut products.

Furthermore, a report by James T. Parker of the Division of Adult Education of the U.S. Office of Education finds that the level of general competency in selecting a nutritious diet decreases as the levels of education and income decline. The report also finds "the older the individual, the more likely that he/she is incompetent" to choose a well-balanced set of foods.

In a test gauging knowledge of nutrition, 71% of respondents correctly selected tuna when asked to choose an item for its protein content from the list: tuna, macaroni, peaches, or spinach. The subset of individuals with the lowest percentage of correct answers was the lowest income group.

Correct scores by age grouping were: ages 18 to 29 years, 62% correct; 30 to 39 years, 79%; 40 to 49 years, 80%; 50 to 59 years, 72%; 60 to 65 years, 66%. This suggests that nutrition education might best be directed to the young and elderly.

In another test related to nutrition, only 56% of respondents correctly estimated the number of calories in question. Again lowest scores fell in the lowest-income and highest-age groups. In the lowest income group, only 38% chose the correct answer.

The problem of appropriate food selection is further confounded by labeling that is incomplete, unhelpful, or unavailable on many food items. Currently labeling of nutritional compo-nents is voluntary and therefore not available on many food packages. Labels often provide little or no information as to types of fats and amounts of sugar, cholesterol, or calories. Food additives are listed for some foods but not for others.

The Senate Select Committee recommended food labeling for all foods, containing the following information to enable the customer to make informed comparisons between foods:

1. Percentage and type of fats
2. Percentage of sugar
3. Milligrams of cholesterol
4. Milligrams of salt
5. Caloric content
6. Complete listing of food additives for all foods, including those now covered by standards of identity
7. Required across-the-board nutrition labeling

It should be noted that some of our most nutrient-dense plain foods (vegetables, fruits, legumes; fresh meat, poultry, fish; fresh dairy foods, eggs) are single entities and are therefore not labeled, which is unfortunate for the comparative shopper. In the meantime, the present food labels are of some help. They list ingredients in order of the amount present by weight.

Additives *purposely* incorporated are included in the list of ingredients. Some of these may be harmful, such as saccharin, nitrates, or salts; others may be nutrient contributors, such as ascorbic acid, sodium erythrobate, and sodium ascorbate. Unfortunately, substances that accidentally get into foods, such as pesticides, benzopyrene, and packaging components, do not appear on food labels. Although we cannot easily avoid such substances, we may be able to lower our risk of cancer by paying attention to those ingredients listed.

In addition, a shift to the U.S. Dietary Goals offers potential for significant reduction in food costs. Savings may be achieved through home preparation and through reduction of

TABLE 5-2 Cost of one day's protein allowance—at average rates for March, 1983 (Numbers in parentheses indicate cents or dollars and cents.)

Cost	Meat	Dairy products	Legumes	Grains and flour	Seafood	Nuts and seeds
30¢			Split peas and lentils (32)	Wheat bran (28) Whole-wheat flour (30) Rye flour (33) Corn meal (38)		
40¢			Pinto and black beans (43) Soybeans (45)			
50¢		Eggs (46) Dry milk, skim (48)	Black-eyed peas (49)			
	Hamburger (56)	Cottage cheese (63) Milk, whole (72) Buttermilk (88)		Egg noodles (60) Oatmeal (70) Millet (82)		Peanuts, raw or roasted (60)
	Chicken (97)					
$1.00		Ricotta cheese (1.03) Cheddar cheese (1.16)				Pumpkin seeds (1.01)
	Pork (1.17)	Swiss cheese (1.33) Parmesan cheese (1.43)		Wheat bread (1.29) Rye bread (1.32)	Salmon, frozen (1.19) Tuna, canned (1.39) Seabass (1.49)	Sunflower seeds (1.40) Peanut butter; ⅓ lb = 45 g (1.50)
$1.50	Steak (1.53)					
$2.00					Swordfish (1.75)	Cashews (1.85) Walnuts, English (2.10)
$2.50						
$3.00						Brazil nuts (3.00)
$4.00					Oysters (4.38)	
$5.00					Crab, in shell (5.50) Clams, canned (6.30)	Pine nuts (5.25)

Modified from Lappé, F.: Diet for a small planet, New York, 1971, Ballantine Books.

and substitution for fats, refined and processed sugar, and expensive fatty protein sources. For the individual who habitually eats lunch and snacks away from home, great savings can be achieved by taking vegetables, sandwiches, fruits, and other simple foods from home. Restaurants, vending machines, and lunch trucks provide foods that are invariably higher in cost and less nutrient dense.

Table 5-2 compares relative 1983 costs of various food groups.

In the category of grain products, choosing the less processed, more nutritious products may often mean a savings. For instance, in one sampling, brand-name converted rice cost 25% more than the low-priced store brand of instant rice. Slightly processed hot cereals such as oatmeal are generally less expensive than ready-to-eat cereals.

The most dramatic savings made by a reduction in sugar consumption result from cutting back or eliminating purchases of candy, sweet-baked goods, and soft drinks. Costs are also cut when the consumer chooses the unsweetened as opposed to the presweetened version of a particular food item; the prime example is breakfast cereals.

Reducing fat consumption, and particularly consumption of saturated fats, may also yield cost savings in several areas. For example, chicken and turkey, which are lower in saturated fat than most meats, may average less than half the price of the beef, pork, and lamb cuts. Butter, on a per-teaspoon basis, is generally more expensive than even the most costly of the unsaturated vegetable oils. Reduced use of prepared salad dressing, catsup, and sauces can cut expenses and reduce fat, sugar, and salt consumption as well.

Greater home preparation can also yield savings in some areas and greater control over diet composition. A recent study by the Department of Agriculture comparing the costs of various convenience foods with their home-prepared counterparts found that out of 25 meat dishes

tested, 21 were more expensive per serving when purchased ready-made. Many of the cost differences were dramatic. The report said:

> The cost of home-prepared batter-dipped chicken was less than one-third that of the convenience products. Both chicken a-la-king frozen in a pouch and canned chicken salad spread were about 60% more expensive per serving . . . . Consumers paid approximately 40 cents more per serving for frozen turkey dinner or tetrazzini than for the separate ingredients.

Some people will find it difficult or impossible to change food preparation patterns drastically. However, home preparation offers savings as well as nutritional advantages.

RECOMMENDED DAILY DIETARY ALLOWANCES

During World War II a variety of nutrition-related projects were launched in the United States in an effort to keep the greatest number of Americans healthy. These included the push for Victory Gardens and food coupons but also developed a set of guidelines for feeding groups of people called the Recommended Daily Dietary Allowance (RDA). The National Research Council, Food and Nutrition Board (a group of nutrition scientists), established the allowances and to the present continues to convene every few years to review the mass of nutrition research and reissue the RDA accordingly. The 1980 RDAs are shown in Table 5-3.

An individual of a given age does *not* necessarily need the RDA for each specific nutrient listed. These are recommended allowances for feeding *groups*. Hence the recommendations for vitamins and minerals are set slightly above the average allowance for a given nutrient (for example, vitamin A in the 25-year-old male).

The U.S. RDA for energy requirements is different in that no "cushion" is provided for calories. Calorie levels are thus considered to be those for the typical person with an average height, weight, and activity level. (See Tables 5-4 and 5-5.)

The protein requirements (see Table 5-3) are set at grams/day/kilogram of body weight. Your kilogram weight equals your weight in pounds divided by 2.2.

Many other nutrients, particularly trace elements such as chromium, selenium, and manganese, have no established standards for intake because the level of research does not allow a definitive statement regarding requirements for intake. There are also limited data regarding levels of these elements in our food supply. This is one of the best reasons for the consumption of a *variety* of foods.

The U.S. RDAs are found on food labels in markets and are there to help guide people's food choices. They are a regulatory standard derived by the Food and Drug Administration (FDA) *from* the initial RDA. The U.S. RDAs are set at the highest nutrient levels required for any group (according to age and sex) on the RDA table, which allows a cushion for most individuals, as does the original RDA.

Since the U.S. RDAs define levels well *above* probable requirements in order to include almost all of those individuals who might have increased need for a particular vitamin or mineral, they are often higher than a typical individual's actual daily intake. Therefore, most of us do quite well with one-half less than the U.S. RDA. The exception is for calories, which does not include a safety factor. Calorie and protein intake should be evaluated per kilogram of body weight. With these limitations in mind, the RDAs can be used to roughly evaluate an individual's diet.

Foods required to conform with the U.S. RDAs labeling regulations include those for which the manufacturer makes nutritional claims, such as vitamins or products to which the manufacturer adds nutrients. Many other foods are voluntarily labeled by the producer. The manufacturer is required to list calories per serving, protein, carbohydrate, and fat content in grams per serving and the percentage of RDA for protein, vitamin A, vitamin C, thiamin, riboflavin, niacin, calcium and iron. There are 12 other nutrients that the manufacturer may elect to show. Cholesterol, saturated and polyunsaturated fats, and sodium are also often listed, since many consumers want this information. Special RDAs have also been established for infants, children under age 4, pregnant women, and nursing mothers. These RDAs are listed on the labels of vitamin and mineral supplements and on infant and toddler foods.

The U.S. RDAs can be very helpful to consumers in comparing and evaluating individual servings of food products for both their nutrient density and caloric value.

Other nutrients exist for which no U.S. RDA has yet been established because research is still "in progress." The RDA has only established required levels of calories and 17 well-known nutrients for the various categories of persons according to age and sex; there are at least 50 nutrients that should be considered. We do not yet know the needs for some of these nutrients, particularly the trace elements.

When shopping and checking food labels, you can simplify the job of assuring a good nutrient intake by looking at what nutritionists call the *indicator nutrients*—protein, calcium, iron, vitamin A, thiamin (vitamin B_1), riboflavin (vitamin B_2), niacin, and vitamin C (see Table 5-6). These nutrients must be listed on a labeled product; they have been shown, when all are taken in ample amounts, to provide good nutrition in terms of other unlisted nutrients such as vitamin B_6. To use the indicator nutrients as a guide, however, your foods must be from natural or only slightly processed sources. Highly processed or synthetic foods that have been fortified with a few nutrients cannot be included, since the presence of certain added nutrients does not necessarily mean that other accepted nutrients are also present. For example, a synthetic, powdered, orange-flavored fruit

TABLE 5-3 Recommended daily dietary allowances (designed for the maintenance of good

	Age (years)	Weight		Height		Protein (g)	Fat-soluble vitamins		
		(kg)	(lb)	(cm)	(in)		Vitamin A (μg RE)†	Vitamin D (μg)‡	Vitamin E (mg α-TE)§
Infants	0.0-0.5	6	13	60	24	kg × 2.2	420	10	3
	0.5-1.0	9	20	71	28	kg × 2.0	400	10	4
Children	1-3	13	29	90	35	23	400	10	5
	4-6	20	44	112	44	30	500	10	6
	7-10	28	62	132	52	34	700	10	7
Males	11-14	45	99	157	62	45	1000	10	8
	15-18	66	145	176	69	56	1000	10	10
	19-22	70	154	177	70	56	1000	7.5	10
	23-50	70	154	178	70	56	1000	5	10
	51 +	70	154	178	70	56	1000	5	10
Females	11-14	46	101	157	62	46	800	10	8
	15-18	55	120	163	64	46	800	10	8
	19-22	55	120	163	64	44	800	7.5	8
	23-50	55	120	163	64	44	800	5	8
	51 +	55	120	163	64	44	800	5	8
Pregnant						+30	+200	+5	+2
Lactating						+20	+400	+5	+3

From Food and Nutrition Board, National Academy of Sciences–National Research Council, Washington, D.C., 1980.
*The allowances are intended to provide for individual variations among most normal persons as they live in the United States under usual environment stresses. Diets should be based on a variety of common foods in order to provide other nutrients for which human requirements have been less well defined. (See also Tables 5-4 and 5-5.)
†Retinol equivalents. 1 Retinol equivalent = μg retinol or 6 μg beta-carotene.
‡As cholecalciferol. 10 μg cholecalciferol = 400 IU vitamin D.
§Alpha-tocopherol equivalents. 1 mg d-α-tocopherol = 1 α TE.

nutrition of practically all healthy people in the United States)*

Water-soluble vitamins							Minerals					
Vita- min C (mg)	Thia- min (mg)	Ribo- flavin (mg)	Niacin (mg NE)‖	Vita- min B₆ (mg)	Fola- cin¶ (μg)	Vita- min B₁₂ μg)	Cal- cium (mg)	Phos- pho- rus (mg)	Mag- ne- sium (mg)	Iron (mg)	Zinc (mg)	Iodine (μg)
35	0.3	0.4	6	0.3	30	0.5#	360	240	50	10	3	40
35	0.5	0.6	8	0.6	45	1.5	540	360	70	15	5	50
45	0.7	0.8	9	0.9	100	2.0	800	800	150	15	10	70
45	0.9	1.0	11	1.3	200	2.5	800	800	200	10	10	90
45	1.2	1.4	16	1.6	300	3.0	800	800	250	10	10	120
50	1.4	1.6	18	1.8	400	3.0	1200	1200	350	18	15	150
60	1.4	1.7	18	2.0	400	3.0	1200	1200	400	18	15	150
60	1.5	1.7	19	2.2	400	3.0	800	800	350	10	15	150
60	1.4	1.6	18	2.2	400	3.0	800	800	350	10	15	150
60	1.2	1.4	16	2.2	400	3.0	800	800	350	10	15	150
50	1.1	1.3	15	1.8	400	3.0	1200	1200	300	18	15	150
60	1.1	1.3	14	2.0	400	3.0	1200	1200	300	18	15	150
60	1.1	1.3	14	2.0	400	3.0	800	800	300	18	15	150
60	1.0	1.2	13	2.0	400	3.0	800	800	300	18	15	150
60	1.0	1.2	13	2.0	400	3.0	800	800	300	10	15	150
+20	+0.4	+0.3	+2	+0.6	+400	+1.0	+400	+400	+150	**	+5	+25
+40	+0.5	+0.5	+5	+0.5	+100	+1.0	+400	+400	+150	**	+10	+50

‖ NE (niacin equivalent) is equal to 1 mg of niacin or 60 mg of dietary tryptophan.

¶The folacin allowances refer to dietary sources as determined by *Lactobacillus casei* assay after treatment with enzymes ("conjugates") to make polyglutamyl forms of the vitamin available for the test organism.

#The RDA for vitamin B₁₂ in infants based on average concentration of the vitamin in human milk. The allowances after weaning are based on energy intake (as recommended by the American Academy of Pediatrics) and consideration of other factors such as intestinal absorption.

**The increased requirement during pregnancy cannot be met by the iron content of habitual American diets nor by the existing iron stores of many women; therefore the use of 30 to 60 mg of supplemental iron is recommended. Iron needs during lactation are not substantially different from those of nonpregnant women, but continued supplementation of the mother for 2 to 3 months after parturition is advisable in order to replenish stores depleted by pregnancy.

TABLE 5-4   Suggested desirable weights for adult males and females according to height*

Height (inches)*	Weight (pounds)†	
	Men	Women
58		102 (92-119)
60		107 (96-125)
62	123 (112-141)	113 (102-131)
64	130 (118-148)	120 (108-138)
66	136 (124-156)	128 (114-146)
68	145 (132-166)	136 (122-154)
70	154 (140-174)	144 (130-163)
72	162 (148-184)	152 (138-173)
74	171 (156-194)	
76	181 (164-204)	

From Food and Nutrition Board, National Academy of Sciences–National Research Council: RDA, ed. 9, Washington, D.C., 1980
*Without shoes.
†Without clothes. Average weight ranges in parentheses.

TABLE 5-5   Mean heights and weights and average recommended energy intake (calories/day)

Category	Age (years)	Weight (kilograms)	(pounds)	Height (inches)	Energy needs (kilocalories)	(range)	(MJ)
Infants	0.0-0.5	6	13	24	kg × 115	(95-145)	kg × 0.48
	0.5-1.0	9	20	28	kg × 105	(80-135)	kg × 0.44
Children	1-3		29	35	1300	(900-1800)	5.5
	4-6		44	44	1700	(1300-2300)	7.1
	7-10		62	52	2400	(1650-3300)	10.1
Males	11-14		99	62	2700	(2000-3700)	11.3
	15-18		145	69	2800	(2100-3900)	11.8
	19-22		154	70	2900	(2500-3300)	12.2
	23-50		154	70	2700	(2300-3100)	11.3
	51-75		154	70	2400	(2000-2800)	10.1
	76+		154	70	2050	(1650-2450)	8.6
Females	11-14		101	62	2200	(1500-3000)	9.2
	15-18		120	64	2100	(1200-3000)	8.8
	19-22		120	64	2100	(1700-2500)	8.8
	23-50		120	64	2000	(1600-2400)	8.4
	51-75		120	64	1800	(1400-2200)	7.6
	76+		120	64	1600	(1200-2000)	6.7
Pregnant					+300		
Lactating					+500		

From Food and Nutrition Board, National Academy of Science–National Research Council: RDA, ed. 9, Washington, D.C. 1980.

TABLE 5-6 Example of food label according to indicator nutrients

Indicator nutrient	Percentage of U.S. RDA*	Amount present*
Protein	25% of 65 g	16 g
Calcium	10% of 1 g	100 mg
Iron	10% of 18 mg	1.8 mg
Vitamin A	25% of 1000 μg RE or 5000 IU	250 μg RE or 1250 IU
Thiamin	10% of 1.5 mg	0.15 mg
Riboflavin	10% of 1.7 mg	0.17 mg
Niacin	25% of 20 mg	5 mg
Vitamin C	25% of 60 mg	15 mg

*Abbreviations: g, grams; mg, milligrams; μg, micrograms; RE, retinol equivalents—1 RE equals 1 μg retinol or 6 μg beta-carotene; IU, international units.

drink may be "fortified" with vitamin C, but that is about its only nutritional selling point. By comparison, real orange juice supplies folacin, potassium, vitamin A, and some calcium and niacin as well as vitamin C.

Finally, one critical problem is that some of our most nutritious foods—fresh produce and high protein foods—are unlabeled. This underemphasizes their critical role in providing dietary balance.

There is a major distinction between the RDA and the Dietary Goals. The U.S. RDAs are determined from basic research on animals and metabolic studies in humans that examine the particular micronutrients (vitamins, minerals, and water) presently considered to be essential to normal human development. Because of the current state of nutrient research, nutritionists have greater confidence in their conclusions concerning micronutrients than in their observations about macronutrients (carbohydrates, fats, and proteins).

The U.S. Dietary Goals, which primarily examine macronutrients, are derived from basic research on animals, metabolic and clinical studies with humans, and epidemiologic investigations. In addition, and unlike the RDA, the Dietary Goals compare food consumption patterns between one decade and another, using

one or more of three data bases, none of which has the accuracy relative to individuals provided by the detailed studies from which RDA recommendations arise. These data bases of the Dietary Goals include:

1. *Food disappearance* looks at levels of food that disappear into civilian households and is sometimes referred to as the U.S. per capita food supply. The data are collected annually by the Economic Research Service of the United States Department of Agriculture; the nutritive value of these amounts of foods is estimated by the Agricultural Research Service.

2. *Household food consumption* comes from data collected approximately every 10 years from representative samples of households across the United States by the Agricultural Research Service. These data are determined by food used in households over a 7-day period, whether purchased, obtained from home gardens, or as a gift or payment. Nutritive values of these amounts of foods are estimated and compared to the RDAs for family members.

3. *Food intake*, or food actually eaten by individuals, is determined from data usually collected by recall methods for a day or a

few days, including amounts of food eaten at home and away from home.

Nevertheless, the U.S. Dietary Goals, when analyzed, generally provide almost 100% of the RDA on a daily basis. By following this approach to food intake, you can achieve a diet based on good nutrition. In looking at any such data on food requirements, remember that the conclusions of research are only as good as the tools used to define that information. Table 5-7 gives some idea of the degree of certainty regarding research data for various nutrients. In the sections of this chapter dealing with specific nutrients, such as fats, protein, vitamins, and minerals, more guidelines for assessing food intake are described.

FAT

Fat is a concentrated energy-storing substance designed in nature as a means of providing long-term energy to the animal or seed that stores it. Also called lipids, fats are found in all food groups but are much more common among some meat and dairy foods. The simplest dairy product, milk, contains fat to provide energy for the baby mammal being fed.

All fats are insoluble in water. The most common fats, triglycerides, are combinations of glycerol and fatty acids, which are stored and transported in the body as needed for fuel. Another category of fats is the steroids, which have ring structures. These often become hor-

TABLE 5-7 State of development of methods for the analysis of nutrients in foods*

Factors	Sufficient	Substantial	Conflicting	Fragmentary	Little to none
Carbohydrates			Fiber Starch	Individual sugars	
Lipids		Cholesterol Fatty acids	Other sterols Total fat	Trans-fatty acids	
Minerals and trace elements	Calcium Copper Magnesium Phosphorus Potassium Sodium Sulfur Zinc	Iron Selenium	Arsenic Chromium Fluorine Iodine Manganese	Molybdenum	Cobalt Silicon Tin Vanadium
Vitamins		Vitamin C Niacin Riboflavin Thiamine	Vitamins A, B$_6$, B$_{12}$, D, and E Folacin Pantothenic acid ~~Available calories~~	Biotin Choline Vitamin K	
Protein		Most amino acids	Total protein Some amino acids		
Calories			Available calories		

From Stewart, K. K.: Nutrient analysis of foods: a reexamination. In Hertz, H. F., and Chester, S. N., editors: Proceedings of the 9th Research Material Symposium, Apr. 10-13, 1978, National Bureau of Standards, Washington, D.C., 1979.
*Food composition analysis is ongoing at the USDA Food Composition Laboratories as well as other laboratories throughout the United States. The table represents the status of food composition data and that likely to be generated in the near future. The results of these assays are the basis for composition tables.

mones in our bodies, which in turn are derived from the common steroid, cholesterol.

Other, more complex forms of triglycerides include phospholipids (lecithin is a good example) and sphingomyelins (which become parts of the brain and nervous system myelin sheaths). Wax, such as earwax (called cerumen), is also a sphingomyelin.

Fats in foods include the visible forms (oils, solid fats like butter or margarine, lard, or other fats covering meat) or the hidden fats such as those within olives, nuts, seeds (including avocados), meat muscle "marbling" of fat, or processed items such as chocolate milk, pastries, potato chips, candies, sauces, and other such items.

Scientific studies

Overwhelming evidence now shows that we have the strongest association to date between habitual and long-term fat intake and the development of various kinds of tumors, particularly in those persons with a family history of cancer. The major problem with this association is that dietary fats and fats stored in the body carry certain other associations with them. For example, certain nutrients are fat soluble, certain substances in our environment are fat soluble, and some of these environmental substances may be harmful in their own right. In addition, many of our protein sources are very high in fat, and it is possible that some of the association between increased fat and increased tumor incidence is related to the intake of protein and not fat itself.

Total fat intake in the diet has been correlated to various degrees with an increased development of breast, prostate, endometrial, and ovarian reproductive organ cancers and to gastrointestinal tract cancers, particularly of the colon. The evidence for breast and prostatic cancer is stronger than that for colon cancer.

One review of epidemiologic studies showed that cholesterol may be somewhat linked with the incidence of some cancers in women, but several other studies have not drawn this conclusion. Inverse relationships between cancer and cholesterol (e.g., low serum cholesterols are often seen in advanced cases of colon cancer) seem not to be causative or predictive of the development of these tumors. It is not clear whether this is a precedent finding or whether the serum cholesterol level becomes lower once the tumor is established because of metabolic changes within that individual. Until this and a variety of other studies are undertaken in a more controlled fashion, it is not possible to conclude anything specific regarding levels of dietary or serum cholesterol and subsequent or concurrent development of cancers. Again, cholesterol often goes hand in hand with total fat intake, which confounds the issue. It has already been detailed in the section on Dietary Goals, how you can establish a more prudent fat intake in your diet (see also Fig. 5-5). However, to recapitulate this information, Table 5-8 and the boxed material following provide streamlined guidance to those wishing to reduce overall fat in the diet.

In terms of dietary cholesterol, which many people wish to avoid because of a family history of heart disease, an intake of less than 300 milligrams a day has been recommended in the U.S. Dietary Goals. A relatively small number of foods contribute a major portion of the cholesterol and saturated fat in a typical American diet. The average American daily cholesterol intake was found to be approximately 600 milligrams. A single egg yolk contains 250 milligrams of cholesterol, which is nearly the daily allowable. Table 5-9 can help you make sensible cholesterol choices.

Table 5-10, the outlined material, and Fig. 5-6 depict certain important concepts that are needed to understand the sections on protein, fat, and carbohydrate. Since foods are mixtures, we need to know more about them to decide whether their calories are what we want for a given level of nutrients included with those calories.

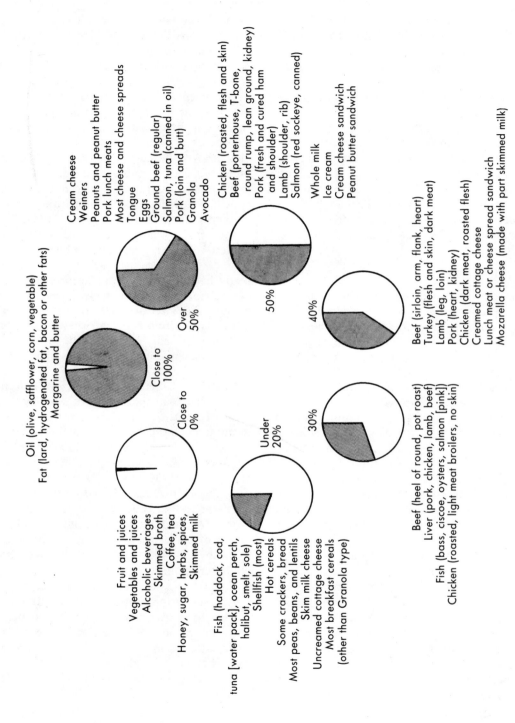

FIG. 5-5 Percentage of calories derived from fat in foods. (Developed from data in Pennington, J.A., and Church, C.F., editors: Bowes and Church's food values of portions commonly used, ed. 13, Philadelphia, 1980, J.B. Lippincott Co.)

TABLE 5-8 Percentage of calories derived from fat in foods

Percentage	Food	Percentage	Food
Close to 100	Oil (olive, safflower, corn, vegetable) Fat (lard, hydrogenated fat, bacon or other meat fats) Margarine and butter	40	Beef—sirloin, arm, flank, heart Turkey—flesh and skin, dark meat Lamb—leg, loin Pork—heart, kidney Chicken—dark meat, roasted flesh Creamed cottage cheese Lunch meat or cheese spread sandwich Mozzarella and Parmesan cheese (part skim milk)
More than 50	Cream cheese Weiners Peanuts and peanut butter Pork lunch meats Most cheese and cheese spreads Tongue Eggs Ground beef—regular Salmon, tuna (canned in oil) Pork—loin and butt Granola	30	Beef—heel of round, pot roast Liver—pork, chicken, lamb, beef Fish—bass, ciscoe, oysters, salmon (pink) Chicken—roasted, light-meat broilers, no skin
50	Chicken—roasted flesh and skin Beef—porterhouse, T-bone, round rump, lean ground, kidney Pork—fresh and cured ham and shoulder Lamb—shoulder, rib Salmon—red sockeye, canned Whole milk Ice cream Cream cheese sandwich Peanut butter sandwich	20	Fish—haddock, cod, tuna (waterpack), ocean perch, halibut, smelt, sole Shellfish—most Hot cereals Bread Most peas, beans, and lentils Skim-milk cheese Uncreamed cottage cheese Most breakfast cereals (other than Granola type)
		Close to 0	Fruit juice Vegetable juice Alcoholic beverages Broth, skimmed Coffee, tea, herbs, and spices

Adapted from Fremes and Sabry: Nutriscore, 1976.

Recommendations regarding high-fat foods

1. See Table 5-8 for relative percentages of fat in foods. In general, eat those foods listed in the lower part on the chart.
2. Use skim milk or buttermilk.
3. Restrict the intake of hard cheeses, which are high in fat and cholesterol; 75% of the calories in cheddar, Muenster, Camembert, and most hard cheeses come from fat. Swiss Criss and Swiss Lorraine are low in cholesterol but are not low-fat cheeses. Even some of the part-skimmed-milk cheeses may have some fat content, since fat is added during the cheese-making process. Processed cheeses are all high in salt and often high in fat and should be avoided.
4. Emphasize the use of parmesan, part-skimmed mozzarella, low-fat cottage, and ricotta cheeses, which have only 20% to 24% fat.
5. Instead of cream cheese use Neufchatel cheese, which has 37% fat content by weight.
6. If you use imitation (processed) cheese spreads, read the label carefully to be sure that palm oil or coconut oil is not used.

TABLE 5-9 Cholesterol content of common measures of selected foods (in descending order)

Food	Amount	Cholesterol (milligrams)
Brains	3 oz, raw	>1700
Kidney, sweetbreads (pancreas)	3 oz, raw	680
Liver beef, calf, hog, lamb	3 oz, cooked	370
Egg	1 yolk or 1 egg	250
Heart, beef	3 oz, cooked	230
Shrimp	3 oz, cooked	130
Lobster, cooked, meat only	145 g	123
Tuna, canned in oil, drained solids	184 g	116
Lamb, veal, crab	3 oz, cooked	85
Beef, pork, lobster, chicken, turkey, dark meat	3 oz, cooked	75
Chicken, turkey, light meat	3 oz, cooked	67
Clams, halibut, tuna	3 oz, cooked	55
Oysters, salmon	3 oz, cooked	40
Cake, baked from mix, yellow 2-layer, made with eggs, water, chocolate	75 g (small serving)	36
Beef and vegetable stew, canned	1 cup	36
Butter	1 tbs	35
Sausage, frankfurter, all meat, cooked	1 frank	34
Milk, whole	1 cup	34
Cheese, cheddar	1 oz	28
Ice cream, regular, 10% fat	½ cup	27
Cream, half and half	¼ cup	26
Cheese, pasteurized processed Swiss	1 oz	(26)*
Cheese, pasteurized processed American	1 oz	(25)*
Cottage cheese, creamed	½ cup (4 oz)	24
Cream, light table	1 fl oz	20
Yogurt, made from fluid and dry nonfat milk, plain or vanilla	carton (227 g)*	17
Lard	1 tbs	12
Mayonnaise, commercial	1 tbs	10
Cottage cheese, uncreamed	½ cup (4 oz)	7
Milk, skim, fluid or reconstituted dry	1 cup (8 oz)	5

From Freeley, R. M., Criner, P. E., and Watt, B. K.: Cholesterol content of foods. Reprinted from Journal of the American Dietetic Association, Vol. 61:134, 1972.
*Estimates in parentheses imputed.

TABLE 5-10 Nutrient density of foods, examples

Food	With high nutrient density	With lower nutrient density	With lowest nutrient density
Orange	Fresh orange Fresh juice	Canned juice (some vitamin C lost in heating)	Screwdriver cocktail (juice, vodka or gin) Tang (orange juice, sugar additive mixture)
Potato	Fresh baked, skin eaten	French fry (fried in fat)	Potato chip (very little potato; high in fat, low in nutrients)
Wheat	Wheat kernel Steamed whole (cereal) Ground whole (100% extraction—wheat flour)	Ground (refined, 50% extraction—white flour) White bread Saltine crackers	Twinkie (white flour, sugar, creamy filling) Brownie (high in fat and sugar; low in flour content —white)

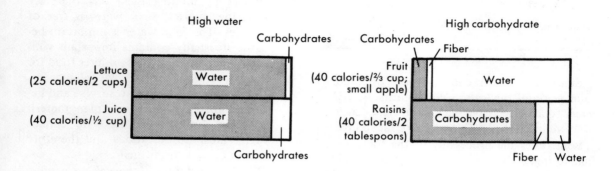

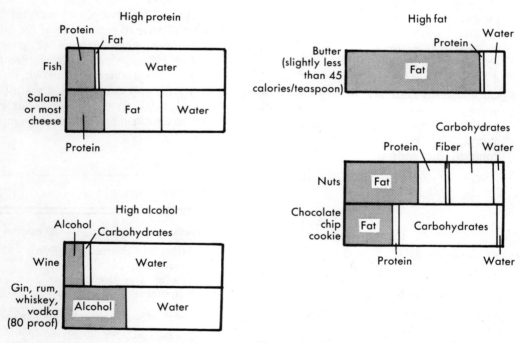

FIG. 5-6 Water, carbohydrate, fiber, protein, and alcohol content of various foods and beverages. Bars represent percentage of total volume of food supplied by the nutrient or by water. (Developed from data in Pennington, J.A., and Church, C.F., editors: Bowes and Church's food values of portions commonly used, ed. 13, Philadelphia, 1980, J.B. Lippincott Co.)

Nutrient density (see Table 5-10) is a concept promoted by Garth Hansen at the University of Utah to describe:

Numerator = Nutritional value (vitamins, minerals, protein*)
_____
Denominator = Calories

Since the water fraction of foods often contains many of the water-soluble nutrients, high-water foods often have the best nutrient density. Only vitamins A, D, E, and K are fat soluble.

Sometimes the processing of the food (drying, frying, pulverizing, storage) is responsible for much of the loss of nutritional value. Note also the following:

1. *Calories come from* (calories/gram if pure):
   a. *Carbohydrate*, 4 cal/g
   b. *Protein*, 4 cal/g
   c. *Fat*, 9 cal/g
   d. *Alcoholic drinks*, 9 cal/g
2. *Only a few foods are free of water or other substances.* Hence very few foods are "purely" one thing and this easy to calculate. The few examples of such one-composition foods are:
   a. *Carbohydrate* (sugar) = 17 cal/5 cc (1 tsp) (about 4 g)

   Sugar or honey = 4 cal/g
   _____
   Carbohydrate

   b. *Protein* (egg white, dried solids) = 17 cal/5 cc (1 tsp) (about 4 g)

   Protein powder = 4 cal/g

   c. *Fat* (oil or solid lard) = 45 cal/5 cc (1 tsp) (about ⅙ oz or 5 g)

   Oil or fat = 9 cal/g

_____

*We only *require* what we cannot make in our own bodies; we require a certain level of protein in our diets so that this is included. Our carbohydrate requirement is only 30 to 40 grams per day—to keep our brain and thyroid gland happy. Only infants require certain fat components.

3. *Most foods contain water*, which changes the basic calories/gram of these substances by diluting them and therefore lowering calories, since water is free of calories. The food water is important because it usually contains important vitamins and minerals. It also dilutes food for a purpose, since living things (plants, fertilized eggs) need water to survive and become a food for us. Fibrous plant materials also diminish calories—we cannot digest most fibrous foods and therefore get no calories from them.
4. When we eat foods, the *calorie content* depends on the food mixture contained in that food.

The boxed material shows calories in milk products relative to percentage of fat. Milk is a complex food and contains 12 grams carbohydrate (48 calories), 8 grams protein (32 calories), and variable fat as shown.

Skim milk and dairy products are the best choice of dairy foods. These foods provide more than a protein and calcium source; impor-

---

Milk exchange
═══════════════════════════════════

Nonfat milk: 1 exchange = 80 calories

Skim (fluid), buttermilk, plain unflavored yogurt—1 cup
Powder, dry—⅓ cup
Evaporated, skim—½ cup

Low-fat milk: 1 exchange = 120 calories

2% fat fluid, 2% unflavored yogurt—1 cup

Whole milk: 1 exchange = 180 calories

Fluid, whole buttermilk, whole plain yogurt—1 cup
Evaporated, whole—1 cup

tant B vitamins are contained as well, which could be insufficient in the diet of the non-milk-drinker.

Some foods contain relatively pure fat and are listed in the following boxed material. The nuts are included here because of their high fat content, but they also contain protein.

Other foods not listed in the box are relatively mixed foods, with fat providing more than 50% of the total calories relative to protein and carbohydrate. These include:

Buttered popcorn	Some cakes, cookies, pies,
Potato chips	and pastries
Fritters, croissants	Cheesecake
Doughnuts	Some pizza, fried chicken,
Piecrust	and fried wonton
Baklava	

High-fat foods

═══════════════════════

Fat exchange: 1 exchange = 45 calories

Butter, margarine, oil, mayonnaise, lard, *bacon fat*—1 tsp
Diet margarine, diet mayonnaise—2 tsp
French or Italian dressing (commercial)—1 tbs
Low-calorie salad dressing—2 tbs
Avocado (4-inch diameter)—⅛
Olives—5 small
Almonds*—10 whole
Pecans*—2 large
Peanuts (unsalted)†: Spanish—20; Virginia—10
Walnuts and other nuts—6 small
Bacon, crisp—1 strip
Cream, light or sour—2 tbs
Cream, heavy—1 tbs
Cream cheese—1 tbs

NOTE: *Italics* indicate foods high in salt.
*Some protein.
†High iron.

Recommendations

By using the lists here and on p. 106 you can lower the fat in your diet. You can also cut down on dietary fat by the way you cook: bake, broil, or boil meats, and when frying, use non-stick cookware to eliminate the need for oil or butter. A nonstick spray for skillets may be made by combining 1 tbs lecithin (granular or liquid) and 1 cup vodka, blending this mixture, and placing it in a spray bottle to lightly coat the skillet before sauteeing or frying a food without fat.

PROTEIN

The protein in our diets comes from various foods. These include, in descending order of protein content: eggs; meats, fish, and poultry; milk and other dairy products; legumes; and storage vegetables such as potatoes, sweet potatoes, turnips, peas, and so on. Finally, grains have important protein levels and include foods such as rice, wheat, millet, buckwheat, rye, oats, and barley.

The highest-protein foods are those from animal sources listed first; Americans often eat these foods in excess. This practice, as mentioned before, is a problem primarily because these foods carry fats to varying degrees with the protein. For those people with severe illnesses of major organ systems such as the liver or kidneys or for the tiny infant or elderly individual, excessive protein intake can burden the kidneys and liver unnecessarily.

The important feature of proteins, unlike the carbohydrate and fat in our diet, is that it is made up of small units called *amino acids*, which contain nitrogen. Some amino acids cannot be manufactured in the human body or are made in insufficient amounts, and these are especially important for growth in youngsters and for tissue repair. They include phenylalanine, tryptophan, tyrosine, valine, methionine, histidine, leucine, lysine, and isoleucine.

A healthy adult requires approximately 0.8

Overall recommendations for decreasing dietary fat

Choose more of	Choose less	Choose much less
Vegetables, including dry peas, beans, tofu		Fried vegetables (potato chips, french fries)
Fruits		
Cereals, all		Granola
	Shelled nuts	Oil-roasted nuts, peanut and other nut butters
Skim (nonfat) milk	Lowfat cottage cheese; lowfat milk, cheese	Creamed cottage cheese; full-fat milk, condensed milk, butter
Fruit ices	Sherbet, ice milk	Ice cream
Egg white	Egg (yolk)*	
Lean meat	Corned beef, ground round (15% fat)	Full fat ground beef (20% fat)
beef (flank steak, round, rump)		*Rib roast*
veal		Lamb breast, mutton
lamb (leg, loin, rib)		
poultry (white meat, no skin)	Poultry, dark meat (chicken, turkey) (no skin or white meat with skin)	Duck, capon, goose
fishes (white, plain)	Salmon	Breaded, fried fish
	Crab,* lobster, oysters, shrimp	
		Cold meats, frankfurters, paté
		Organ meats, liver,* brains,* sweetbreads,* kidneys,* heart
	Fats, oil, butter, margarine	Lard*

*Higher in cholesterol.

grams of protein per kilogram of desirable body weight. Remember: to calculate your daily requirement of protein in grams, divide your desirable body weight in pounds by 2.2 to determine kilograms. Then multiply this number by 0.8 to obtain grams of protein that you need per day. This number has cushion in it; you probably require something less than this amount. Most adults can achieve their protein needs by eating as described in the section on Dietary Goals, that is, two small servings of meat or high-protein vegetable foods, two servings of the dairy products per day, and a variety of vegetables, grains, and cereals. The boxed material on p. 108 gives a breakdown of the highest-protein foods, with progressively higher amounts of fat contained in those foods farther down the list. Note the difference in calories. The excess calories in the medium-fat and high-fat categories come from extra fat. It should be remembered that this group of foods is high in a variety of vitamins and minerals in addition to their amino-acid content.

There has been wide publicizing of the concept of complementary protein, which describes combining certain foods with insufficient levels of one amino acid with those that have insufficient levels of another to provide the full range of amino acids in the intestinal tract at the same time, during a particular meal. These combinations include using milk products with rice, wheat, or other grains; or using milk products with wheat, rice, other grains, plus various kinds of seeds and nuts such as peanuts or sesame. Only rice and sesame seeds do not work well. Other complements combine brewer's yeast with rice or various grains with beans, such as rice plus black beans, corn plus beans, and wheat plus beans. However, for an adult who has not been ill, stressed, or lost a great deal of weight, the ongoing tissue repair requirements for complementary or complete proteins are quite small; what we need primarily in our diets is simply the nitrogen that comes from a whole range of protein foods not necessarily provided

in "optimum" levels. In other words, our protein requirement may be fulfilled with really modest amounts of complete proteins; most of us could get by very nicely with grain, legume, and vegetable sources of protein as the primary items in our diet, with only occasional meat or dairy product proteins.

Despite this, the Senate Select Committee did not recommend a reduction in overall protein intake; they left this at approximately 12% of the total dietary calories. They did recommend that people increase the ratio of proteins coming from vegetable sources and reduce those coming from animal sources to improve the type and level of fat eaten in association with that protein. In addition, the vegetable sources of protein include important amounts of fiber — undigestible carbohydrate substances that probably serve to diminish levels of cholesterol and fat absorbed by the individual. This is dealt with more fully in the section on fiber.

As stated in the section on Dietary Goals, it is recommended that a healthy adult consume two small servings of the high-protein foods per day and two servings of the high-calcium, high-protein foods to obtain the protein necessary for a complete, nutritious diet.

Scientific studies

Cursory studies have correlated the incidence of cancer with those populations of people consuming a high-protein diet. As is true in other areas of nutrition research, the evidence comes from both epidemiologic and laboratory studies, specifically those done with animals. As noted earlier, the difficulty in looking at dietary protein is that most of the high-protein foods in the human diet also contain substantial amounts of fat. Because fat is strongly correlated with the development of cancers of various types, it is very difficult to separate these two major components of foods to investigate whether or not the protein content per se is

High-protein foods with protein-rich exchanges

Lean meat: 1 exchange = 55 calories

Beef*: baby beef, *chipped beef*, chuck, flank steak, tenderloin, plate ribs, plate skirt
    steak, round, rump, spare ribs, tripe—1 oz
Lamb*: leg, rib, sirloin, loin, shank, shoulder—1 oz
Pork*: leg, *ham, smoked*—1 oz
Veal*: leg, loin, rib, shank, shoulder, cutlets—1 oz
Poultry*: chicken, turkey, cornish hen, guinea hen, pheasant (all without skin)—1 oz
Fish: any fresh or frozen—1 oz
        mackerel, crab, tuna, lobster, canned salmon†—¼ cup
        clams, oysters†, scallops, shrimp—1 oz or 5
        sardines*, drained—3
Cheese†: containing less than 5% butterfat (Baker's cheese)—1 oz
        cottage cheese*, dry or 2% butterfat—¼ cup
Dried beans and peas*, cooked—½ cup
Tofu†—2 oz

Medium-fat meat: 1 exchange = 78 calories

Beef*: ground (15% fat), *corned beef,* rib eye, round (ground commercial)—1 oz
Pork*: loin (all cuts tenderloin), shoulder arm (picnic), shoulder blade, boston butt,
    Canadian bacon, boiled ham—1 oz
Liver*, heart, kidney, sweetbreads—1 oz
Cottage cheese†: mozzarella, ricotta, farmers, Neufchatel, Lorraine, Swiss Criss,
    Parmesan—3 tbs
Egg*—1
Peanut butter*, unsalted—2 tbs

High-fat meat: 1 exchange = 100 calories

Beef*: brisket, *corned beef* (brisket), ground beef (more than 20% fat), hamburger
    (commercial), chuck (ground commercial), roasts (rib), club and rib steaks—1 oz
Lamb*: breast—1 oz
Pork*: spareribs, loin (back ribs), pork (ground) *country style ham, deviled ham*—1 oz
Veal*: breast—1 oz
Poultry*: capon, duck (domestic), goose—1 oz
Cheese†: *cheddar types*—1 oz
Cold cuts—4½ x ⅛ inches
Frankfurters—1

NOTE: *italics* indicate foods high in salt.
*Iron-rich foods.
†High in calcium.

causing cancers to some extent independent of fat content.

In one exhaustive epidemiologic study conducted in 1975, a retrospective analysis was made of the incidence of 27 types of cancer in 23 countries and the mortality rate for 14 cancers in 32 countries. These numbers were correlated with per capita intake of many dietary substances and other environmental factors. It was found that total protein and animal protein correlated to a great extent with total fat. Then, looking repeatedly at dietary influences and breast cancer, endometrial cancer, and other tumor types that could occur, it was found over and over that fat correlated as strongly or more strongly with the onset and incidence of those cancers than did protein in the diet.

Most laboratory studies have looked more extensively at the relationship between animal intake of fat and subsequent tumor development than between animal protein intake and tumors. However, a few interesting studies concluded that if an animal receives the minimal protein required for optimum growth, fewer tumors develop than in those animals who receive excessive levels of protein. Some difficulties creep in immediately, since animal requirements for amino acids are varied and depend on the animal, as are human requirements. In addition, these requirements change through the life cycle, depending on the level of amino-acid synthesis that the body of the developing or adult animal is able to sustain in the face of a limited or absent amino acid in the diet. In one study done in 1951, a strain of mice bred for its development of spontaneous liver tumors was subjected to various levels of and various degrees of adequacy of protein. Some protein may supply higher levels of nitrogen that is insufficient in terms of the amino acid required for growth and thus not supply extra protein that can be used by the animal. In juggling various amino acids, it was discovered that the lower the total protein available to a certain

animal—that is, the lower the total adequate protein—the fewer the liver tumors in that animal. If the diet was then supplemented with a poor-quality amino acid such as gelatin, no increased level of tumor growth was seen. However, if two essential amino acids, methionine and cystine, were added, it was found that hepatomas (liver tumors) did occur at a greater rate.

Another animal study looked at the level of protein in the diet as it related to the development of liver tumors that were deliberately induced by adding to the animal's diet various aflatoxins—powerful substances known to induce hepatomas. (More data on aflatoxins are found in the section on extrinsic carcinogens.) In this study researchers studied young rats who were fed casein as 5% or 20% of their diets for 1 year, after aflatoxins had been introduced at equal levels in both groups of animals; the incidence of hepatoma was much higher in the animals with high-protein diets. Another study, done in 1976, confirmed the previous information by looking at increasing levels of hepatomas developing under the circumstances just outlined, at dietary levels of 8%, 22%, and 30% casein in three different groups of animals. The hepatoma development was 0% at the lowest protein intake, 80% at the highest. Other animal studies have shown similar results in the development of a variety of tumors by inducing various chemical substances. In rats with induced adenocarcinomas of the small and large intestine and in rats given a chemical to promote lung tumors, the animals on a lower-protein diet developed fewer of these cancers.

Another study investigated the rate of growth of tumors implanted into various kinds of animals who were then fed various levels of protein, starting with 0% and working up to levels much higher than would normally be found in the diet of that particular animal. In general, these studies have shown that tumors grow less well and sometimes are completely encapsulated by the animal's response to the tumor at lower levels of protein in the diet; the higher the protein content of the diet, the more tumors tend to flourish.

In all of these studies the mechanism for the inhibition of tumor growth at low levels of protein is probably quite complicated; it may occur at several steps in the process of host defense and will not be commented on here. In general, it seems that dietary protein is probably of less importance to the development of various cancers in humans and in animals than is the associated fat content.

In summary, it can probably be said at this time, although we do not have any firm recommendations in terms of a desirable level of protein, that the dietary level should not be excessive relative to the remainder of the diet. It is prudent to suggest that the protein in the diet should be sufficient for growth during pregnancy and for growth of children and adolescents, but it should not be excessive, particularly during the adult years.

CARBOHYDRATES

Carbohydrates are foods produced in plants by the action of sunshine on plant leaves, specifically on the chlorophyll in the leaf. This process generates *glucose*, a six-carbon unit known as a simple sugar; other six-carbon sugars are formed in other ways and are called galactose and fructose. Glucose is then hooked up in various ways to other sugars to form two-sugar units, sucrose and lactose. *Sucrose*, the primary sugar in beet and cane sugar products, which are used in various sweetened foods in the United States, is the primary sugar found in our diet. In infants drinking milk, whether cow or human, the primary two-sugar unit taken in is *lactose*, which comes from the glucose and galactose manufactured in the mammary gland of the human or other mammal. The complex carbohydrate called *starch* is made from units of glucose hooked together with bonds that our digestive tracts are able to digest. The other complex carbohydrates, as mentioned before, include such substances as cellulose and other fibers that are undigestible by the human. Certain advantages and disadvantages are derived from ingestion of these "fiber carbohydrate sources."

The Senate Select Committee has recommended an increase in consumption of complex carbohydrates in our diets from a present level of 28% to approximately 48% of the total energy or calories. The consumption of complex carbohydrates has progressively fallen during the 20th century, as reported to the Senate Select Committee, with intake of simple sugars increasing.

A Department of Agriculture report published in 1972 found that nutrient availability from fruits and vegetables had declined with increased use of canned, frozen, and dried produce and that shifts in consumption had occurred away from such vegetables as white and sweet potatoes, dark-green and yellow vegetables, dry beans and dry peas, and grain products.

The shift from the uses of fresh fruit and vegetables to processed, as well as changes in selection among different fruits and vegetables, have resulted in some significant trends in nutrients obtained from this food group. The amount of vitamin A obtained from fruits and vegetables has declined 11 percent since 1925-29, and 18 percent since 1947-49. Vitamin B_6 and magnesium declined by nearly 20 percent since 1925-29, while the amount of thiamin obtained from fruits and vegetables declined almost 10 percent.

It appears that increased consumption of fresh fruits and vegetables, particularly the high nutrient forms, would be beneficial for many persons in need of dietary improvement.

The type and degree of milling of the wheat berry or kernel to produce flour is important to the level of nutrients retained in that flour. The percentage of the original kernel kept in flour is called the extraction rate. A 90% extraction flour, for example, only deletes 10% of the kernel, primarily the bran and germ (see Fig. 5-7). The greater the extraction rate, the more

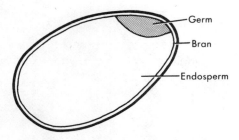

FIG. 5-7   Components of wheat kernel.

nutrients one loses, since most of the nutrients are present in the outer layers in close association with the bran coating, and very little is formed in the endosperm, or flour fraction of the kernel (Fig. 5-8). The germ has a different set of nutrients, a high proportion of fat, and is routinely removed in milling to prevent spoilage from rancid changes in the fat.

Scientific studies

Carbohydrates have not been linked with increasing levels of cancer development in either human epidemiologic studies or animal studies. This can never be a blanket statement, since carbohydrates contribute calories to the diet, and we know that the total caloric content of the diet has been linked with increased incidence of certain kinds of cancers. However, more calories per gram are derived from fat, which is much more strongly correlated with total caloric content of the diet and with the incidence of cancer.

In two epidemiologic studies researchers found an increased incidence of breast cancer in women taking in a high level of refined sugar. A different study reported that breast cancer was inversely related to the intake of complex dietary carbohydrates such as starch. This may be in some way related to the kinds of substances (fat) that are associated with these kinds of dietary substances. For example, many sugary foods, whether coffee with cream and sugar or a cookie, have fat associated with the sugar. One could argue that many complex-carbohydrate foods such as bread, rice, and potatoes are often eaten with a fat such as mayonnaise or butter—but this fat is generally taken in smaller quantities on a piece of bread than in a cookie or piecrust.

A second issue with some complex carbohydrates involves the extrinsic carcinogens introduced with the food. For example, aflatoxin, which is a mold and a carcinogen, is sometimes seen growing in grains that are stored under highly moist, warm conditions. In this case it would be expected that increased levels of liver tumors might be seen in those people consuming high levels of this moldy grain. The starchy food itself is not the culprit.

Experimental animal evidence is limited in terms of starchy or sugary foods. In some cases the tumor development must be looked at in terms of another substance in addition to the sugar. One such study was done with rats who had no genetic predisposition to cancer of the bladder. These animals were given either high levels of dietary lactose (milk sugar) or sucrose, then they received either adequate or deficient levels of vitamin A. With lactose, if sufficient vitamin A was given, very few kidney or bladder stones developed; if insufficient vitamin A was given, about 60% of the rats developed bladder stones. Along with stone development, the wall of the bladder developed many little areas of transitional cell hyperplasia, and approximately 30% of the stone-containing bladders had evidence of early carcinoma. In animals receiving sucrose, however, whether given high or low levels of vitamin A, no stone formation or cancerous changes occurred. Another study looking at chemically induced tumors in rats compared rats receiving diets with either refined sugar or complex starch as a source of carbohydrate. Many more breast tumors were seen in the rats fed refined sugar than in those receiving starch as their dietary carbohydrate.

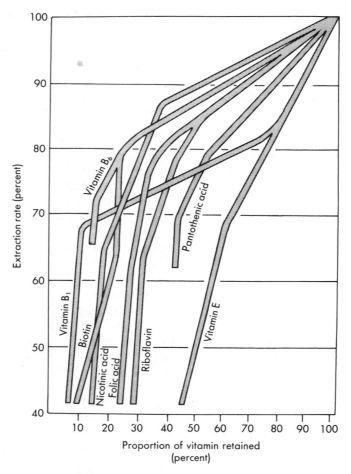

FIG. 5-8 Percentages of nutrients retained in milled flour of different extractions. (Data from McCance and Widdowson: Medical Research Council Special Report Series 235, 1940.)

The difficulty with any of these studies is that when one dietary component is increased, another may or must be decreased; this in itself causes another variable in the incidence of the cancer being studied. The overall summary drawn by the Diet, Nutrition and Cancer Review Committee has been that there is too little evidence from epidemiologic human studies and laboratory studies regarding carbohydrate to suggest a clear conclusion in the incidence or promotion of cancer growth.

However, since high-sugar foods are very often high in fat, additives, and empty (low-nutrient-density) calories, these foods should be deemphasized. The goal, instead, should concentrate on the intake of higher levels of high-fiber, low-sugar, and low-fat foods such as grains, cereals, legumes, and starchy vegetables.

The following boxed material lists high-carbohydrate foods—fruits, breads and cereals. Vegetables are given as well, although they contain little or no starch.

High-carbohydrate foods

Fruit exchange: 1 exchange = 40 calories

Apple—1 small
Apple juice, apple cider—⅓ cup
Applesauce (unsweetened)—½ cup
Apricots, fresh—2 medium
Apricots*, dried—4 halves
Banana—½ small
Berries:
   strawberries—¾ cup
   blackberries, blueberries—½ cup
   raspberries—½ cup
Cherries—10 large
Cranberries—1 cup
Dates*—2
Figs, fresh or dry—1
Grapefruit—½
Grapefruit juice—½ cup
Grapes—12
Grape juice—¼ cup

Mango—½
Melon
   cantaloupe—¼ medium
   honeydew—⅛ medium
   watermelon*—1 cup
Nectarine—1 small
Orange—1 small
Orange juice—½ cup
Papaya—¾ cup
Peach—1 small
Pear—1 small
Pineapple—½ cup
Pineapple juice—⅓ cup
Plums—2 medium
Prunes*—2 medium
Prune juice*—¼ cup
Raisins*—2 tbs
Tangerine—1 medium

Bread exchange: 1 exchange = 70 calories (Includes bread, cereal, and starchy vegetables)

Bread: whole wheat, white, rye, pumpernickel, raisin—1 slice
Rolls: bagel, English muffin, frankfurter or hamburger roll—½
Plain dinner roll—1
Tortilla†, 6 inches (corn)—1
Pita bread (pocket bread)—½
Bread crumbs, dried—3 tbs
Crackers:
   graham—2 squares
   rice crackers—2 round
   matzo 4 x 6 inches—½
   oyster—20
   Ritz—5
   Saltines—6
   pretzels, 3⅛ x ⅛ inches—25
Cereal:
   ready to serve, unsweetened variety—¾ cup
   cooked—½ cup

Pasta, cooked: spaghetti, noodles, macaroni, rice, barley, grits—½ cup
Popcorn (popped, no fat added, unsalted)—3 cups
Cornmeal, dry—2 tbs
Flour—2½ tbs
Wheat germ—¼ cup
Legumes*:
   baked beans, *canned*—¼ cup
   dried beans, kidney, lima, navy, pinto, red, chickpeas (garbonzo), black-eyed peas, split peas, sprouted legumes—½ cup
Starchy vegetables:
   corn—⅓ cup
   corn on the cob—1 small
   lima beans, mashed potatoes, winter squash—½ cup
   parsnips—¾ cup
Green peas*—¾ cup

NOTE: *Italics* indicate foods high in salt.
*High iron.
†High calcium.

Continued.

High-carbohydrate foods—cont'd

Bread exchange: 1 exchange = 70 calories (Includes bread, cereal, and starchy vegetables)—cont'd

Potato, white or sweet—1 medium
Pumpkin—¾ cup
Yams—¼ cup
Prepared foods:
  biscuit or muffin, 2 inches (115 calories)—1
  cornbread, 2 x 2 x 2 inches (115 calories)—1

potatoes, french fried, 2 x 3½ inches (115 calories)—8
potato or corn chips (160 calories)—15
pancake or waffle, 5 x ½ inches (115 calories)—1

Vegetable exchange: 1 exchange = 25 calories
Group A—½ cup serving

Artichokes, hearts
Asparagus
Bean sprouts
Beets
Broccoli
Brussels sprouts
Cabbage
Carrots
Chinese pea pods
Eggplant
Green pepper
Greens*

Kohlrabi
Okra
Onion
Rutabaga
String beans, green or yellow
Summer squash
Tomatoes (1 small)
Tomato juice (commercial)
Turnips
Vegetable juice (commercial)
Water chestnuts
Zucchini

Group B—approximately amounts shown

Cauliflower—1½ cups
Celery—1 cup
Chicory—2 cups
Chinese cabbage—2 cups
Cucumbers—2 cups
Endive—1½ cups
Escarole—1½ cups

Lettuce, spinach*—2 cups
Mushrooms—1 cup
Parsley—2 cups
Radishes—2 cups
Rhubarb—1 cup
Sauerkraut—1 cup
Watercress—2 cups

Some carbohydrate foods are snacks or desserts and not "substantial" foods, including:

Hard candy or caramel—1, 50 calories

Sugar, syrup, honey, jam, jelly, cocoa—1 level tsp, 50 calories

Frozen low-fat yogurt—6 oz, ¾ cup, 150 calories

Ice cream—4 oz, ½ cup, 150 calories

Angelfood cake, no icing—1/16, 110 calories

Wine, dry—6 oz, 150 calories

Wine, sweet—4 oz, 150 calories

It is useful to note that a few foods contain almost no calories. Those few calories present are generally derived from carbohydrates. Such "free" foods with miscellaneous exchanges include (italics indicate foods high in salt):

Bouillon, broth (commercial)

Coffee, tea

Herbs, spices

Gelatin, plain

Rennet tablets

Lemon juice, lime juice

Club soda—Perrier, Belfast (lowest in sodium)

Pickles (unsweetened)

Dry mustard, vinegar

Soy sauce

Diet soda

Saccharin

SUGAR

Sugar is a refined carbohydrate. In 1875 Americans used 40 pounds of sweeteners annually. This became 70 pounds by 1910, and by 1980, 128 pounds. The American craving for sugar remained high even when the price of sugar quadrupled in 1974—there was only a 3% drop in total sugar consumption. Some of our sugar-coated cereals have over 50% of their total weight as sucrose. Even granolas have a sugar content that ranges from 22% to 32%, and these usually contain significant fat as well.

Perhaps the most important problem is the danger in displacing complex carbohydrate, which is high in micronutrients, with refined sugar, which is essentially an energy source offering little or no nutritional value. This not only increases the potential for depriving the body of essential micronutrients, but sugar calories may actually increase the body's need for some B vitamins. As stated by Dr. Jean Mayer in 1976 in the *New York Times Magazine*:

(Sugar calories) increase requirements for certain vitamins, like thiamin, which are needed (for the body) to metabolize carbohydrates. They may increase the need for the trace mineral, chromium, as well . . . . Thus, a greater burden is placed on the other components of the diet to contribute all the necessary nutrients—other foods need to show extraordinary "nutrient density" to compensate for the emptiness of the sugar calories.

Since the average American eats 128 pounds of sugar per year, this translates into almost 600 empty calories each day.

The greatest increase in sugar use apparently has come from the addition of refined sugar (cane and beet) to process foods, whereby the consumer is unaware of the total sugar consumed each day. According to the U.S. Department of Agriculture:

Use in processed food products and beverages has increased more than threefold, from nearly 20 to 70 lbs., while household purchase has dropped one-half from a little more than 50 to about 25 lbs. Currently, food products and beverages account for more than two-thirds of the refined sugar consumed—70 lbs. out of a little over 100 lbs.

Beverages now comprise the largest single industry use of refined sugar, accounting for over one-fifth of the total refined sugar in the U.S. diet, or nearly 23 lbs. Furthermore, the amount used in beverages has increased nearly sevenfold since early in the century when 3½ lbs./person/year was used in these products. Use of refined sugar in beverages is now second only to household use.

Unfortunately, many of these products are in high use among members of society who can ill afford the low nutrient density contributed—children, the elderly and low-income families.

Sucrose is the medium required in the mouth

for the onset of tooth decay and thus should be limited in the diet for this reason as well. The bacteria that begins the decay process in dental plaque must have sucrose bonds for its own energy needs. Eating honey (fructose) or the vegetable and grain starch forms of carbohydrate does not provide this bond.

Sticky, sugary foods (taffylike candies, sugar-coated cereals, granolas, peanut butter and jelly, raisins and other dried fruits), are particularly implicated in tooth decay. Dr. Jean Mayer, citing a government survey, said in a *New York Times* article:

> In nations of the Far East, where sugar intake per person per year ranged (at the time) from 12 to 32 pounds, the national averages for decayed, missing or filled teeth in adults 20 to 24 years old, ran from 0.9 to 5. By contrast, in South American nations, where sugar intake was high (44 to 88 pounds per person annually) the averages for decayed, missing or filled teeth in the same age group ran from 8.4 to 12.6. As for the United States today, it has been estimated that 98 percent of American children have some tooth decay; by age 55 about half of the population of this country have no teeth.

Cavities can be reduced by flossing, tooth care, and drinking water or other unsweetened drinks after meals.

Honey is of no particular benefit in the diet. There is some evidence that honey may contain a cancer-causing substance that bees extract from flowers. Molasses, a concentrate of sugar impurities, does have more nutrients than table sugar, but it and honey may be more caries-producing because of their stickiness.

Contrary to widespread opinion, too much sugar in the diet does not directly cause diabetes, except insofar as it contributes to excess calories, obesity, and the adult-onset form of the disease.

To review recommmendations from the Dietary Goals, the McGovern Committee recommends that carbohydrates comprise 55% to 60% of our caloric intake and that we should drop our sugar from the current 18% to 10%, substituting the bulk of these calories with complex starchy foods and naturally occurring sugars in fruits and vegetables.

VITAMINS

Vitamins are potent, essential, noncaloric organic compounds needed in very small amounts in our diet on a regular basis. They perform specific functions that promote growth for reproduction or maintain health in life. We need vitamins in milligram or microgram doses each day, from 0.001 to 0.0001 of a gram of each vitamin. Sometimes the vitamins come to us in the form of *provitamins*, that is, the form that precedes the actual vitamin that is active in the body. This means that in measuring the vitamins in food, the provitamin form as well as the vitamin itself must be measured. The term "vitamin*e*" was given initially to these dietary substances by Kasamir Funk in 1912, when he first discovered thiamine, which contains an amine and which Funk thought was a component of each of these substances. It was later realized that most vitamins are not amines, and the *e* in vitamin*e* was dropped. The known vitamins are divided into those that are fat-soluble (vitamins A, D, E, and K) and those that are water soluble (which includes the range of B vitamins and vitamin C).

Although we discuss only those few vitamins and minerals believed to be anticarcinogenic, there are some general principles that need to be described about all vitamins. For example, vitamins occasionally have pharmacologic, druglike roles that provide much higher levels than those small concentrations that prevent vitamin deficiency diseases. Two examples are the use of a vitamin A analog for treatment of cystic severe acne and the use of vitamin C at relatively high doses on frequent occasions throughout the day for prevention of bacteria buildup during a urinary tract infection.

The role and recommended levels of most vitamins for cancer protection are still being studied. In general, however, a vitamin is given at a dose much higher than that required in the U.S. RDA. A second general principle is that as a vitamin is provided by diet or by pills, many things can happen in the intestinal tract that may result in different levels of absorption of that vitamin. In general, the food form of the vitamin is the best in terms of absorption and availability. If you did an experiment and mixed four solutions—(1) freshly squeezed orange juice; (2) frozen orange juice, reconstituted; (3) Tang, which provides a certain level of vitamin C; and (4) vitamin C tablets crushed up to a certain known concentration in water—and then measured the vitamin directly, the vitamin is at a particular level. If you stored these four solutions both at refrigerated and at room temperatures for 2 days and then remeasured the vitamin levels, the orange juice retains vitamin C to the best degree, particularly if fresh. The frozen juice retains it to the next degree, and Tang retains it quite poorly, comparable to the vitamin C mixed in water. The reason for this is that antioxidants naturally available in the food itself (in this case the orange juice) prevent some of the deterioration of vitamin C.

In general, when we eat foods containing vitamins we absorb those vitamins best. Absorption is usually poorer from vitamin pills. In addition, pills listed as containing "natural" vitamins generally contain only a tiny proportion of the food-derived vitamin; most of the vitamin in that pill is synthetic.

The overall reason for eating a good diet with its complement of good vitamins is that we generally are healthier and our bodies are better able to perform an immune role throughout our lives, which may be generally preventive of cancer. In terms of specific anticarcinogenic vitamins, very few fill this role. These include vitamins A, C, E, and perhaps some B vitamins, which are discussed in the section on lipotropes.

Potentially anticarcinogenic vitamins

Anticarcinogens are substances that either directly oppose the effect of carcinogens or prevent their activation. Some anticarcinogens may be present naturally in food, whereas others are chemical additives. Anticarcinogens often act by preventing enzymatic oxidation of carcinogens to their ultimate form; most anticarcinogenic vitamins are antioxidants. There are other substances that may act like antioxidant vitamins in this regard. We now look with special interest at vitamins and minerals that are considered to be anticancer substances.

During the 1970s, data from research on both animals and humans implied that vitamins A, C, and E may play an anticarcinogenic role in prevention and treatment of some forms of cancer. It will take many years to determine the nature and extent of this relationship and to provide guidelines on doses of these vitamins with respect to cancer. This is an exciting area of research, however, and requires some forbearance on the part of general physicians and the public, since it may eventually be shown that high-dose vitamins do help under carefully controlled circumstances.

Of all of the vitamins with known or potential anticarcinogenic effects, the most strongly linked in this regard is vitamin A. A growing set of epidemiologic evidence has suggested that there is an inverse relationship between the risk of cancer development and the long-term dietary intake of foods containing either preformed vitamin A such as liver or provitamin A, the beta-carotenes found most readily in dark-green leafy vegetables and yellow fruits and vegetables. A variety of studies has shown that an inverse relationship exists in humans between the characteristic intake of vitamin A substances and the ultimate development of cancers, particularly those of the lung, urinary bladder, and larynx. No studies have adequately identified whether there is any difference between preformed or precursor vitamin A substances in terms of this effect.

Vitamin A. Vitamin A, or retinol, is a fat-soluble organic compound derived from vegetable and fruit carotenoids called beta-carotenes. Considerable beta-carotene is directly converted to vitamin A and stored in the liver. But some beta-carotene is absorbed intact, allowing beta-carotene dioxygenase to convert it to vitamin A. We may ingest vitamin A directly from animal source foods such as liver or from capsules.

Moreover, in several areas of the world—India, the Middle East, and Africa—there is no increase in the number of cases of cancer in general, or of squamous lung cancer in particular, in spite of a diet deficient in vitamin A.

The epidemiologic evidence for an inverse relationship between vitamin A consumption and development of various forms of tumors is very good. These types of studies are either prospective—observing food intake and waiting for the incidence of tumors in that population—or retrospective—comparing information about diet based on histories of how people had eaten with the incidence of tumor development. Most of these studies primarily observed intake of beta-carotenes in the form of fresh fruits and vegetables rather than attempting to assess milk-and liver-derived vitamin A sources as well. In one long-term study in Chicago with a 19-year follow-up, 1954 men were observed. The development of lung cancer was inversely associated with beta-carotene intake from fresh products, whether cigarette smoking was taken into account or not. No significant association was found between the development of lung cancer and the intake of preformed vitamin A.

Another study, which compared men who had developed cancer of the larynx or throat with control groups and which controlled for cigarette smoking and alcohol, showed an inverse relationship between the level of both vitamins A and C in the diet and the development of cancer.

The London-based International Cancer Research Fund reported a 5-year investigation of 16,000 British men, 86 of whom developed cancer. Blood samples from the 86 were compared with those from men of similar age and habits who had not developed cancer. The men with the lowest vitamin A levels in the blood were more than twice as likely to develop cancer, especially lung cancer, as men with higher blood levels of vitamin A.

Other studies have corroborated this International Cancer Research Study; cohort studies in the United States and England have shown an inverse relationship between blood serum levels of vitamin A and subsequent risk of cancer. The relationship between dietary vitamin A and its level in the blood serum, which is homeostatically controlled, is not very clear.

Some interesting studies on prevention of cancer of the skin have been done with hairless mice. Hairless mice given beta-carotene, one fraction of the carotene category of substances, were shown to have a lower development of ultraviolet light–induced skin tumors. It is known that one of the roles of vitamin A is to protect and repair mucous membranes throughout the intestinal tract and lung as well as the skin epithelium. It may be that this predisposition to protecting those areas is somehow involved in this phenomenon.

In the studies of oral cancer in India and Pakistan, lower serum concentrations of beta-carotene, as well as of retinol, were observed more frequently in the cases than in the controls. As the amount of beta-carotene eaten increases, the proportion converted to vitamin A decreases and the serum concentration of beta-carotene rises steadily. But because massive doses of vitamin A are toxic, it cannot as such be used as a anticarcinogen. Instead, studies are currently under way testing nontoxic chemical cousins of vitamin A as possible cancer suppressors. These chemicals are not currently available for purchase, and the first results of the tests will not be known for several years.

Vitamin A toxicity observed after massive intakes of preformed retinoids, called *hypervitaminosis A*, is characterized by changes in the skin and mucous membranes, liver dysfunction, and headache. This has limited their systemic use in clinical practice.

At this time beta-carotene and vitamin A are considered safe for humans at doses of 30 milligrams and 10,000 IU (international units) a day, respectively. Beta-carotene can be taken at much higher levels than 30 mg/day. However, large doses of beta-carotene from vegetables and fruit turn the skin yellow (called *carotenemia*), and preformed vitamin A in high doses can produce toxic side effects such as blurred vision or blindness and liver and bone damage. Therefore, when doses of vitamin A in experimental programs average as high as 100,000 IU, periodic chemical analyses of the blood are performed to monitor toxic side effects. The following list* shows IU of vitamin A (in parentheses) in 100-gram helping of various foods.

Liver — lamb, calf, beef, turkey, hog, chicken (34,220)
Hot red chili pepper, raw (21,000)
Dandelion greens
   raw (14,000)
   cooked (11,700)
Carrots
   raw (11,000)
   cooked (10,500)
Dried apricots, uncooked (10,900)
Hot chili sauce, canned (9500)
Kale, leaves only
   raw (10,000)
   cooked (8300)
Parsley, raw (8500)
Spinach
   raw (8100)
   cooked (8100)
Sweet potato, cooked (7900)

*From Doll, R., and Peto, R.: Your Patient and Cancer, January 1983.

Liverwurst (6530)*
Pumpkin, canned (6400)
Greens (collards, turnip, beet, mustard, watercress)
   raw (6980)
   cooked (6250)
Chicken giblets (5760)*
Sweet red pepper, raw (4450)
Winter squash, cooked (3500)
Cantaloupe (3400)
Egg yolk (3400)
Endive (3300)
Butter, margarine (3300)

Until the results of research tell us otherwise, consumption of vitamin A through foods in which it naturally occurs is recommended (see boxed material). These foods include butter, margarine, milk products, and liver; beta-carotenes are seen in green and leafy vegetables (especially spinach and Swiss chard), green peppers, carrots, sweet potatoes, pumpkins, yellow squashes, and yellow-orange fruits. Vitamin A foods to be avoided include vitamin A supplements and highly fortified, processed foods such as breakfast bars and powdered breakfast drinks, which usually have poor nutrient density, high sugar and fat content, and additives.

*High iron

Recommended vitamin A foods with beta-carotene

Dark-green vegetables, such as broccoli, Swiss chard, kale, spinash, green peppers, and collards
Turnip greens
Yellow-orange vegetables, such as carrots, sweet potatoes, pumpkin, winter squash, and red peppers
Yellow-orange fruits, such as peaches, cantaloupe, and apricots

To summarize, there is some interesting data to suggest that carotenoids and retinol or vitamin A itself do act to reduce the incidence of carcinoma at several sites, including the lung, larynx, and urinary bladder. They may also be shown to have some role in the development of skin cancers.

Vitamin C. Vitamin C has several interesting roles. It is known to be required for the production and maintenance of *collagen*, which is a protein substance forming the basis for all connective tissues in the body, including those in bones, skin, teeth, and tendons. Collagen provides the support material for capillaries and thereby prevents bruises. Ascorbic acid promotes the absorption of iron, especially from vegetable sources, and protects against infections. The vitamin is depleted from the cortex (outer portion) of the adrenal gland, where it is involved in the release of stress hormones, *epinephrine* and *norepinephrine*. This is the basis for the belief that increased levels might be required in times of stress. Vitamin C also is required for production of *thyroxine*, the hormone produced by the thyroid gland.

Vitamin C helps to prevent the transformation of nitrates and nitrites plus amines into carcinogenic nitrosamines in the intestinal tract, which is discussed further in the section on nitrates. Since this is known to occur, some manufacturers of ham and bacon, sausage, and other cured meat products have begun including vitamin C in their meats. However, as shown later, cured meats are generally not the major source of nitrates and nitrites in the diet.

A variety of studies have looked at the development of cancer as it relates to vitamin C in the diet. Epidemiologic evidence is indirect, but several studies have shown that cancer of the stomach and esophagus develops with greater frequency in those individuals who characteristically ingest a low vitamin C diet than a high one. The difficulty with this retrospective view of food intake is that many of the foods containing high levels of vitamin C are also very high in vitamin A, so it is somewhat hard to separate the two vitamins to determine their impact on the development of various cancers. It should be recalled also that the roles of the two vitamins overlap in terms of epithelial integrity (the intestinal tract mucosa is a form of epithelium). One study, for example, looked at vitamin A and vitamin C consumption in relation to esophageal cancer. The study was done observing male cases with esophageal cancer and controls, with smoking and alcohol use held constant in both groups. Vitamin C was even more strongly linked than vitamin A as being protective against cancer of the esophagus.

A variety of experimental studies have attempted to demonstrate the effect of vitamin C on tumors implanted in animals, various kinds of induced tumors, and tissue cultures. These often conflict with one another. Basically, the addition of ascorbic acid to tissue culture cells prevented chemically induced transformation of cells and sometimes caused reversion of transformed cells, but this is preliminary data. Various human studies have been done with patients dying of an assortment of cancers. Large doses of oral vitamin C were given in one study on 1100 patients; despite the massive doses the patients ultimately died of their cancers. However, a delay in death was noted for those patients receiving megadoses of vitamin C, although *a more recent study has failed to confirm this deferred death in patients with known tumors taking large doses of vitamin C.*

One interesting study regarding vitamin C may have a bearing upon the kind of immune surveillance that is important in avoiding certain cancers. This study looked at 279 healthy individuals over the age of 60, many of whom were taking macrodoses of various vitamins and minerals. It was found that those people taking large amounts of vitamin C (defined as ≥355 mg/day for women, ≥500 mg/day for men) had increased cell-mediated immune responses, as measured in vivo by skin test reactivity. This may be important in avoiding the development of certain specific cancers.

The following list gives milligrams of vitamin C (in parentheses) in 100-gram servings of various foods.

*Vegetables**
Hot red chili pepper, raw (369)
Hot green chili pepper, raw (235)
Sweet red pepper, raw (204)
Currants, raw (200)
Kale, leaves only
  raw (186)
  cooked (93)
Parsley, raw (172)
Collards, leaves only
  raw (152)
  cooked (76)
Turnip greens
  raw (139)
  cooked (69)
Sweet green pepper
  raw (128)
  cooked (96)
Broccoli
  raw (113)
  cooked (90)
Brussels sprouts
  raw (102)
  cooked (87)
Mustard greens, raw (97)
Pimento, canned, solids and liquid (95)
Cauliflower, raw (78)

Fruits (all fresh)†
Guava (180)
Papaya (170)
Mango (81)
Orange (66)
Grapefruit (54)
Orange juice (50)
Cantaloupe (45)
Watermelon (45)
Strawberries (44)
Lemon (39)

---

*From Doll, R., and Peto, R.: Your Patient and Cancer, January 1983.
†Adapted from Pennington, J. A., and Church, C. F., editors: Bowes, Church's food values of portions commonly used, ed. 13, Philadelphia, 1980, J. B. Lippincott Co.

Some problems arise with megadoses of vitamin C; these include gastrointestinal distress, diarrhea, possible kidney oxalate stones with doses of more than 10 grams a day, and the theoretical possibility of iron toxicity in some people as a result of enhanced iron absorption. In summary, the various evidence (which is somewhat limited) suggests that vitamin C may very well inhibit the formation of some carcinogens and that consumption of vitamin C–rich foods may be associated with a reduced risk of cancers of the stomach and esophagus.

For some people vitamin C supplements used at certain times of the year—when stresses are high, food supply is marginal, or levels of sleep or rest are insufficient—may be a useful adjunct to the food sources of vitamin C. In theory it is better to include natural vitamin C in the diet rather than resorting to supplementation. Some hazards exist with supplementation on a general level: if one uses high-level supplementary vitamin C over a long period and then stops, the enzymes that metabolize and alter the vitamin C in the body have adapted to high levels and tend to deplete those lower levels supplied in the normal diet at much greater speed than usual. This has occasionally been seen to cause problems in the babies of women who have taken high-dose vitamin C throughout a pregnancy. When the baby begins to breast-feed and very little vitamin C is available in the breast milk, the infant can actually develop scurvy.

The recommendation has been made by a number of researchers that even though the evidence has not been confirmed in terms of optimum levels of vitamin C, it is generally considered prudent for smokers to include vitamin C supplements in their diets because of the preventive role of vitamin C in cancer of the esophagus.

Vitamin E. Vitamin E, also known as alpha-tocopherol, is a fat-soluble vitamin. Like vitamin C, it also has a role in blocking the production of nitrosamines in the intestinal tract. It also plays an antioxidant role in many systems

insert #9 cont'd

of the body and may retard the action of free radicals called superoxides, which can adversely affect metabolic changes in the body. Superoxides may also induce genetic DNA change and may thus lead to cancer.

There are little epidemiologic data associating vitamin E with the risk for cancer development. Part of the difficulty arises because of its widespread availability in a variety of foods. Vitamin E is unstable during storage, which means it is often impossible to tell what level of vitamin E has been ingested in an epidemiologic retrospective study.

The major known effect of vitamin E in preventing cancer is linked with nitrites, which is discussed in the section on nitrites and nitrates. Although there are a few animal studies that hint at a possible protective effect of vitamin E when fed to mice who had ingested various substances to induce cancers, the data are not widespread or conclusive enough to draw any strong recommendations. Nevertheless, vitamin E–rich foods are good for other reasons and should be eaten on a daily basis. The primary sources are listed below. Other more saturated oils contain lesser amounts of vitamin E.

The following list gives milligrams of vitamin E (in parentheses) in 100-gram helpings of various foods.*

Cottonseed oil (43.6)
Walnuts (22.0)
Almonds (15.0)
Olive oil (14.4)
Wheat germ, crude, commercially milled (13.5)
Margarine (12.5)
Soy bean oil (12.1)
Mayonnaise (11.9)
Italian salad dressing (9.1)
Cabbage
  raw (7.8)
  cooked (7.6)
Peanuts, peanut butter (6.6)

---

*From Doll, R., and Peto, R.: Your Patient and Cancer, January 1983.

Collards, leaves only, cooked (5.9)
Salad dressing, mayonnaise type (5.3)
Cashews (5.1)
Cream (4.9)
Popcorn (4.4)
Potato chips (4.3)
Spinach, raw (2.9)
Summer squash, cooked (2.4)
Vegetable fat (2.3)

Another issue concerns the use of vitamin E in the remission of *mammary dysplasia* (lumpy breasts). Two different studies have shown that giving approximately 600 IU of vitamin E per day for cystic mastitis causes a remission in about one third of the women receiving this

---

Disorders associated with vitamin E

Thrombophlebitis (inflammation and clotting in veins)
Pulmonary embolism (obstruction or clotting in pulmonary arteries)
Hypertension
Fatigue
Gynecomastia (enlargement of male breasts) and breast tumors
Vaginal bleeding
Headache
Dizziness
Nausea, diarrhea, and intestinal cramps
Muscle weakness and myopathy (abnormal muscle condition)
Visual complaints (large doses of vitamin E can oppose the action of vitamin A)
Hypoglycemia (reduced blood sugar levels)
Stomatitis (inflammation of mucous membrane in mouth)
Chapping of lips
Urticaria (skin eruptions)
Apparent aggravation of diabetes mellitus
Apparent aggravation of angina pectoris
Disturbances of reproduction
Decreased rate of wound healing (in laboratory animals)

*refuted by JAMA council report, 252 8/10/84, 803.

Love et al
307: 1010
1982

level for 4 to 6 months. However, a recent article in the *New England Journal of Medicine* has shown statistically that there is no increased incidence of breast cancer in women with lumpy breasts when controlling for those who actually went on to have a biopsy of one or both breasts. This means that although it may help to examine one's breasts more readily if the breasts are less lumpy, the chances for cancerous change are not necessarily improved by the vitamin E; it is simply easier to examine one's health and note changes in the breasts.

A variety of problems may be caused or aggravated by self-medication with vitamin E in high dosages.The more serious ones include those listed in the boxed material.

MINERALS

Minerals provide an important role in nutrition; they comprise approximately 5 pounds of the total body weight of an adult. Three fourths of this comes from calcium and phosphorus in approximately a 2:1 ratio. The remaining minerals in descending order include potassium, sulfur, sodium and chloride in equal amounts, magnesium, iron, manganese, copper, iodide, fluorine, silicone, vanadium, chromium, cobalt, nickel, molybdenum, and tin. Of these, only a few have been linked with the development of or protection from cancer, and these are all confined to the category of trace minerals rather than major minerals. All minerals are at some time dissolved in a water medium for transport via the blood or extracellular fluid in and out of cells. Trace metals, including selenium and zinc, are important in maintaining good health. Only these last two will be discussed in connection with their possible roles in cancer prevention.

Selenium

Selenium forms a part of large enzyme molecules. Its primary role is as an antioxidant, preventing breakdown of fats and other body chemicals; it also interreacts with vitamin E. A selenium deficiency is unknown in humans, but in animals pancreatic degeneration can occur. Parts of the United States where selenium is present in low amounts have higher cancer rates and more deaths from high blood pressure. Seafoods and organ meats can be rich in selenium, depending on the selenium content of the soil or water milieu.

Epidemiologic data recently collected by G. N. Schrauzer at the University of California, San Diego, suggest that selenium may protect humans against cancer. These multicountry data show that an inverse relationship exists between selenium consumption and death from several forms of cancer, including those of the breast, colon, rectum, and prostate. Other studies compiled from national and international sources also suggest that the level of selenium consumption is directly related to cancer. In Bulgaria, for example, where the annual per capita consumption of selenium is relatively high—107.6 milligrams—the incidence of death from breast cancer is one of the lowest of the countries examined. On the other hand, in the United States, where annual selenium intake is relatively low—61 milligrams per person—the mortality rates for breast cancer are among the highest.

Although these data suggest that selenium may play a role in preventing human cancer, a cause-and-effect relationship is not obvious.

The results of two Canadian studies have shown a correlation between increased selenium levels and decreases in cancer mortality. However, similar studies in 22 other countries do not corroborate these results. Special studies are needed that control for other factors, such as total calories and dietary fat intake, to get a clear idea of the role of selenium.

Although there is extensive speculation that selenium may prevent the production of active carcinogens, the studies are just beginning. For example, recent studies in mice show that the addition of selenium to the drinking water reduced the incidence of breast cancer and preneoplastic (precancerous) tumors such as colon cancer. Thus, selenium given to an animal before inducing the development of cancer cells by viral or chemical means appears to prevent the formation of cancer. However, selenium supplementation did not inhibit the growth rate of established mammary tumors induced by viral and chemical carcinogens.

Clinical trials are now underway in the United States, China, and Finland on the use of selenium supplements in the prevention and treatment of cancer. These trials will require many years of research because the mechanisms of the metabolic interactions for selenium are not well understood. At this time there is no evidence that selenium has any effect on a cancer that has already developed.

While it is known that toxic levels of selenium are undesirable, in some areas of the Orient selenium intake is as high as 500 micrograms per day with no apparent ill effects. Selenium consumption therefore could probably be doubled in the United States without any adverse consequences.

Good food sources of selenium, along with microgram amount of selenium per gram of food, include the following:

Fish (sardines, especially)—0.75
Whole wheat—0.50
Barley—0.50
Oats—0.50
Rye—0.50
Rice—0.38
Beef—0.25
Lamb—0.25
Pork—0.24
Eggs—0.20
Whole milk—0.01

While tea is often listed as a good source, the level is difficult to set, for it depends on the type of black tea, amount used, and time for steeping.

Selenium can be harmful in large quantities. The current Food and Nutrition Board's recommended selenium intake is 50 to 200 micrograms daily. As yet there are no recommended dietary allowances. Toxicity, or chronic selenosis, has resulted from doses of approximately 2400 micrograms a day. Data from animal research show that high intake of selenium can result in weight loss and death.

From both epidemiologic and laboratory studies it seems that selenium offers some protection against cancer. It is still too soon to draw conclusions from the available data. However, it should be noted that excessive selenium is inadvisable, and an intake greater than 200 micrograms per day in supplements has not been shown to provide benefits.

Zinc

Zinc is another essential body mineral and is found in 95 of the enzymes involved in cell division. In the body high levels are found in the eyes, reproductive organs, with lesser amounts in the liver, muscles, and bone. Deficiency in zinc can cause retarded male sexual development and loss of taste.

Both epidemiologic and animal studies regarding zinc and other trace minerals, such as copper, molybdenum, and iodine, are extremely limited. One interesting zinc study observed the mineral content of the soil in vegetable gardens cultivated by patients and control subjects in and around the area of Cheshire and Devon, England. The patients all had gastric cancer. In the zinc and zinc/copper ratios studied, it was found that the zinc levels in the gardens of those patients with gastric cancer were higher than in the control subjects' gardens or in gardens of patients who had developed other forms of cancer. To underscore these findings, animal studies have shown that if 200 parts per million of zinc are available in the water, small amounts of selenium uptake are prevented in the face of these high zinc levels, and that the problem with zinc may be one of selenium unavailability. Since selenium acts as an antioxidant, it may prevent production of carcinogens. This is probably the mechanism for the previous finding.

Zinc-rich foods (amount of zinc in milligrams)

Legumes

Black-eyed peas, 1 cup—3.0
Peas, green, 1 cup—2.1
Garbanzos, lentils, 1 cup—2.0
Beans, common, 1 cup—1.8
Beans, lima—1.7

Grains

Soy meal, 3½ oz—5.9
Wheat bran, 1 cup—5.7
Rice bran, 1 cup—3.1
Wheat flour, whole, 1 cup—2.9
Cornmeal, bolted, 1 cup—2.1
Oatmeal, brown rice—1.2

Dairy products

Milk, dry, nonfat, 1 cup—3.1
Milk, fluid, 1 cup—0.9
Cottage cheese, 1 cup—1.04
Cheddar cheese, slice—0.5
Egg, whole—0.5

Meats

Beef, 3 oz—3.8-5.0
Organ meats, ½ cup—3.5-5.0
Lamb, 3 oz—3.9
Veal, 3 oz—3.5
Turkey, 3 oz.
   Dark meat—3.7
   Light meat—1.8
Pork, 3 oz—2.6-3.8
Chicken, ½ cup—2.5

Seafood

Lobster, ½ cup—7.9
Crab, ½ cup—3.8
Oysters, ½ cup—3.0
Fish, deep-sea, ½ cup—0.6-1.5

Other foods

Cocoa powder, 1 oz—1.6
Spinach, raw, boiled, 1 cup—1.3
Peas, green immature, 1 cup—1.2
Wheat bran flakes—1.0
Banana—0.3

For Recommended Daily Allowances of zinc, see Table 5-3.

However, the Diet, Nutrition and Cancer Review Board has concluded that the variability and study results regarding zinc do not provide sufficient evidence for them to make a recommendation regarding zinc intake. They have made similar conclusions for iron, copper, molybdenum, and iodine. Nevertheless, a list of selected zinc-rich foods is provided in the boxed material.

LIPOTROPES AND B VITAMINS

There are a variety of B vitamins, all water soluble and many of them available together in foods and interrelated in terms of metabolic actions within the body. It is very difficult to control for intake of a single B vitamin to determine its effect on the incidence of cancer. In one study the intake of B vitamins was found to have either no effect or at most a minimal one on the occurrence of cancer. In terms of animal studies, it has sometimes been found that the promotion of increased levels of cancer occur at one level of intake of a particular B vitamin and not at another. This may be related to the role of those vitamins in many metabolic processes. In any case, it is premature to provide any specific recommendation for the B vitamins.

An interesting side issue concerning B vitamins is the role of certain B vitamins and a few other metabolic substances as *lipotropes*. These include methionine, an essential amino acid, choline (usually thought not to be a nutrient, since the body is able to manufacture this substance), and folic acid, one of the B vitamins. A variety of animal studies have shown that there is an important protective influence on the incidence of cancer when one observes a high ratio of these lipotropes to the fat in the diet. Since the word "lipotrope" implies the movement of fat, the protective role of lipotropes in cancer development may stem from the alteration in fat metabolism and movement. Other substances can also act as lipotropes, including vitamin B_6, vitamin B_{12}, and a substance called inositol.

It is not recommended at this time that any drastic changes be made in the level of B-vitamin or overall lipotrope intake. However, returning to the U.S. Dietary Goals and the Recommended Daily Allowances, it must be remembered that it is important to get a full range of the B vitamins and that these are widely distributed in the meat and milk groups, in the bread and cereal group, and in a number of vegetables.

FIBER

Dietary fiber, which is derived from plants, is that material not digested by the enzymes of the human intestinal tract. These materials are structural components of the cell wall of the plant. As can be seen from Table 5-11, the fibrous components of our foods range widely. Not all of these fibrous components are effective in terms of providing residue or bulk in the diet. A major problem with the controlled measurement of fiber is that laboratory-derived results concerning levels of crude fiber are strikingly different from the amount of fiber actually excreted from the gastrointestinal tract. Crude fiber analysis involves acid and alkali treatment, and other laboratory analyses are done in various ways and yield various percentages of fiber in a total amount of food. The table attempts a reasonable correction for the body's handling of fiber (see legend).

One source of fiber is agar and psyllium-seed colloid, the basis of commercial laxatives. The best forms of food fiber come from such wholegrain items as wheat bran, and fiber levels are also high in such fruits as pears, blackberries, and persimmons. Many legumes and a variety of vegetables have significant amounts of fiber as well. These levels are listed in Table 5-11.

Fibrous foods have been in the limelight for the last 12 to 13 years, largely for their possible effect on such diseases as diverticulitis, gallstones, and lipid metabolism. Other diseases are thought to be possibly treatable via a high-fiber diet; one important example is diabetes mellitus. It has been amply demonstrated that the introduction of significant fiber into the diet will lower the blood sugar level, often into the normal range, thereby allowing for a more normal diet requiring less medicines. Fiber is also useful in the treatment of irritable bowel syndrome, which affects about 5% of the population and is characterized by alternating loose and hard, constipated stools and abdominal cramping. Bran is particularly helpful in improving this problem.

The main concern in this section is the role of fiber as it relates to cancer of the bowel. The issue was first popularized in the late 1960s and early 1970s by Burkitt, a British physician. He noted in some of his work in Africa that the African stool was much bulkier than the typical British stool; generally, more than 450 grams (1 pound) a day of feces was produced by the African adult, whereas the typical British cohort produced less than 200 grams of stool per day. He related this to the fact that Africans had virtually none of the degenerative diseases just mentioned and almost no incidence of colon carcinoma, whereas in British subjects colon cancer is very common.

It is theoretically thought that the fiber may decrease transit time, making for a fast transit of stool through the colon and therefore allowing less exposure of colon mucosa to various

TABLE 5-11 Approximate fiber in commonly used food portions*

Fiber group	Breads and cereals	Fruits	Vegetables	Legumes, nuts, and seeds	Miscellaneous
Group 1 (less than 1.5 g DF†)	White flour Plain white bread, crackers, etc. Pastas White rice Cheerios Rice Krispies Special K Plain cooked refined cereals Oatmeal	Strained clear fruit juices	Peppers, cooked	Most texturized vegetable protein entrees Split peas, cooked	Jam Jelly Marmalade
Group II (1.6-1.99 g DF)	Brown rice Most cold cereals‡	Applesause Avocado Banana Cantaloupe Plums, canned	Asparagus, cooked Cucumber, peeled Lettuce Tomato, canned		
Group III (2.0-2.99 g DF)		Most canned, cooked, and fresh fruits‡	Most canned or cooked vegetables without peelings or seeds‡ Cucumber, unpeeled Turnips, fresh Tomato, fresh	Smooth peanut butter Cashews	
Group IV (3.0-3.99 g DF)	Whole-wheat and rye flour, bread, etc. Cereals with dried fruits or nuts Granola Grapenuts	Raisins Oranges, fresh Figs, fresh Dates Prunes Apples, fresh Blackberries, fresh	White potato Beet greens Beets Green beans Sweet potato Wax beans Pumpkin, canned	Kidney beans	Popcorn
Group V (4.0-5.99 g DF)	Shredded wheat	Raspberries, fresh and canned Guava, fresh Boysenberries, fresh	Broccoli Corn Parsnips Green peas	Lima beans Lentils Soybeans Most nuts‡	
Group VI (greater than 6.0 g DF)	Bran, bran cereals, bran muffins, etc.	Pear, fresh Figs, dried Persimmon, fresh Currants, dried Elderberries, fresh Strawberries, fresh	Artichoke Winter squash	Chick peas Baked beans Filberts Sunflower seeds	

Adapted from Pennington, J. A., and Church, C. F., editors: Bowes and Church's food values of portions commonly used, ed. 13, Philadelphia, 1980, J. B. Lippincott Co.

*Foods which are generally not restricted for Minimal Residue Diets, but for which actual figures for dietary fiber or residue were unobtainable are: cereal beverages, coffee, tea, bouillon, broth, margarine, butter, vegetable oil, shortening, whipped cream, eggs, tender meats, poultry, fish, strained vegetable juices, and seasonings. Dietary fiber includes all the indigestible substances in food; crude fiber is the residue remaining after treatment with boiling sulfuric acid, sodium hydroxide, water, alcohol, and ether. Although some sources state that crude fiber is approximately 50% of dietary fiber, comparison of foods for which both figures are available yielded estimates of 20% to 30%. Most vegetable portions equal ½ cup, all legume portions are ½ cup, and portions of nuts and seeds are 60 grams.

†Dietary fiber. Based on value for dietary fiber when available or estimated from crude fiber as follows:

Dietary fiber = 5 × Crude fiber for breads, cereals, and grains

Dietary fiber = 3.5 × Crude fiber for legumes, nuts, seeds, and vegetables

Dietary fiber = 4 × Crude fiber for fruits

‡Unless specified elsewhere.

carcinogenic substances in the stool. Carcinogens are believed to arise from high-fat diets. During the course of transit, gut bacteria act on the fat, and carcinogenic fatty subcomponents are formed that promote cancerous change in the colon. Another possibility is that fiber simply dilutes the carcinogens or perhaps promotes higher levels of bile acid excretion via the stool. (These are known to be procarcinogens.) It is thought that the undesirable metabolic activity of the fecal bacteria may be reduced with high levels of fiber. In most of the following epidemiologic studies that explored the issue of fiber and colon cancer, it must be borne in mind that fiber is often analyzed and defined differently from study to study, accounting for the variable study results in correlating "fiber" with the development of colon cancer. A variety of other studies, such as Burkitt's, have simply compared stool *bulk* with the incidence of colon cancer. Similarly, another study in 1978 compared low stool bulk in men from Copenhagen, Denmark, who have a higher risk for colon cancer, compared with men from Kuopio, Finland, who have larger stools and a low risk for colon cancer. In Great Britain a 1979 study calculated the average fiber intake by populations in different areas of the country. No good correlation between total fiber and deaths from colon and rectal cancer were seen, but the mean intake of pentosans (a group of five-carbon sugars) and vegetables besides potatoes was inversely correlated with death from colon cancer. This supported the previous suggestion that the specific components of fiber must be observed as they correlate with the incidence of colon cancer.

One interesting study, done by G. A. Glober and associates and reported in 1974 and 1977, investigated whether transit time or stool weight was more important in the development of cancer of the colon by examining Japanese men in Japan and Hawaii and Caucasian men in Hawaii. Table 5-12 gives the results of their findings. As can be seen, the more important factor was the total stool weight rather than the transit time. Another study reported in 1978 looked at the incidence of colorectal cancer in black subjects in United States. By assessing dietary intake from selected food items on a checklist, it was found consistently that those developing colorectal cancer consumed fewer fiber-containing foods than did the control group, and there was a dose/response relationship. In addition, the diet of those developing colorectal cancer was significantly higher in saturated fat than that of the control group. In these studies it must be remembered that total fat should be observed in the diet in addition to total fiber. Several studies have shown a positive correlation between the intake of fat and the development of colorectal cancer, whether or not fiber correlated. Finally, if we are suggesting that bile acids may play some role in the development of colorectal cancer, the total intake of fat, which influences the level of bile acid seen in the colon, must be one of the considerations in any study.

Various animal studies have also been done to clarify our knowledge of fiber and of colon cancer. Many have been based on the introduction of known carcinogens into the animal's body, either by feeding or providing it intrarec-

TABLE 5-12 Comparison of bowel transit time and stool bulk with the development of colon cancer

Male group	Colon cancer	Transit time	Stool weight
Japanese in Japan	Low	Faster	High
Japanese in Hawaii	High	Faster	Lower
Caucasians in Hawaii	High	Slower	Lower

tally or intravenously. Findings have indicated that bran protects rats against certain induced colon cancers whether or not the carcinogen is given orally or under the skin. It has no effect on the incidence or number of tumors in the duodenum or cecum of the small intestine. Cellulose, another fibrous component, has been found to protect rats against certain induced tumors, but pectin does not have the same effect. Indeed, with a different kind of tumor-promoting chemical, cellulose does not protect against the induced tumor, and agar, another fibrous substance, actually enhanced one type of induced colon cancer in mice.

Furthermore, it is possible that certain substances irritate the mucosa of the colon or small intestine and provide an impetus for development of cancer that is not strictly related to fiber. One such substance, which comes from alfalfa, possesses a binding capacity that disrupts the topography of the colon mucosa, making it susceptible to the action of a locally administered carcinogen (or some substance in the diet that is potentially carcinogenic). Saponins from bean sprouts may have a similar action on the mucosa of the gastrointestinal tract.

In conclusion, the *Diet, Nutrition and Cancer* report suggests that, because of the vagaries of reporting methodology in these summarized studies and because of our inability to relate the complexities of the diet to the dose/response results between fibrous components and incidence of colorectal cancer, no recommendation can be made regarding fiber intake. The report did strongly suggest that more work be done on specific components of fiber as these relate to

---

Recommendations for increasing dietary fiber

Choose more of	Choose less	Choose much less
Vegetables, including dry peas, beans, variety of fresh vegetables cooked and raw	Canned vegetables	
Fruits, especially berries, pears, apples, persimmons, dried fruits, pineapple	Juices	Canned fruits Fruit drinks
Cereals, breads, whole grain products, hot cereals, wheat crackers, bran muffins		*Snack* items made with refined flour (e.g., cookies, cupcakes, cakes, pies) Refined (often highly sweetened) cold cereals
Nuts, seeds, popcorn (use lower fat forms of these)		
		*Dairy products** *Eggs** *Meats,** including poultry and fish have negligible fiber Fats*

*Negligible or no fiber, but important foods.

various processes in the colon. Despite these conclusions vis-a-vis colon cancer, it is the belief of most nutritionists that including fibrous foods as a major component of the diet is an appropriate recommendation. These foods are described in the Dietary Goals section; in addition, Table 5-11 serves as a guideline for inclusion of some of the components listed in the daily intake of foods. Certainly, fiber is helpful in terms of ameliorating constipation, hemorrhoids, diverticular disease, diabetes, and possibly cancer of the colon. The foods that would be included are those complex carbohydrates such as beans, peas, nuts, seeds, fruits and vegetables, whole-grain breads and cereals, and bran itself. It must be recalled that there is a minor hazard to eating excess levels of these fiber-containing foods, since the metals in our diet—zinc, calcium, and several others—are probably absorbed to a slightly lesser degree with the intake of a high-fiber diet.

The food lists in the boxed material on p. 129 can help you increase the fiber in your diet.

HEALTHY FOOD SELECTION, STORAGE, AND PREPARATION

In this era of modern food storage and widespread food availability, it seems obvious that somebody must be watching the levels of nutrients that we get in our foods. However, this is not always the case. The individual must accept the final responsibility, since we have charts and tables that tell us how to best preserve the nutritional value of our foods.

This level of nutritional value with respect to vitamins is best when the food is freshly picked; when a plant such as an orange is picked off the tree, the enzymes that produce vitamin C in that fruit stop working. The vitamin C can be maintained best if that orange is frozen quickly, thawed quickly, and consumed or refrigerated for a brief period and then consumed. The specific level of the vitamin may depend on the variety of orange and how ripe it is when picked,

but storage is generally thought to be the more important factor in the final level of vitamin C in that orange. If done correctly, freezing preserves the vitamin C best; the lowest level of preservation arises in a canned version of that fruit, for example, canned orange juice. However, if freezing is going to be the best, this presumes that the manufacturer, the transporting vehicle, the market, and the consumer have correctly handled this frozen product to keep it frozen. The B vitamins are similarly labile in varying degrees and under varying forms of treatment. One of the worst things we can do with thiamine, for example, is to dry heat or "brown" a rice product for a recipe called "feathered rice." The B vitamins survive best in vegetables if the vegetable is heated very quickly and barely cooked. The fat-soluble vitamins are less destructible, and minerals in foods are generally preserved throughout the life of that food before consumption.

To summarize, healthy food selection would ideally include gardening our own fruits and vegetables. Many of us cannot do this for various reasons, but we can find the stores that offer a good selection of fresh fruits and vegetables and we can choose vegetables and fruits on a seasonal basis, selecting those items that are fresh and in abundance, when they possess optimum vitamin levels. The best frozen foods are those in their original form; simple frozen fruits or vegetables should be selected rather than those altered by a high-sugar content or a high-salt or high-fat content, as is the case with buttered and seasoned mixed vegetables. These mixtures tend to be much higher in cost for the level of nutritional value obtained, and the nutrient density is obviously less than in a simple food. Canned foods should be reserved for the most part for use during emergencies. Dried foods, such as those used on camping trips, generally have much less in the way of nutritional value than their fresh counterparts; it might be advised that one take vitamin pills while on a lengthy camping trip for this reason.

The principles of storage are basic; refrigeration is the mainstay for many foods. Dried, canned, or boxed products that are dry by nature should be kept in a cool, dry, semidark area. Keeping the freezer at an appropriate temperature is ideal for frozen foods, and transferring those frozen foods from freezer to pan with the least delay possible is also advisable. Even a frozen chicken or turkey can be quick-thawed at a very low setting in the oven and then prepared in whatever fashion one wishes rather than letting it sit for a full day before cooking while it thaws. This is particularly important in preventing bacterial contamination or proliferation of that food while it remains at room temperature.

In terms of carcinogenesis, the Ames test has been mentioned as a means of identifying certain carcinogens or procarcinogens in our foods. The Ames test has disclosed some interesting features regarding food preparation, suggesting that browning should be avoided whether done over dry heat (such as feathered rice) or over direct heat with fat involved (such as grilling meats). The fat, as well as the browning itself, introduces changes that cause positive Ames test results with foods such as grilled barbecued, or charbroiled hamburgers, steaks, and other meats or corn and other products browned over an open fire. Ideal food preparation methods include stewing, baking with a cover on the pan, and steaming, for example, vegetables in a basket. For the most part, those foods that can be eaten fresh should be. The only exceptions are raw grains containing phytic acid, which interferes with iron absorption, and raw egg whites, which contain avidin, a protein that interferes with absorption of biotin, one of the minor B vitamins.

Barbecued, open-grilled, and smoked foods

When meats are cooked over a wood or charcoal fire, they are exposed to high amounts of polycyclic aromatic hydrocarbons (PAHs), which come from the smoke formed when fat from the meat drips onto the hot coals. One of these PAHs is benzpyrene, which is a potent carcinogen. Lesser levels of PAH are found in foods exposed to these chemicals in water, air, and soil; smoked foods, however, are much greater contributors of these PAHs to our diets. When foods are smoked, benzpyrenes permeate the food fully during the smoking process.

In addition to PAHs, protein foods undergo a process called *pyrolysis* when cooked. Many pyrolysins are mutagenic and these most likely contribute to carcinogenesis in barbecued meats.

To avoid major levels of PAHs, don't eat barbecued or smoked foods. To limit these substances, the measures given on p. 132 will help.

Frying and flat grilling of foods can lead to very high temperatures. This can increase the level of pyrolysin (mutagen) formation in high-protein meat foods. The level of these substances tends to be greater in browned meats.

INTRINSIC CANCER-PROMOTING SUBSTANCES IN FOOD

Many intrinsic cancerous substances have been identified, particularly through animal studies. The more important members of this group are listed in Table 5-13. Only a few of these are detailed here, since generally we are not exposed to such substances as bracken fern in our diets. One of these substances is *cycasin*, which is a potent plant carcinogen. It occurs in palm cycad trees, which provide food for the natives in a variety of tropical and subtropical areas of the world. The cycad nut is generally treated by extracting it with water before consumption, but despite this treatment, acute poisonings with cycasin have occurred.

Hydrazine derivates of two different mushrooms, *Agaricus bisporus* and *Gyromitra esculenta*, both of which are consumed in many parts of the world, appear to be carcinogenic in mice and hamsters and are mutagenic in bacte-

When selecting or preparing high-protein foods

Choose more of	Choose less	Choose much less
Steamed, braised, baked, low-temperature roasted meats	Low-fat meats, barbecued over a pan to catch the fat, cooked far from coals	High-fat, smoked meats and fishes
		Meats that have been oil-basted during barbecue cooking
Fresh, lower fat fish	Barbecued fatty fish or chicken; remove skin before eating (this greatly limits benzpyrene intake)	Smoked salmon (lox), white-fish, other fish
		Smoked hams and other meats treated with hickory or other wood chip smoke
Cheeses, especially lowfat		Smoked cheese

When selecting or cooking high-protein (meat) foods

Choose more of	Choose less	Choose much less
Microwave-cooked meats, poultry, fish, other meats without ceramic browning plate	Microwave with ceramic browning plate	Meats fried at temperatures over 300°
	Meats fried in electric skillet (temperatures less than 300°)	
Braised, stewed meats	Low-temperature, oven-roasted meats	
Unbrowned meats	Lightly browned meats	

TABLE 5-13   Intrinsic food substances that promote cancer

Food	Substance	Possible tumor promoter	Possible mutagen in vitro	Possible carcinogen in vivo
Cycad Nut	Cycasin		X	X
Coltsfoot				
Comfrey (tea)	Pyrrolizidine alkaloid		X	X
Rutin plant	Flavanoid from quercetin		X	
Astralgin*	Flavonoid from Kaemp ferol		X	
Braken fern (eaten in Japan)	Flavonoids			X
Alcohol				
Red wine mutagens	Flavonoids†	X (esophagus)	X	
Whiskey mutagens	Flavonoids		X	
Brandy mutagens	Flavonoids		X	
Coffee (brewed†, instant, regular, or decaffeinated)			X	
Sumac	Flavonoid (quercetin)		X	
Dill weed	Flavonoid (quercetin and others)			
Japanese pickles	Flavonoids		X	
Seaweed ingredients	Indole alkaloids	X		
Tryptophan		X		
Saccharin		X		

From Sugimura, T.: Mutagens, carcinogens, and tumor promoters in our daily food, Cancer **49**: 1970, 1982.
*Sometimes added to "high-potency vitamins."
†Sulfite may be added to the beverage to decrease/abolish mutagenicity.

ria. No epidemiologic data has been provided in terms of human cancer.

Pyrrolidine alkaloids occurring in the *Senecio crotalaria heliotropium* plants have long been known to include a number of substances that cause liver cancer. These substances cause acute poisonings as well as liver cancer in the long-term exposed animal. It is known that acute poisoning has also occurred in humans; whether these agents cause liver cancer in humans is not known. Another substance called *safrole* is found in several spices and is a major component of sassafras tea. It was used in the United States as a flavoring agent until it was found that small levels fed to adult rats caused liver tumors in those animals. Safrole has also been shown to cause liver tumors in mice who receive the substance before weaning. *Bracken fern*, when fed as several percent of the diet by weight, can cause urinary bladder cancer in cat-

tle and rats and intestinal cancer in rats and Japanese quail. In some parts of the world bracken fern is consumed in the human diet but may never be eaten to the extent that cancer is induced. Certain foods contain trace amounts of polycyclic aromatic hydrocarbons, particularly land plants and marine flora and fauna. These may be by-products of heating, or they may occur by synthesis in the plant itself. This is the same substance that is produced in higher levels when a food is broiled and when pyrolysis (changes resulting from heating) causes burning fat to be altered and deposited back on the food. These fatty breakdown products are thought to be the primary carcinogens seen when the Ames test is done on a broiled hamburger, for example. Nitrates are discussed in a later section.

In summary, very few of the substances just listed have been included in the diets of most

Americans to any degree. In general, the Diet, Nutrition and Cancer Report Committee has concluded that the significance of various plant constituents—including the substances mentioned plus methylxanthines derived from coffee, tea, cocoa, and cola products; thiourea; tanins from tea; cumerin; parascorbic acid; estragol; eugenol; and plant estrogens—is not clear in relation to human cancer. We do know that each of these substances is either carcinogenic in laboratory animals or mutagenic in bacteria or mammal cell systems.

EXTRINSIC CANCER-PROMOTING SUBSTANCES IN FOOD

The main categories of extrinsic cancer-promoting substances in food are pesticides, molds and fungi (aflatoxins) and hormones introduced during the growing process in animals before slaughter.

Pesticides

Pesticide residues often remain on the fruits and vegetables that we find in the marketplace. They may also find their way into processed foods derived from these commodities. It is thought that some of these residues, many of which are fat soluble, may be removed by using a process of rinsing the vegetables or fruits in citric acid or some other weak acid before consuming the food. However, since much of the pesticide seeps through the skin to the level of the fruit or vegetable just underlying the skin, it may be important to peel these products fairly deeply to avoid pesticide consumption. This, however, also often removes a major proportion of the nutrients found in that food, and since much of the fiber is often contained in the skin as well, this is not necessarily an acceptable solution to the problem. Since the early 1960s Market Basket Surveys have been conducted by the Food and Drug Administration as a means of checking the levels of pesticide found in the general food supply. They have found that

these levels tend to vary only slightly between one region of the United States and another and that the levels tend to be low overall. A general principle is that *organochlorine* compounds tend to accumulate in fat-containing foods (meat, fish, poultry, dairy products), whereas *organophosphates* generally are more common in cereal products. However, not every product is monitored by the Food and Drug Administration, and anyone who views such television programs as *60 Minutes* becomes concerned about pesticides in food; their recent coverage of the temex question in Florida's citrus fruits is a good example. The problem with many of the epidemiologic studies regarding various pesticides is that they are often done with a very brief follow-up after the exposure to the substance, and there is the difficult problem of controlling for other substances in the environment that may act as cocarcinogens and of missing late-developing problems. In terms of experimental evidence, the *organochlorine* pesticides are known to cause liver cell tumors in mice. Some major organochlorines include toxaphene,* DDT, Captan, PCNB, methoxychlor, chlordane, kepone, heptachlor, hexachlorobenzene,* and lindane.* The * substances have all been linked with aplastic anemia (where bone marrow fails to produce blood cells) in humans. The next category, *organophosphates*, includes malathion, parathion, methyl parathion, and diazinon. Some have been shown to be carcinogenic in animal model studies and others have not. Parathion, for example, resulted in adrenal tumors in one strain of rats. It also causes chromosome changes in guinea pigs but has been shown in bacterial tests not to be mutagenic. This is one example where the bacterial tests may not be of much value in screening organochlorine compounds for potential problems in animals or humans. The conclusion of the Diet, Nutrition, Cancer, and Research Committee was that certain pesticide substances, specifically kepone (Chlordecone), toxaphene, and hexachlorobenzene and possibly heptachlor and lindane, may very well pose carcinogenic hazard to humans.

Another environmental contaminant is the mixture of chlorinated hydrocarbons, called *polychlorinated biphenyls*, or PCBs. These are found widely in the environment as a result of industrial contamination over the last 50 years. They tend to concentrate in animal foods such as fish, milk, cheese, and eggs and in animal feed such as fish meal. One worrisome epidemiologic study was done in Japan over a 9-year period during which people were observed following the accidental consumption of contaminated rice oil. The substance was called Kanechlor 400, and it was found that 41% of the deaths reported during the follow-up were caused by cancers. One problem with the study is that controls were not compared for their incidence of cancer over a similar period. Experimental evidence from animal studies with mice and rats show that various PCBs do cause cancers in these animals. The summary of the Diet, Nutrition and Cancer Committee is that PCBs, if taken in high levels, could lead to the development of malignancy in humans, possibly malignant melanoma in particular. PCBs may also act as tumor promotors, but this role is hard to evaluate. It is believed that the levels of PCBs in the environment in general are much lower than would be required to cause cancer outright. Other possible food contaminants that fall in a similar category to PCBs, that is, probably carcinogenic at high levels in the diet in animals and possibly in humans and possibly carcinogenic in humans at the current level of exposure in the "typical" diet, are the polybromenated biphenyls (PDBs).

The *polycyclic aromatic hydrocarbons (PAHs)* are another varied set of compounds — more than 100 have been identified. About 20 of these have been shown to cause cancer in laboratory animals, and only five of those induced cancer with oral administration. The nonfood sources of these substances include contaminated soil, air and water pollution, and the production by plants and the bacteria within the plants. PAHs are widely found in fresh and grilled, roasted, and smoked fish and meats, roasted foods, leafy and root vegetables, vegetable oils, grains, fruits and vegetables, seafood, and whiskey. Shellfish are particularly high in PAHs and seem unable to metabolize them further. Leafy plants such as spinach, kale, and tobacco contain high levels relative to other vegetables. Very little has been done in the way of epidemiologic studies, and the information is confounded; although with PAHs one would check for smoking of meats, the nitrates introduced by the curing part of most smoking procedures distort the issue. Nevertheless, studies have been done in West Hungary and Iceland in which meats were smoked without nitrate preservation, and in both places cancer of the stomach was found to occur at higher levels than in other population groups. PAHs shown to be carcinogenic when eaten by animals include benzpyrene, dibenzanthracene, benzanthracene, 3-methylcholanthrene, and 7-12-dimethylbenzanthracene. The last two are not normally found in the diet of humans.

Molds and fungi: aflatoxins

The next category of extrinsic cancer-promoting substances — mold and fungus — is best exemplified by the most potent and well known of this group, the aflatoxins.

Aflatoxins are highly potent carcinogens produced by the fungus *Aspergillus flavus*. They commonly develop in most carbohydrate foods in hot, humid climates. Therefore, nuts, grains, seeds, and rice should be kept dry after being harvested and stored. In the United States peanut and grain storage is carefully checked during the drying process. However, the drying procedure is not always as strictly monitored in Southeast Asia and Africa. In these areas hepatitis B virus is common and may act together with aflatoxins to produce liver cancer, as indicated in a 1979 study. Aflatoxins have been shown to produce liver and kidney tumors and

---

Recommendations concerning avoidance of aflatoxins

Choose	Never eat
Fresh dry nuts, grains, seeds, corn	Moldy nuts, especially peanuts, grains, seeds, corn
	Moldy bread, crackers, cereal, beans
	Peanut and cottonseed oils with a moldy flavor

---

to a lesser extent colon cancer in rats and zoo bears fed stale peanuts. Males seem to have a greater predilection for this cancer than females.

It is recommended that·when in areas such as Southeast Asia, China, and Africa, one try to avoid eating nuts, rice, grains, and seeds that are not properly dried and show signs of mold.

Moldy breads should also be avoided. Many species of fungi have been isolated from moldy bread, and three strains have been found to cause cancer in rats.

Of all the naturally occurring carcinogens that contaminate human food, aflatoxins appear to be the most potent carcinogens in humans. Several other fungal carcinogens have been discovered as well. Aflatoxins may be avoided by keeping nuts, grains, and seeds including dry corn in a dry place. If they become damp or develop a moldy flavor during storage, they should not be eaten.

Hormones in animal flesh

The third major representative of extrinsic cancer promoters are the various hormones added to animal flesh to induce growth spurts, specifically through laying down a final amount of fat in an animal just before slaughter. The most well-known substance in this category is *diethystilbestrol* (DES). The Food and Drug Administration has required that the manufacturer wait 72 hours before slaughter to theoretically clear this substance from the flesh to which humans will be exposed in eating the meat, but this is not always well monitored. As

a result, there have been a few instances of gynecomastia in males, believed to be caused by the DES levels in a man who eats large amounts of meat. However, controls are getting more rigid over time, and this should assume a lesser degree of importance in the future. What role this level of DES might play in a subsequent development of tumors is unknown.

• • •

To summarize the role of extrinsic cancer-promoting substances in our food supply, it can only be said that this depends on the intake peculiarities of the individual or family. A vegetarian would be exposed to a different range and concentration of pesticides or added substances, for example, than would the individual with a high-meat intake. In addition, food handling in the home can alter the levels of these substances; it is prudent to suggest that one might seriously consider having one's own garden as a means of controlling these levels to some extent. However, the role of airborne pesticides is not easy to explore, since there are no supporting data.

FOOD ADDITIVES

For several decades the U.S. public has been very concerned about "food additives" as a possible source of carcinogens in our diet. Any ingredient with a name five syllables long arouses suspicion, and not without reason. Over the years the Food and Drug Administration (FDA) has banned more than 25 food additives that proved to be toxic to man and/or animals. Fully half of the banned additives have been coaltar dyes, usually shown as "artificial colors" on labels.

A food additive is any substance or combination of substances intentionally added to food in order to improve it in some way. Food additives may preserve freshness, heighten taste or nutritive value, or act as coloring, thickening, or stabilizing agents. The 1300 food additives approved by the FDA include the following classifications:

1. *Antioxidants.* These are used to prevent the oxidation that leads to the rancidity of fats and browning of fruits. These include BHA (butylhydroxanisole), BHT (butyl-hydroxytoluene), tocopherols, ascorbic acid, and citric acid.

2. *Stabilizers and thickeners.* The substances are used to give processed foods a uniform texture. They include agar, cellulose, guar gums, gelatin, pectin, and dextrin, all of which are derived from natural sources.

3. *Emulsifiers.* These blend liquids together for more uniform appearance. They include phosphoric acid and phosphates; polysorbate 60, 65, and 80; sorbitan monostearate; and lecithin.

4. *Nitrates and nitrites.* These have been used to preserve meats since the last century. They inhibit the growth of *Clostridium botulinum* and enhance the pink color of meat. Although they are not harmful themselves, they may combine with other chemicals in food to form nitrosamines, which are known to cause cancer. *Nutriscore* recommends that their addition be limited to the minimum necessary level to check the growth of bacteria. The food industry should look for safer preservatives.

5. *Coloring agents.* These include some natural substances (chlorophyll, beet or tomato powders, caramelized sugar or carotene) and others that are synthetic.

6. *Flavoring agents.* These also include natural products (cocoa, lemon, orange, vanilla) and some synthetic ones (mostly fruit flavors).

7. *Miscellaneous agents.* This category includes anticaking agents and antifoaming agents (sodium salicoaluminate), flavor enhancers (MSG), and various firming, bleaching, and maturing agents, as well as nutritional supplements.

Some non-nutritive additives may be hazardous, and their use shall be (or has been) discontinued. Many additives, however, perform important roles in preserving foods until they reach the table and in enhancing taste, texture, and appearance.

Although some food additives have been shown to cause cancer in animals, generally at very high levels relative to what would be consumed in a typical human diet, there is no evidence that they play a direct role in the development of any specific human cancers. The safety of all food additives is now under review by the FDA. Under current laws, known carcinogens must be banned from food, under the Delaney Clause of the Federal Food, Drug and Cosmetic Act.

A list of "generally recognized as safe" substances (called the GRAS list) includes all food and drug items consumed by humans in various amounts. Some groups of people, however, may be ingesting levels of substances that vary widely from the "typical" U.S. consumer. Children and generally older individuals taking increasing levels of prescribed medicines are two such groups. In terms of children of different ages, Table 5-14 shows the ratio.

More than 2500 different additives have been used at various times in the United States. Despite the banning of certain carcinogenic additives, some equivocally safe items remain on the GRAS list. These include nitrates, nitrites, and saccharin. A new sweetener, aspar-

TABLE 5-14   Average amount of all FD and C colors in food intake by food category among two groups of children

	Color intake (milligrams)			
	Average diet age-group only (years)		Diets of total age-group (years)	
Food category	1-5	6-12	1-5	6-12
Candy and confections	5.2	6.0	0.9	1.2
Beverages	21.1	29.3	8.5	13.6
Dessert powders	18.0	20.7	1.8	1.9
Cereals	8.4	10.6	3.8	4.6
Maraschino cherries	—	8.4	—	*
Bakery goods	3.5	5.1	2.5	3.8
Ice cream	2.6	3.6	0.8	1.3
Sausage	7.5	9.2	1.6	2.3
Snack food	3.0	3.4	0.5	0.8
Miscellaneous	48.6	55.4	38.8	46.4
Food with color, less miscellaneous	21.3	30.3	20.5	29.3
Food with color, including miscellaneous	60.0	76.2	59.2	75.5

From Food and Drug Administration memorandum, 1976.
*Less than 0.05 milligrams.

tame, has also been questioned in terms of carcinogenicity, despite its recent availability on the market.

In 1977 a ban on *saccharin* was proposed. Canadian researchers have reported that three of 100 rats fed huge saccharin loads (at 5% of their total diet) developed bladder cancer. In several studies the habits of large groups of people with bladder cancer were compared with case controls; those with bladder cancer had a higher intake of saccharin, in general. In one large National Cancer Institute study, it was found that no association existed between level of artificial sweetener intake and bladder cancer except for white nonsmoking women, who did show dose-related bladder cancer increases after heavy saccharin use.

The ban on saccharin has been deferred, but its use by pregnant women is discouraged because we do not know whether it poses a risk to the fetus. The use of saccharin by young people is also discouraged to avoid prolonged exposure over a lifetime.

Cyclamates were introduced in the United States in the 1950s. In a study in the 1960s four of 240 rats on a high-cyclamate diet developed cancer. Cyclamates were banned in 1969; however, subsequent tests have failed to produce the same results as the initial study. Thus cyclamates, with no clearly demonstrated evidence of cancer risk, are banned in the United States, whereas saccharin, which poses a small cancer risk, is used in the United States and banned in Canada. However, the risk of developing cancer from saccharin is minimal as long as the exposure is limited. A 12-ounce bottle of diet soda contains $\frac{1}{200}$ ounce of saccharin, which only becomes important if diet soda is consumed in large amounts. Americans, particularly children, consume large amounts of saccharin in prepared foods; many children drink several bottles of diet soda a day.

After some controversy, the FDA has approved *aspartame* (a derivative of an amino acid from protein) as a low-calorie sweetener. It is 180 times sweeter than table sugar and is free

Recommendations for intake of saccharin and aspartame	
Choose more of	**Choose less** (Two or less servings per day as a guide)
Foods without saccharin or aspartame	Saccharin in "diet" fruits, drinks, juices,
Fresh fruit, juices	desserts, chewing gum
Fruits canned in their own juices	Aspartame in similar items

of the bitter aftertaste found in saccharin. It cannot be heated, so that its main role will be as a table addition and as an additive to dry substances such as fruit drink mix, dry pudding mix, gelatins, toppings, cold cereals, and chewing gum. It is presently available as an over-the-counter item in pharmacies, and it will soon be found on grocery shelves.

Aspartame, like saccharin, is capable of causing cancer in animals when fed at very high levels. Like saccharin, one should limit intake.

Immunotoxicity (causing toxic reactions in the immune system) seems on its way to joining carcinogenicity and teratrogenicity (producing physical defects in the embryo) as parameters used to assess food additives, drugs, pollutants, and other modifiable elements of the environment. Our environment is now apparently laced with a variety of incidental modifiers of the immune response mechanism, with the list ranging from food additives and antioxidants to ionizing and microwave radiation, heavy metals, pesticide residues, alcohol, and tobacco smoke. There is also agreement that the total impact of unintentional modification of the immune response mechanism on human health is unknown and that determination of both the extent and the consequences of the danger will require considerable improvement in tests used for assessing immunotoxicity as well as more widespread application of such tests.

In a report dealing with what had been assumed to be completely innocuous substances

(at least in the quantities used), D. L. Borcher of the FDA's Bureau of Foods, suggested that a reevaluation of the antioxidant compounds butylated hydroxyanisole (BHA) and propyl gallate may be in order. Both are phenolic antioxidants widely used in a variety of foods to retard rancidity of fats and oils caused by the oxidation of unsaturated fatty acid chains.

Evidence drawn from studies of another food additive, *carrageenan*, by H. J. Schwartz of Case Western Reserve University in Cleveland emphasized that carrageenan may pose an immunotoxic threat. This compound, a non-nutritive polysaccharide derived from several species of red algae, is widely used as a filler, suspending agent, gelling agent, and bodying or conditioning agent for a wide variety of foods and medicines, including infant foods, ice creams, canned meats, beer, wine, and vinegar. It is used in a wide range of lubricating jellies, mineral oil emulsions, tablet binders, and hand lotions. From laboratory studies Schwartz concluded it is clear that "carrageenan . . . has profound effects on experimental inflammation, both of an immunologically and nonimmunologically mediated variety." He believes further studies should be done to determine whether any of these effects occur in man.

The food-coloring agent *tartrazine* (FD&C Yellow No. 5) merits further study but not only for its immunotoxic potential. This substance has long been known to result in severe adverse reactions in susceptible individuals. Some and

TABLE 5-15   Example of dye-free diet

Category	Dye-free examples
Beverages	Milk, tea, coffee, cognac, water
Cereal	Homemade bread with unbleached flour, using yeast cake (not dried yeast); no store products; cream of rice, cream of wheat, oatmeal
Fats	Olive oil, Wesson oil, Ferncrest butter
Fruit	Grapefruit, Sunkist oranges*
Meat	Any fresh meat, fish, shellfish, eggs
Miscellaneous	Salt, sugar
Vegetables	Any fresh vegetable except sweet potatoes or yams
Toothpaste	Salt and baking soda

Prohibited items
Any medication without approval of physician
Lipstick, colored nail polish
Soft drinks, powdered drinks
Candy, ice cream, desserts
Mouthwashes, toothpastes, tooth powders, vaginal douches

*Many fruit skins, especially oranges, are dyed prior to marketing.

perhaps all of these reactions involve allergylike symptoms that are not mediated by an immunologic response. Tartrazine is widely used in soft drinks, bakery products, candy, dessert powders, cereals, sherbert, ice cream, and other dairy products, as well as in analgesics, antihistamines, cough remedies, and other nonprescription and prescription drugs. Recently the FDA has begun requiring that all food and drug products containing tartrazine carry a notice to the effect that some individuals may be sensitive to this substance.

For the sensitive or cautious individual, Table 5-15 is included as a means for avoiding all dye substances, whether added or intrinsic to the food.

In summary, eating a diet that follows the U.S. Dietary Goals, with few or no processed foods and a variety of fresh, whole foods, is the best protection against the consumption of excess levels of "additives." Over-the-counter

medicines and vitamins, as well as prescribed medication, should also be scrutinized for possible additives.

NITRITES, NITRATES, AND NITROSAMINES

Nitrite, when used as a food additive, may have a more important impact than might be expected because it reaches the stomach in concentrated amounts and reacts chemically in proportion to its concentration. The National Research Council's 1978 Panel on Nitrates was unable to reach any conclusions about the quantitative effect of nitrate, but advised that reasonable measures be taken to minimize human exposure to nitrosocompounds, including the restriction of the amounts of nitrate and nitrite added to meat products. Gastric cancer, for example, is more common in areas where drinking water contains much nitrate. Because of the uncertainty regarding the effect of nitrites and the possibility that other additives might have unsuspected effects, researchers have not excluded such food additives as a source of cancer risk but have attributed to them a token proportion of being potentially related to less than 1% of cancers.

Despite its decline, stomach cancer still must be reckoned with in the United States. The American Cancer Society projects 23,900 new cases a year with 13,900 deaths. The incidence of stomach cancer remains high in such parts of the world as Japan, Ireland, Chile, Colombia, and eastern Europe. Evidence points to nitrosureas or related chemical compounds as etiologic agents for at least some stomach cancers.

Nitrites represent a class of chemical additives that are fairly nontoxic by themselves, but they may interact with other chemicals or even with normal constituents of food to form carcinogens. Most importantly, nitrites interact in the gastrointestinal tract with amines—byproducts from the breakdown of proteins—to

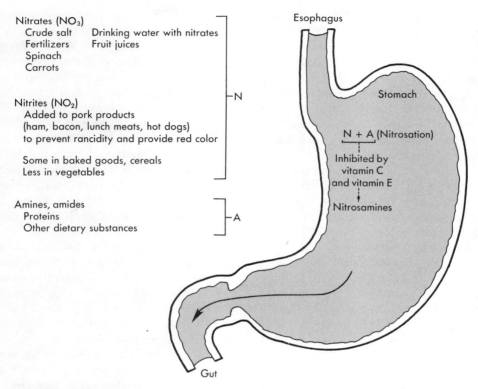

Nitrates (NO₃)
Crude salt   Drinking water with nitrates
Fertilizers   Fruit juices
Spinach
Carrots

Nitrites (NO₂)
Added to pork products
(ham, bacon, lunch meats, hot dogs)
to prevent rancidity and provide red color

Some in baked goods, cereals
Less in vegetables

Amines, amides
Proteins
Other dietary substances

Esophagus

Stomach

N + A (Nitrosation)

Inhibited by
vitamin C
and vitamin E

Nitrosamines

Gut

FIG. 5-9 Interaction of nitrates and nitrites with amines to form nitrosamines.

form nitrosamines. Nitrosamines are compounds that are highly carcinogenic in animals, and possibly in humans, as evidenced by epidemiologic studies. Fig. 5-9 depicts the nitrate and nitrite interaction with aminos to form nitrosamines. The helpful aspects of dietary vitamin-C and vitamin-E intake are also shown.

Nitrates occur throughout nature, with especially large amounts in some vegetables such as spinach, beets, radishes, lettuce, and collard greens. But these foods are not known to form nitrosamines, either in cooking or when eaten. Many fresh vegetables contain substantial vitamin C, which inhibits nitrosamine formation.

Nitrates from all these sources are absorbed into the bloodstream from the stomach and the intestine. When these nitrates reach the mouth, they are reconverted, by bacteria in saliva in a recycling process, to nitrites and are again ingested in the gastrointestinal tract. Acidic stomach fluids at each stage in the cycle enhance the transformation of the nitrites into nitrosamines, the carcinogens that ultimately form stomach cancer.

Nitrosamines are also found in increased levels in association with beer drinking. Many beers contain preformed nitrosamines developed during the heat-drying process of green barley. Beer companies have now reduced the level of nitrosamines by improving the drying process and by using sulfur, which interferes with the formation of nitrosamines.

The switchover to new methods was industry-wide by January 1980, and now any malt beverages that contain nitrosamines at levels that can be reliably be detected—above 5 parts per billion—are subject to regulatory action. However, trace amounts of nitrosamines below that level may still be present in beer and scotch.

Sodium nitrite is still used to preserve foods such as hot dogs, salami, bacon, ham, and cured fish. It is known to prevent botulism, a deadly bacterial poison.

Nitrates and nitrites have been used as curing agents for meat for more than 2000 years. Although they both have the ability to retard the growth of microorganisms, notably the potentially lethal botulism bacteria, they are primarily used for coloring and flavoring. They give hot dogs, cold cuts, and ham their characteristic pink color. Without these additives, these meats would have a brownish hue similar to that of bratwurst. They may also have a slightly different flavor, although meat products free of nitrates and nitrites have been produced that taste nearly the same as their chemically treated counterparts.

In a risk/benefit analysis, the FDA calculated that of 135 cases of cancer a year related to nitrites, only six of these cases would be the result of nitrites in cured meats. If these meats were not cured with nitrites, 22 cases of fatal botulism would occur, even with an intensive public education program. Without a public education program, the occurrence of botulism would be even higher. The six cases of cancer that result from the use of nitrites seem insignificant in comparison not only to the 22 cases of botulism, but to 100,000 new cases of lung cancer, caused primarily by cigarette smoking, such as developed in 1979. Paradoxically, the amount of nitrosamines in a 3-ounce portion of nitrite-preserved bacon is roughly the same as that absorbed in smoking a pack of cigarettes.

Although the risk of cancer from nitrites in cured meat is low, consumption of fresh meats, poultry, and seafood are recommended over ham, bacon, sausage, hot dogs, corned beef, and smoked seafoods.

During the last 5 years, the federal government has tried to decrease public exposure to nitrites, nitrates, and nitrosamines. The levels of nitrite used in cured meats have been reduced, and with a few exceptions, the use of nitrate in cured meats has been banned. Nitrosamines in beer and bacon have been reduced significantly. The manufacture and sale of nitrite-free processed meats has gained limited acceptance. Americans have reduced their consumption of meats cured with nitrites from 50 grams per person a day in the 1950s to 30 grams in the 1970s.

Although the disagreements over the relative dangers of these chemicals probably will go on for years, consumers can take measures such as the following to reduce their exposure to nitrosamines:

1. Take vitamin C. Since the vitamin ascorbic acid is a proved inhibitor of nitrosamine formation if it is ingested at the same time nitrites are consumed, drinking a glass of orange juice when eating ham and eggs is a prudent measure. The tomato in a bacon, lettuce, and tomato sandwich not only makes the sandwich taste better, but it is a form of preventive medicine. Other good sources of vitamin C include grapefruit, cabbage, potatoes, cantaloupe, strawberries, peppers, and lettuce. Stomach cancer shows a negative correlation with consumption of fresh (citrus) fruit and vegetables that contain vitamin C.

2. Take vitamin E. Some scientific reports have shown that naturally occurring vitamin E, found in cereal grains and vegetable fats, prevents the formation of nitrosamines.

3. Care for and store vegetables properly. This can considerably reduce the formation of nitrites. Once vegetables are cooked, bacteria act to reduce nitrates to nitrites. Only the amount of vegetables

that will be eaten immediately should be cooked. Once vegetables are cooked, they should not be left at room temperature. If there are leftovers, they should be stored for no more than a day or two in the refrigerator. Since freezing stops the bacterial action, commercially frozen cooked vegetables are not a problem.

4. Use low-nitrate fertilizers. For those who grow their own vegetables, a switch to fertilizers that contain less nitrate will reduce its concentration in the vegetables. In a study on spinach, researchers showed that harvesting the spinach at the end of a day, after it has been exposed to daylight for 12 hours, reduced the levels of nitrate by more than 20%. Many scientists believe this may well be true of other vegetables.

5. Eat meats that are cured differently. Alternatives to meats cured with sodium nitrite include bratwurst, color-free hot dogs, and fresh sausage. There also are a number of specially processed nitrite-free meats, including bologna and salami. They are available in natural food stores. Many of them do not have the color and flavor associated with traditionally cured meats, however. Nitrite-free meat prod-

ucts should be kept frozen until they are cooked, to keep them from spoiling.

In summary, the boxed material will help you avoid nitrosamines resulting from nitrate and nitrite in cured meats and seafood.

CAFFEINE, COFFEE, AND TEA

Coffee, tea, cocoa, and cola drinks contain caffeine; however, it must be noted that other substances are also found in these beverages and that caffeine itself has not been clearly implicated as a cancer-causing chemical. More than 50% of the world's coffee is consumed in the United States; only Sweden consumes more. On a yearly basis each of us drinks about 20 pounds of coffee—approximately three cups per day per person. Coffee is low in calories, with only 5 per cup. In a 6-ounce cup, ground-roast coffee averages 83 milligrams of caffeine, instant coffee averages 60, and decaffeinated contains about 3. Leaf tea has 41 milligrams of caffeine, instant averages 28, and other teas vary (Tetley, 18; Red Rose, 90). Table 5-16 shows caffeine levels in various beverages.

Caffeine is a stimulant that alters heart rate, respiration, muscular coordination, central nervous system activity, wakefulness, and blood

---

Recommendations regarding nitrites, nitrates, and *N*-nitroso compounds in foods

Choose more of	Choose much less
Fresh foods without nitrates or nitrites	Foods containing nitrates or nitrites (all develop a pink color when nitrates are added to meat)
Fresh meats, poultry, seafood	
Fresh vegetables and fruits	Cured bacon, sausage, ham
Foods containing ample vitamin C and/ or E (best vitamin E from wheat germ, almonds, filberts, walnuts; sunflower seeds; asparagus, greens, leeks, spinach, sweet potato; blackberries)	Hot dogs, frankfurters, bologna, luncheon meats, corned beef, turkey
	Some beers

TABLE 5-16   Caffeine content of beverages

Beverage	Caffeine (milligrams)		
	mg/1 oz	mg/5 oz	mg/12 oz
Carbonated			
Mello Yello			53
Coca-Cola, Diet Coca-Cola*			46
Dr. Pepper*			40
Mountain Dew*			54
Diet Dr. Pepper*			40
Tab*			47
Pepsi-Cola*			38
RC Cola*			36
Shasta Cola, Cherry			44
Diet Rite*			36
Canada Dry Cola, diet			1
Diet Mr. Pibb			59
Coffee			
Instant‡		40–108	
Percolated‡		64–124	
Dripolated‡		110–150	
Coffee: decaffeinated			
Infused‡		2–4	
Instant‡		1–2	
Decaf†		2–5	
Nescafe†		5–8	
Sanka†		3	
Tea, bagged			
Black, 5 min brew‡		20–50	
Black, 1 min brew‡		9–33	
Tea, loose			
Black, 5 min brew‡		20–50	
Green, 5 min brew*		37.5	
Green, Japan, 5 min brew*		22.5	
Cocoa; baking chocolate‡		6	
Ovaltine‡	35		

*Bunker, M. L., and McWilliams, M.: Caffeine content of common beverages, J. Am. Diet. Assoc. **74**:28, 1979.
†Nutritional analysis data supplied by the manufacturer.
‡Caffeine, Scientific Status Summary, Institute of Food Technologists' Expert Panel on Food Safety and Nutrition, published by the Institute of Food Technologists, 221 N. LaSalle St., Chicago, Illinois.

pressure (upward) in some people. Its major hazards are those associated with heart and cardiovascular disease.

The possibility for an association between bladder cancer and coffee drinking (especially in concomitant saccharin users) has been explored. Thus far, no evidence can be shown to link caffeine and coffee with bladder cancer.

Benign breast lumps (called mammary dysplasia) have also been related to caffeine. In many instances eliminating tea, coffee, chocolate, and cola from women's diets has resulted in complete disappearance of long-standing breast disease. (Remember, as noted earlier, that breast lumps are *not* associated with an increased risk of breast cancer.)

In the laboratory caffeine can cause cancer-like changes in cells at doses 20 to 40 times higher than the highest blood level ever measured in an habitual coffee drinker. At lower doses, however, caffeine seems to inhibit the cancer-inducing effects of other chemicals. Thus, in ordinary amounts, caffeine may actually protect against cancer.

Concern that caffeine may cause birth defects has led the Food and Drug Administration to caution pregnant women to limit their caffeine intake. Little is known about whether caffeine is indeed a human teratogen. A case-control study of 2000 malformed infants indicated that caffeine is not a major teratogen with regard to six defects evaluated.

Herbal teas have enjoyed increasing popularity in recent years and can now be purchased in supermarkets as well as health food and specialty food stores. We are unaware of many constituents of herbal teas, however, and these can potentially contain harmful substances. Herbal teas in many instances are toxic: some cause watery diarrhea, and if they contain senna leaf in combination with other contents, abdominal cramps may result. Others contain chemicals that affect both physical and mental functions.

Cancer-causing substances are present in tea made from sassafras root bark. Tannins in tea, including ordinary tea and peppermint tea, have been linked to high rates of cancer of the esophagus and stomach. Adding milk to the tea binds the tannins and presumably protects the digestive tract from their effects.

If one is interested in removing caffeine from the diet, steam-processed decaffeinated coffee is an appropriate choice. None of the typical supermarket decaffeinated brands use this method. Decaffeinated coffee may be substituted for one or two of your cups of regular coffee each day until you are drinking nothing but decaffeinated. Or you can mix decaffeinated and regular coffee in various proportions to reduce your total caffeine intake.

Other alternatives to caffeine are the grain-based beverages, such as Postum and Pero. These are very low in calories—12 per cup for Postum, which is made from bran, wheat, and molasses, and 7 per cup for Cafix, a West German product made from barley, rye, chicory, and beets. If not in your supermarket, such products can usually be found in health food stores. Another beverage, Wilson's Heritage, a 100% barley product made in Kansas, can even be brewed like coffee and perhaps mixed with your favorite coffee. However, excessive consumption of such grain products may have a laxative effect or cause flatulence (gas).

BREAST MILK

During the last decade, women in the United States have increasingly chosen breast-feeding, often for prolonged periods, as the major source of nutrition for their babies during the first months of life. This is laudable and ideal for a variety of reasons, including the enhancement of bonding between mother and infant and the appropriateness of breast-milk components in the diet of the newborn.

However, many environmental agents specifically known to be stored in the fat of both animals and humans are also stored in the breast, which itself has a large supply of fat tissue. The question is whether or not some of these substances creep into the milk and may pose a risk for the infant. One might think that the hazard would be greater in the infant of an elderly mother or a primipara (first-time mother). A study in the *American Journal of Clinical Nutrition* noted that levels of harmful environmental substances such as vinylchloride and dieldrin were indeed found in breast milk in levels much greater than those seen in the comparable infant formula. The effects of this can only be surmised.

Very little is known and little can be recommended with certainty with respect to cancer and the breast-versus-bottle-feeding issue. Carcinogenesis is not clearly demonstrable from the levels of breast milk contaminants; however, in several instances these levels were shown in the study mentioned to be higher than levels allowed in the environment by various agencies monitoring our food and water supply. It seems prudent to suggest that elderly primipara females consider nursing their babies for a limited time, perhaps 1 to 2 months, rather than for some prolonged period, as a hedge against the level of these toxins in the infant's diet.

OBESITY

The alarming prevalence of obesity in the United States is partly attributable to the steadily declining energy requirements of Americans over recent decades — a decline in energy expenditure that has not been paralleled by a decrease in food intake. Our level of physical activity in the United States is generally considered to be light to sedentary rather than heavy, as was true earlier in this century.

Obesity from the overconsumption of calories is a major risk factor in many killer diseases. It is extremely important either to maintain an optimal weight or to alter weight to reach an optimal level. Altering calorie consumption is not the only way to control weight and lessen the risk factors associated with obesity; exercise can and should play an integral role as well. Even if dietary patterns remain the same, the influence of an increasingly sedentary life-style may turn what was previously a diet adequate in calories into one with too many calories. According to a Senate Select Committee, the first goal in avoiding possible obesity involves the following:

> To avoid being overweight, consume only as much energy (calories) as is expended; if overweight, decrease energy intake and increase energy expenditure.

Fifteen million Americans are obese to an extent that seriously raises their risk of ill health. Obesity is associated with the onset and clinical progression of diseases such as hypertension, diabetes mellitus, heart disease, joint problems, endometrial cancer, and gallbladder disease. It may also modify the quality of one's life.

According to B. Winikoff of the Rockefeller Foundation:

> With increasing affluence, we have also increased our bodily weights. Obesity is probably the most common and one of the most serious nutritional problems affecting the American public today.
>
> Over 30 percent of all men between 50-59 are 20 percent overweight, and fully 60 percent are over 10 percent overweight. About one-third of the population is overweight to a degree which has been shown to diminish life expectancy. In the United States, this type of malnutrition is a more common burden among the poor than among the wealthy.
>
> Obesity has the effect of increasing blood cholesterol, blood pressure and blood glucose levels. Through these effects, it is an important risk factor for coronary disease.
>
> Reductions in obesity improve the condition of hypertensives and diabetics, and thereby reduces the risk of heart disease and stroke. Data from the Framingham study examined by Ashley and Kan-

nel in 1973 indicate that each 10 percent reduction in weight in men 35-55 years old would result in about a 20 percent decrease in incidence of coronary disease.

Conversely, each 10 percent increase in weight would result in a 30 percent increase in coronary disease.

In light of the fact that *decrease* close to 700,000 Americans die of coronary disease every year, the staggering implication of these figures become apparent: if a 20 percent increase in incidence did occur throughout the population and were reflected in a 20 percent decrease in overall mortality, about 140,000 lives would be saved per year. Since at least one-half of the coronary deaths — almost one-third of a million — occur before reaching a hospital, prevention is not only cheaper, but clearly more effective than cure.

With respect to weight control, it should be recalled that fat is the most concentrated source of food energy. As pointed out previously, fat supplies 9 calories per gram; alcohol, 7 calories; and protein and carbohydrates, only 4 calories per gram.

Fat and obesity

As already discussed, research has linked a high consumption of saturated and unsaturated fats with cancers of the colon, breast, rectum, and endometrium. In the West, where 40% of daily caloric intake is from fats (meat, cheese, butter, margarine, oils, whole-milk products), the incidence of colon and breast cancer is high. In Japan, Thailand, and India, where fat comprises only 12% of daily caloric intake, the incidence of these two cancers is low.

The higher levels of colon cancer among Japanese migrants to the United States then those in Japan lends further support to the environment, rather than genetic factors, being implicated in colon cancer.

Women with a large body mass (obesity), high-fat intake, and a high-cholesterol level have a greater risk of developing breast cancer and an increased rate of cancer recurrence than the general population. Of interest is new information on cholesterol that suggests an inverse relationship between cholesterol and cancer; two papers have reported that a lower blood cholesterol level is related to an increased incidence of colon cancer in men.

In the clearest link between obesity and cancer, heavier women are much more likely to develop endometrial cancer and breast cancer postmenopausally, because increasing obesity increases the synthesis of estrogen and exposure of tissues to this hormone. Estrogens are growth-promoting substances for the uterine endometrium and the breast ductal epithelium.

In animal studies, enhanced tumor development has been seen in rats fed 20% corn oil or sunflower seed oil, and with slightly less tumor enhancement with 20% lard. When fed beef tallow or coconut oil, however, there has been no enhancement unless the diet was supplemented in essential fatty acids, and even *intact* rats had fewer tumors and longer latent periods than did the rats fed the same total amount of corn or sunflower seed oil.

Evidently, there are also differences in fats in whether they are tumor initiators or promoters. Corn and sunflower seed oils influence tumor formation even if fed after carcinogen exposure, which suggests that these oils are promoters and not initiators. However, studies using lard indicated an effect if lard was fed before or before and after carcinogen exposure, but no effect if it was fed *only after* exposure. Therefore, lard appears to influence tumor development at initiation and not to be effective at later stages; the effects of dietary fats may be both qualitative and quantitative. Fat may alter the endocrine system, directly affect mammary gland growth and body responses to hormonal influences, induce membrane abnormalities, influence carcinogen metabolism or DNA repair processes, or possibly have other effects.

In humans hormonal imbalance may be one pathway by which dietary fat promotes tumor development. Prolactin and estrogen are the two hormones with the strongest links to cancer development; however, the evidence has been stronger in animals than humans. Animal investigations have shown that suppression of prolactin levels reduces tumor growth and number.

Losing weight

If you need to lose weight, do so gradually. Steady loss of 1 to 2 pounds a week until you reach your goal is relatively safe and more likely to be maintained. Long-term success depends on acquiring new and better habits of eating and exercise, which is why "crash" diets usually fail in the long run.

Do not try to lose weight too rapidly. Avoid diets that are severely restricted in the variety of foods they allow. Diets containing fewer than 800 calories may be hazardous. Some people have developed gallstones, disturbing psychologic changes, and other complications while following such diets; a few people have even died suddenly.

A pound of body fat provides 3500 calories. To lose 1 pound of fat, you must burn 3500 calories more than you consume. If you burn 500 calories more a day than you consume, you will lose 1 pound of fat a week. If you normally burn 1700 calories a day, you can expect to lose about a pound of fat each week if you adhere to a 1200-calorie-per-day diet.

Do not attempt to reduce your weight below the acceptable range. Severe weight loss may be associated with nutrient deficiencies, menstrual irregularities, infertility, hair loss, skin changes, cold intolerance, severe constipation, psychiatric disturbances, and other complications. If you lose weight suddenly or for unknown reasons, see your physician. Unexplained weight loss may be an early clue to an unsuspected underlying disorder.

Elderly or very inactive people may eat relatively little food. They should pay special attention to avoiding foods that are high in calories but low in other essential nutrients such as fat, oils, alcohol, and sugars. Infants also have spe-cial nutritional needs. Healthy full-term infants should be breastfed unless there are special problems. The nutrients in human breast milk tend to be digested and absorbed more easily than those in cow's milk.

In summary, do the following to lose weight:
1. Increase physical activity
2. Eat less fat and fatty foods
3. Eat less sugar and sweets
4. Avoid too much alcohol

Exercise and obesity

Gradual increase of everyday physical activities such as walking or climbing stairs can be very helpful in avoiding obesity. Table 5-17 gives the calories used per hour in different activities. Table 5-18 shows a typical chart that can be used to keep track of calories burned through various activities during a week.

Exercise goes hand-in-hand with the issue of obesity. It also alters a variety of things in terms of total body fat percentage in that aerobic exercise, maintained at a certain level in a person's life throughout the lifespan, can provide an active means of keeping the percentage of total body fat under control. Our cave-dwelling ancestors performed an astonishing array of tasks during a given day: building fires, gathering food, catching live animals, fabricating assorted materials for clothing and shelter, and moving from place to place at regular intervals. Our bodies were not designed to sit to the extent that we do at present, and a variety of studies are beginning to show that this is detrimental in many ways. For example, one compared young men in college who exercised actively and aerobically (running 25 or more miles per week) to other subjects who sat and primarily studied. Those who actively exercised were more efficient in using protein and several other nutrients available in their diets than those who were sedentary. This may be important in terms of increasing the nutrient availability in our diets.

Another interesting study reported in the *American Journal of Clinical Nutrition* in 1981

TABLE 5-17 Approximate energy expenditure by a 150-pound person engaged in various activities

Activity	Calories burned per hour
Lying down or sleeping	80
Sitting	100
Driving an automobile	120
Standing	140
Domestic work	180
Walking, 2½ mph	210
Bicycling, 5½ mph	210
Gardening	220
Golf, lawn mowing with power mower	250
Bowling	270
Walking, 3¾ mph	300
Swimming, ¼ mph	300
Square dancing, volleyball, roller skating	350
Wood chopping or sawing	400
Tennis	420
Skiing, 10 mph	600
Squash and handball	600
Bicycling, 13 mph	660
Running, 10 mph	900

compared three groups of males: the first was required to lose 5 pounds on a calorie-restricted diet, the second group was to lose 5 pounds on a calorie-restricted diet and increased exercise routine, and the third simply exercised and maintained their weight. In the first group, who simply dieted, lipid levels—high-density lipoproteins (HDLs), which promote cardiovascular health, relative to low-density lipoproteins (LDLs), which are associated with more cardiovascular risk—became unbalanced. The second group, who dieted and exercised, had the best improvement in HDLs relative to LDLs. The third group, who exercised alone, also showed some improvement in HDLs relative to LDLs. This suggests that if one is modestly overweight and sedentary and has difficulty losing weight, it is better to exercise and maintain a proper diet to avoid possible heart disease risks than to try a stringent diet without the introduction of exercise.

In summary, no studies have been done on the direct relationship between exercise and cancer, but there could be some added risk for certain types of cancer associated with obesity if dieting and exercise were not used together by individuals wishing to lose weight.

SUMMARY

About 20% of all deaths in the United States are caused by cancer. Of these, approximately 35% of cancers are potentially preventable by diet, including (percentages from Doll, R., and Peto, R.: Your patient and cancer, January 1983, p. 123):

Stomach and large bowel—90%

Endometrium, gallbladder, pancreas, and breast—50%

Lung, larynx, bladder, cervix, mouth, pharynx, and esophagus—20%

Other types—10%

Overall—35%

(Although this figure of 35% is a plausible total, the parts that contribute to it are uncertain in the extreme. We make no pretense of the reliability of this total because of this degree of uncertainty. It is still possible, although unlikely, that no practical modification in diet will be discovered that can reduce total U.S. cancer death rates by more than 10%. However, it is equally possible that a reduction of even *double* our suggested total of 35% might be ultimately achieved.)

A diet appropriate to meet your basic needs, coupled with vigorous daily exercise, can maintain or improve your basic health and reduce the risk of cancer, heart and vascular disease, and other illnesss.

Fat in the diet seems to be most closely linked with cancer, with total calories being related to this.

Cholesterol is not clearly demonstrated to be linked with cancer.

A *high-protein* diet may be associated with cancer incidence, but assessment is difficult,

TABLE 5-18   Chart for expended calories in a week

Name _____

Week of (dates) _____

Activity	Minutes of activity							Total weekly minutes	Calories/ week
	Sat	Sun	Mon	Tues	Wed	Thurs	Fri		
1									
2									
3									
4									
5									
6									

Total calories expended _____ = Total exercise calories

*Basal calories** _____ Basal calories

ADL calories† _____ ADL calories

Total: all calories used _____ Total expended calorie/week

Computations based on (weight): _____

Calories expended this week: _____

*Basal calories: 600/day for women; 700/day for men.
†ADL—activity of daily living calories; normally, Ideal body weight × 10 − Basal calories = ADL calories.

since protein and the implicated fat are closely linked in many foods.

Certain *vitamins* may be useful in helping to prevent certain cancers. These include:

1. Vitamin A (preformed in liver products, liver oils and vitamin pills can be toxic)
2. Carotenoids (water-soluble precursors, found in red, dark-yellow, and green vegetables and fruits) may be especially protective.
3. The vitamin-A substances (retinoids) have major protective effects against lung, bladder, and laryngeal cancer. They may also be important protectors against breast, cervical, and other head and neck tumors, as well as against melanoma.
4. Vitamin C probably protects against development of esophageal and stomach cancer.
5. Vitamin E probably acts in a similar fashion. Both are antioxidants.

Of the various minerals studied, *selenium* acts as an antioxidant and seems protective against some tumors. However, above 200 milligrams a day should be viewed as potentially toxic. Other minerals may protect against cancer, but the information is equivocal.

Certain *cruciferous vegetables* contain components which are held to be protective. These include cabbage, broccoli, brussels sprouts, and cauliflower.

Fiber is a difficult topic, since methods used to determine and report food fiber levels vary. Nevertheless, one important study has shown that colon cancer is lower in those consuming a high-whole-wheat diet that contains pentosan. Pentosans may be the primary protective factor in fiber-containing foods. Some components of fiber bind substances (iron, calcium, vitamin B_{12}) and prevent absorption.

Natural carcinogens are found in some foods. Of these, hydrazines in mushrooms and *N*-nitroso compounds can be a hazard if found in high levels in the diet. Aflatoxin, the primary mold-produced toxin, arises in some foods (grains, nuts) if these are allowed to become stale in a moist, muddy environment. Aflatoxins are thought to be almost a nonexistent problem in the United States food supply.

Food mutagens may or may not be carcinogens in an animal or human, but since these may be detected by using the bacterial Ames test, we are able to check for a food's mutagenic potential. Various vegetables contain naturally occurring mutagens.

Pesticides can cause cancer in animals. Studies in humans are lacking, but individuals can best avoid this potential risk by washing or peeling all commercially grown produce known to be sprayed with pesticides. These include primarily organochlorides. Polychlorinated biphenyls and polycyclic aromatic hydrocarbons are other substances in the environment shown to be carcinogenic in animals.

Food additives (there are approximately 3000 of these in our food supply) are added intentionally or sometimes unintentionally, as with vinyl chloride or acrylonitrate seeping into the food from the package. Very few of these (except saccharin and other non-nutritive sweeteners) have been tested adequately. We do not know whether diets skewed toward repetitive use of limited foods might be a problem. A wide selection of fresh foods, cooked without smoking or broiling, is no doubt the best means of avoiding large levels of additives.

The following recommendations in the boxed material offer a good summary of how best to avoid potential cancer associated with diet; good nutrition is certainly the basis for any preventive measures in the realm of dietary intake.

A dietary approach to cancer prevention

1. **Eat a diet which includes:**

   Low-fat preparation of the following foods:
   Cereal and whole-grain products
   Fresh fruits and vegetables
   Low-fat milk, cheese, or yogurt (or other calcium-rich foods)
   Poultry, fish, lean meats
   Eggs (one or less per day)
   Legumes (dried beans and peas)

2. **Strive for good physical status and normal weight:**

   Reduce:
      Excess calories (calculate your daily needs)
      Sugars and sweets
      Dietary fat intake
      Alcohol, wine, and beer consumption
   Eat slowly
   Exercise regularly

3. **Include fiber in your diet:**

   Select foods that have a high fiber content—fruits, vegetables, and whole-grain bread
   and cereal products
   Peas, dried beans, potato skins, and seeds are also good sources of fiber

4. **Your diet should be low in fat, saturated fat, and cholesterol:**

   Select lean meat, fish, poultry, or peas and dried beans
   Reduce intake of organ meats (liver, etc.) and egg yolks
   Reduce intake of butter, shortening, cream, margarine, coconut oil, and foods containing any of these products
   Avoid frying; try to bake, broil, boil, or braise foods most of the time
   Trim excess fat and skin from meats
   Make yourself aware of amounts and types of fat contained in foods—read labels!

5. **Drink alcohol in moderation:**

   Aim for a maximum of one to two alcoholic drinks per day (mixed drinks, wine, and beer)

6. **Reduce sugar intake:**

   Decrease the amount of all sugars (white, brown, or raw) in your diet including honey and syrups
   Reduce intake of foods containing sugars (candy, soft drinks, ice cream, cookies, cakes, etc.)
   Select fresh fruit when possible; if canned fruit must be used, choose those in light syrup or sugar free (water packed)

7. **Decrease sodium intake:**

   Taste the natural flavors of foods—they are most enjoyable
   Decrease the amount of added salt while cooking
   Keep the salt shaker in the cupboard, not on the table!
   Avoid presalted foods such as lunch meats, pickles, catsup, mustard, relish, garlic salt, steak sauce, soy sauce, potato chips, salted nuts, and pretzels
   Make yourself aware of salt, sodium, or MSG content in foods—read labels!
   Use spices, fresh seasonings, and herbs for flavoring
   Use sour foods such as lemon juice, lime juice, or vinegar for flavoring

8. **Reduce the amount of charcoal broiling.**

CHAPTER 6

Alcohol and Cancer

One swallow does not make a summer, but too many swallows make a fall.

GEORGE D. PRENTICE

ERNEST H. ROSENBAUM

Alcohol has been around for a long time. Archeologists believe that wine was made from fermented grapes 10,000 years ago, and date and palm wine may be even older. Yet only recently has there been conclusive evidence that alcohol has a relationship to cancer, although alcohol has been a suspected carcinogen for more than 60 years. The first indication of a link between alcohol and cancer was through the observation that people who drank excessively or those who work in drinking establishments, such as bartenders, had an increased rate of cancer.

This observation has since been borne out by studies of people who consume alcohol. In 1979 O. M. Jensen investigated brewery workers in Denmark who were given 4 pints of free beer per day as part of their work benefits; Jensen assumed that the workers probably drank the beer, which exceeded the average daily consumption of beer for the Danish male population in general. When death rates of these brewery workers and the rest of the population were compared, the workers showed increased rates of cancers of the esophagus, larynx, lung, and liver.

Findings show that approximately 7% of cancer deaths in men and 3% in women are alcohol-related. There is an increased mortality when one regularly has three to five drinks daily. The risk sharply increases at six or more drinks per day. It is known that cancer of the larynx is 10 times more likely in those who drink than in those who abstain or drink only moderately; cancer of the esophagus is 25 times more common in heavy drinkers than in the general population. Alcoholic cirrhosis is considered a risk factor for liver cancer. For example, France has the highest incidence of upper alimentary tract cancer and cirrhosis when compared with Europe and North America, a finding associated with the wine-drinking habits of the French.

In the United States cirrhosis of the liver is the fourth leading cause of death in persons between the ages of 45 and 65. It occurs more often in men, reflecting the drinking ratio. Liver damage caused by cirrhosis is permanent, although one can improve compensation and ability to function by ceasing drinking. A recent report by M. Leo and C. Liebet found that alcoholic liver disease was associated with severely decreased hepatic vitamin A levels, even though liver injury was moderate and blood vitamin A levels were normal. Vitamin A in high amounts (>10,000 to 25,000 U/day) may be toxic to the liver (New England Journal of Medicine, Sept. 1982). Vitamin A should not be given in high doses with alcohol. A low-dose (5,000 to 10,000 U vitamin D) daily supplement to B-complex vitamins is currently being considered as a therapeutic recommendation.

Some studies indicate that women who drink have about one and a half to two times the breast cancer rate of women who never drink. This seems to hold true regardless of the type of alcohol consumed—wine, beer, or high-proof spirits. However, the evidence of the alcohol/breast cancer relationship is currently *not* conclusive. For example, one of the studies did not include information on the diets of the women studied, and diet has also been implicated in breast cancer. Other studies do *not* confirm the relationship between alcohol and breast cancer. All investigators agree that future epidemiologic studies need to be completed to resolve this issue.

Several studies show that pregnant women who daily drink 1 ounce of hard liquor (3 ounces of wine, 12 ounces of beer)—about one drink of straight liquor or one mixed drink—may have babies with a higher percentage of growth deficiencies, mental retardation, and malformations of the body, including the face, limbs, heart, skin, and lungs.

When pregnant women drink heavily, they risk having babies who have *fetal alcohol syndrome (FAS)*. These children are at risk for all of the symptoms mentioned. There is a relationship between the amount of alcohol consumed and the seriousness of the defects, although ceasing to drink as late as the second trimester decreases the potential number of defects. No one currently knows the quantity of alcohol it takes to cause fetal damage. Therefore, the safest recommendation is to rarely drink or not drink at all during pregnancy.

Another negative effect of excessive alcohol consumption for both men and women is that it depresses the inflammatory response of the body's immunity system. By disturbing and reducing the functions of the immune system, alcohol may make a person more susceptible to cancer and infections.

Groups of people who abstain from alcohol for religious reasons, such as Mormons or Seventh Day Adventists, show a much lower overall cancer rate compared to the general public. This is especially true in cancers that are associated with alcohol consumption—cancers of the mouth, head, and neck.

So far the evidence suggests that the higher incidence of cancer among heavy drinkers is caused by the alcohol itself and that this is largely independent of the *kind* of alcoholic beverage—whether it be wine, beer, a mixed drink, or straight high-proof alcohol. Many people mistakenly believe that they are protecting themselves from the bad effects of alcohol by avoiding the "hard stuff" and drinking wine and beer. Wine and beer are still alcohol in terms of their carcinogenic or cocarcinogenic effects in the body.

Mashberg, Garfinkel, and Harris recently reported that there is a difference in the risk factor for oral cancer, depending on the type of alcoholic beverage consumed. Beer and wine drinkers had a much higher adjusted relative risk factor than whiskey drinkers (20.4 versus 7.3, respectively) for those consuming 10 or more drinks per day.

Under experimental conditions pure alcohol (ethanol) given to laboratory animals did not cause cancer. Humans never consume pure alcohol but use alcoholic beverages containing various chemical compounds, and drinking is usually associated with smoking.

The link between alcohol in any form and cancer has been supported by a 1979 study by Weaver et al. and a 1983 study by Wynder and associates showing higher rates of oral cancer among habitual users of strongly alcoholic mouthwashes. The alcohol may itself be a carcinogen, promoting tumor growth when it comes in frequent contact with body tissue. Most likely alcohol is a cocarcinogen, strengthening the tumor-causing effect of other agents, especially tobacco. The alcohol may act as an effective solvent to carry other carcinogens easily dissolved in it to body tissues, where they are rapidly absorbed. The areas most commonly associated with cancers due to excessive drinking—the head and neck—are the first to come in contact with alcohol when one drinks.

If one drinks and smokes—a common practice—the carcinogenic effects of each substance are multiplied. This interaction greatly increases the chances of getting cancer, especially those of the head and neck (mouth, throat, esophagus, larynx). Someone who drinks moderately but does not smoke still increases the cancer risk rate two or three times the average of one who neither smokes nor drinks. A person who drinks *and* smokes pushes his risk of cancer up to 15 times the average rate.* According to K. Rothman, this is two and one half times the expected risk ratio for oral cancer if the effects of alcohol and tobacco were only additive. *The smoking/alcohol combination accounts for 75% of all oral cancer.* Poor dental

---

*One or two ounces of alcohol plus 40 cigarettes daily increases the cancer risk approximately 10 to 15 times; 3 to 5 + ounces of alcohol plus 40 cigarettes daily increases the cancer risk greater than 15 times.

and mouth hygiene are additional factors contributing to oral cancer.

In one study of people who smoked and drank, those who smoked two or more packs a day and consumed six to eight drinks had a slightly lower death rate than those who smoked the same and drank nine or more drinks. Both groups of smoking drinkers had higher-than-average death rates from cancers of the lung, esophagus, and pharynx. Most of the respiratory deaths in this study were caused by emphysema, which was much more frequent among people who consumed three or more drinks a day, compared to those who had two or less. Liver cirrhosis deaths showed the expected strong relationship to heavy alcohol use. (See Table 6-1 for relative risk from drinking and smoking habits.)

Alcohol may also work in conjunction with poor dietary habits to encourage or promote colorectal cancers. It seems likely to some researchers that the effects of the alcohol do not work independently, but rather as an additional "hit" on top of the negative effects caused by an affluent diet rich in fats and red meats and low in whole-food fiber. This is, of course, further complicated in heavy eaters and drinkers who also smoke.

Beer specifically seems to be associated with rectal cancer, with an increasing death rate depending on the amount of beer consumed. Both

---

TABLE 6-1   Relative risks by smoking and drinking habits

Smoking habit	Minimal drinking*	Less than 6 WEs†	6 to 9 WEs	10 or more WEs
Minimal smoking‡	1.0	9.3	16.9	23.2
Cigar/pipe	13.7	16.9	96.0	80.0
10 to 19 cigarettes a day	4.6	48.0	134.5	27.4
20 to 39 cigarettes a day	7.5	31.0	107.3	92.2
40 or more cigarettes a day	8.0	15.2	149.3	104.7

From Mashberg, A., Garfinkel, L., and Harris, S.: Alcohol as a primary risk factor in oral squamous carcinoma, CA 31(3): 151, 1981.
*Includes nondrinkers, occasional drinkers, and ex-drinkers of 2 or more years.
†WE, whiskey equivalent.
‡Includes nonsmokers, occasional smokers, ex-smokers of 2 or more years, and those who smoked less than 10 cigarettes a day.

beer and scotch are made from malt, which contains *N*-nitrosodimethylamine (NDMA), a known carcinogen. This may be the causative agent, or it might be another as yet unknown component. Recently, the contaminants and carcinogens in beer have been reduced, yet an association of some sort exists between alcohol consumption and cancers of the bowel and rectum; these cancers kill 57,000 people each year.

Alcohol has played a central role in festivals, ceremonies, and religious rites for thousands of years. It is both stimulating and relaxing and can be made by fermenting the sugars that occur naturally in grain, fruits, and vegetables. Today, alcohol is widely accepted as a means of relaxing, brightening one's outlook, or entertaining other people. Drinking is an accepted part of everyday life in the United States and in the rest of the world. Many people who drink alcohol censure others who use drugs such as marijuana and other addicting substances without ever considering how similar the abuse of alcohol is in many respects; alcohol *is* a drug. The same may be said for tobacco smokers.

Although the sale, manufacture, and consumption of alcohol was prohibited in this country from 1919 to 1933, its consumption is currently poorly regulated, although its manufacture and sale is subject to stringent laws. Alcohol consumption is associated with many diseases, including alcoholism itself. Additionally, alcohol has negative social effects, such as the accidents that occur when people drink and drive. Half of all highway deaths are said to involve alcohol. The same statistic applies to incidents of domestic violence, in which half involve excessive alcohol consumption. The costs of alcohol abuse in terms of physical and mental health, time or efficiency lost at the workplace, and family tragedy are difficult to calculate and probably astronomical, yet drinking is widely encouraged through advertising and our social practices. Americans drink three major forms of alcoholic beverages:

Beer is a fermented drink brewed with yeast, using a cereal grain such as corn, wheat, rye, or rice for the basic fermentation process. The alcoholic content is between 3% and 5%, and 12 ounces of regular (nonlight) beer contains 140 to 150 calories.

Wine is an alcoholic beverage usually made from fermented grape juices, although there are fruit wines as well. The alcoholic content of wine varies from around 10% to 18% in fortified wines, and there are approximately 190 calories in an 8-ounce glass.

Spirits involve the distillation of grain products into whiskey or of wine into brandy. These beverages vary in alcoholic content between 25% and 50%, or between 50 and 100 proof. A jigger, or 1½ ounces, of high-proof spirits (86 proof) contains 110 calories.

Beer is the most popular form of alcoholic drink in the United States today, accounting for half the total alcohol consumption. The average alcohol consumption in the United States is 2.8 gallons of alcoholic beverage per year. Men drink roughly three times more alcohol than women.

If you only have an occasional drink with dinner, someone out there is making up for you to reach the average consumption, and that person might well be suffering the many bad effects of drinking too much for too long. A dedicated alcoholic consumes approximately 900 to 1000 calories a day from alcohol. Because of this, he eats less and may suffer the effects of malnutrition, one of the effects of alcoholism. Most alcoholics have a deficiency of the B vitamins because of their poor diet.

About 95% of all the alcohol one drinks has to be detoxified and processed by the liver before it is converted into energy; this puts an extra burden on the liver. This is why chronic drinking leads to degeneration and/or cirrhosis of the liver, which develops in 15% of heavy drinkers. Primary liver cancer occurs more commonly in cases of chronic alcohol abuse. The production of liver cancer is increased in persons who have had hepatitis or toxic exposure to aflatoxins (see Chapters 4 and 10). Thus alcohol is a risk factor for liver cancer in addition to its damaging effects on the liver.

SUMMARY AND RECOMMENDATIONS

Alcohol, like so many substances, is another part of what we take for granted as the "good life." As with smoking and a high-fat diet, it has become implicated in cancer. So far the evidence applies to excessive drinking, more than two drinks per day, consumed regularly over a long period. People who consume three to five drinks daily have a 50% increased mortality rate; those whose drinking exceeds five drinks daily double their mortality rate. Moderation rather than abstinence seems to be a possible choice for good health. The obvious recommendation would be to limit drinks to two or fewer per day and make these two standard-sized drinks. If you drink moderately and smoke, reduce your drinking and stop smoking or avoid drinking and smoking at the same time. Improve your diet, following the general guidelines listed in Chapter 5. Following this moderate, health-oriented approach, you should be able to lift your glass to toast "L'Chaim" (to life) and still be around a long time to enjoy it.

Resource List
Alcoholics Anonymous
General Services Office
P.O. Box 459
Grand Central Station
New York, New York 10063

National Council on Alcoholism
733 Third Avenue
New York, New York 10017

Recommendations regarding alcohol consumption

1. Restrict intake of alcohol to two or fewer average-sized drinks a day. Make an effort to choose nonalcoholic drinks more often and alcoholic drinks less often. If you must drink, maintain good nutritional habits (see Chapter 4).
2. Do not drink alcohol during pregnancy.
3. Abstain from smoking when drinking.
4. Maintain excellent oral hygiene, which is particularly important if you drink and smoke.
5. Work to increase public awareness and reduce apathy and easy acceptance of alcohol.
6. Begin health education on alcohol for children early in school and at home.
7. Be careful not to believe or accept the slick, well-targeted advertising on television and in the news media, which does not tell about the toxicity and dangers of drinking alcoholic beverages but makes drinking a normal, healthy part of everyday adult life. George Hacker of the Center for Science in the Public Interest stated: "The casual Miller Time attitude towards drinking has helped create health and social devastation that claims up to 200,000 American lives each year."
8. Social recommendations would be:
   a. Put strict controls on alcohol advertising, broadcast, and print media.
   b. Require that alcoholic beverages carry labels listing ingredients and warnings.
9. Changes are needed now on the public's perception of the role of alcohol, and a more active and responsible role should be played by both government and industry in preventative measures.

CHAPTER 7

Tobacco and Cancer

ERNEST H. ROSENBAUM

DANGER: SMOKING ZONE

Whenever you light up a cigarette, you are inviting cancer into your life. It is that simple and straightforward. Conversely, the single most effective action you can take to reduce your chances of getting cancer is to never start smoking or to stop smoking. Someone who smokes a pack a day puffs on a lighted cigarette more than 50,000 times a year, delivering a virtual chemical factory of burnt ingredients to the membranes of the nose, mouth, throat, and lungs. One of the primary ingredients, tobacco, is a carcinogen, a substance that produces or incites cancer. This is a fact—whether you wish to believe or accept it is up to you. There is no longer any doubt that you greatly increase the risk of cancer and death when you smoke. The bad news does not stop here; cigarette smoking is also connected to coronary heart disease, pulmonary emphysema, and other serious circulatory illness. A person who smokes one pack of cigarettes per day will live approximately 5 years less than a nonsmoker and 8 to 9 years less if that person smokes two packs per day. Smokers have a 70% greater chance of dying from disease than nonsmokers. For example, the rate of fatal heart attacks between ages 40 and 49, when comparing smokers of more than two packs a day and nonsmokers, is 5.5 times greater for men and 3.6 times greater for women.

Cigarette smoking is the major single cause of death from cancer in the United States, according to a Department of Health and Human Services report. Among all types of deaths from cancer, 30%—one in three—are directly related to smoking. An estimated 180,000 people died in 1983 from some form of cancer associated with cigarette smoking. Approximately 180,000 more died from noncancerous illness attributable to the pursuit of the smoking habit. In addition, the cost of smoking-related illness exceeds $27 billion a year for medical care, absenteeism, accidents, and decreased work productivity in the United States.

159

Habit is one word for smoking; *addiction* is a more accurate description. Smoking can easily become an addiction that is both physical and psychological, complete with its own assortment of withdrawal symptoms, as anyone who has tried to stop smoking can tell you. The U.S. Public Health Service* in March 1983 called smoking "the most deadly form of drug dependence." They further stated that cigarettes cause "more illness and death than all other drugs" and that "smoking was not just a habit, but in fact the most widespread example of drug dependence in our country." Cigarette smokers spend more time "administering" to their habit than any other drug addict. The problem is simple; smoking is as lethal as cyanide, one of the ingredients in cigarette smoke. The solution, however, is difficult: kicking a habit that is socially approved and reinforced and is advertised as glamorous causes personal pain to give up. Yet, the alternative—to keep right on smoking—means you may die unnecessarily from cancer, heart, lung, or vascular disease.

When we look at the specifics of the 1982 Surgeon General's report on the health conse-

*Public Health Service's new report: Office on Smoking and Health, Rockville, Md. 20857.

quences of smoking, an estimated 85% of all lung cancer cases are the result of smoking cigarettes. In 1983 the ACS estimated that 135,000 new cases of lung cancer will be diagnosed, and approximately 117,000 people will die. Smokers are 20 times more likely to get lung cancer than are nonsmokers. This risk increases proportionally with the amount smoked, the amount of time a person smokes, and the frequency and duration of inhalation. There is, in other words, a dose/response relationship among heavy smokers, building to a death rate from lung cancer among heavy smokers that is 25 times greater than that of nonsmokers. The 5-year survival rate of people with lung cancer is less than 10%; this means that of every 10 people with lung cancer, only *one* will survive more than 5 years. This rate has not changed or improved over the last 15 years.

Of cancers affecting the larynx (or voice box) and mouth, 50% to 70% were associated with tobacco smoking; 13,000 people die of these cancers each year. Every year also brings 40,000 new cases with a 5-year survival rate of roughly 50%—half of these cancers were uncured after 5 years and half were cured.

In relation to esophageal cancer, cigarette smoking is estimated to be a factor in more than

TABLE 7-1   Estimated new cancer cases and deaths for sites associated with cigarette smoking (1983)

Site	Estimated new cases			Estimated deaths		
	Total	Male	Female	Total	Male	Female
Oral	27,100	18,600	8500	9150	6300	2850
Esophagus	9000	6400	2600	8500	6200	2300
Pancreas	25,000	12,900	12,100	22,600	11,800	10,800
Larynx	11,000	9200	1800	3700	3100	600
Lung	135,000	94,000	41,000	117,000	83,000	34,000
Bladder	38,500	28,000	10,500	10,700	7300	3400
Kidney and other urinary	18,200	11,400	6800	8500	5200	3300
Totals	263,800	180,500	83,300	180,150	122,900	57,250

half of the 8500 yearly deaths. The survival rate is very low for this cancer—only 4% live 5 years after diagnosis, and most die within 6 months. Of the 56,500 Americans who develop kidney and bladder cancer annually, 30% to 40% are estimated to be smoking related; 20,000 individuals die of these cancers each year.

Approximately 25,000 people developed cancer of the pancreas in 1983, with an estimated 22,600 deaths. As with lung and esophageal cancer, pancreatic cancer is usually fatal. Although few estimates are available, it seems accurate to say that smoking is a contributing factor in 30% of these cancer cases. Pancreatic cancer rates are increasing more rapidly than those of most other cancers.

There also seems to be a link between smoking and stomach and cervical cancers, but the data are as yet too limited to make a specific statement about percentages. More studies need to be done.

Fig. 7-1 shows the risk of male smokers for developing smoke-related cancers.

The evidence is overwhelming that smoking increases the risk of cancer, as well as of other serious and life-threatening diseases. But there are other, more immediate effects that change the quality of a smoker's daily life. For example, French researchers Centron and Vallery-Masson found that men between the ages of 20 to 40 who smoked one or more packs of cigarettes a day showed "a marked decline in sexual activity."

Happily this is reversible. The late Alton Ochsner, renowned as a leader in the antismoking movement, said, "I have seen literally thousands of patients who invariably tell me that they feel more energetic, healthy, and alive after they quit. But many will also say . . . that they are better off in the bedroom. And that you really don't know the difference until you quit smoking."

This reversal process extends to the more serious effects of smoking. As soon as a person quits, the cancer risk begins a slow but progressive return toward normal, until after 15 years, the nonsmoker and the exsmoker are in the same statistical range with respect to risk of cancer. Fig. 7-2 shows cancer risks of male exsmokers. People who smoke more than a pack of cigarettes a day—the heavy smokers—give themselves three to four times the risk of dying from some form of cancer than nonsmokers. It is a sad enough gift to themselves, but they also share the detrimental effects of their smoking habits with others, often the people they care for most.

Secondhand smoke

Secondhand smoke has recently received wide media coverage, and the public has become curious about whether or not a nonsmoker can get lung cancer from someone else's smoking habit. A cigarette usually burns for about 12 minutes, but the average smoker only takes one or two puffs a minute, especially if that person is working or talking while smoking. Most of the smoke from these 12 minutes of burning tobacco is discharged into the air. Called *sidestream smoke*, it contains the same chemicals as mainstream smoke, which the smoker exhales: tar, benzo(a)pyrene, formaldehyde, hydrogen cyanide, oxide of nitrogen, and carbon monoxide, to name a few.

Abnormal blood levels of carbon monoxide (COHb) have been documented in nonsmokers exposed to secondhand smoke in poorly ventilated rooms. Increased levels of carbon monoxide may pose a specific risk for heart patients.

Nonsmokers in a closed room with one or two burning cigarettes are smoking; they are "passive smokers" inhaling the same pollutants as smokers even though they do not actively smoke themselves. After a short time they can experience nausea, headaches, watery eyes, irritation in their small airways, and difficulty in breathing. People with allergies may start wheezing and coughing. Infants and young children are particularly vulnerable to secondhand smoke, partly because they ventilate differently

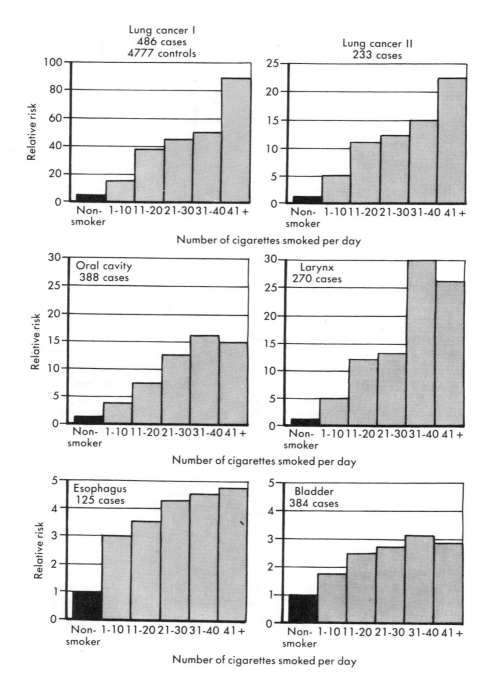

FIG. 7-1 Relative risk of present (10 years) male smokers for tobacco related cancers. In all graphs nonsmokers are assigned relative of one. Lung cancer I—giant cell/large cell, small cell/oat cell, squamous cell/epidermoid, spindle cell, clear cell, large cell undifferentiated; lung cancer II—adenocarcinoma, terminal bronchiolar carcinoma, alveolar cell, bronchial adenoma, acinar, papillary, bronchiolar-alveolar cell. (Modified from Wynder, E.: Your Patient and Cancer, August 1981.)

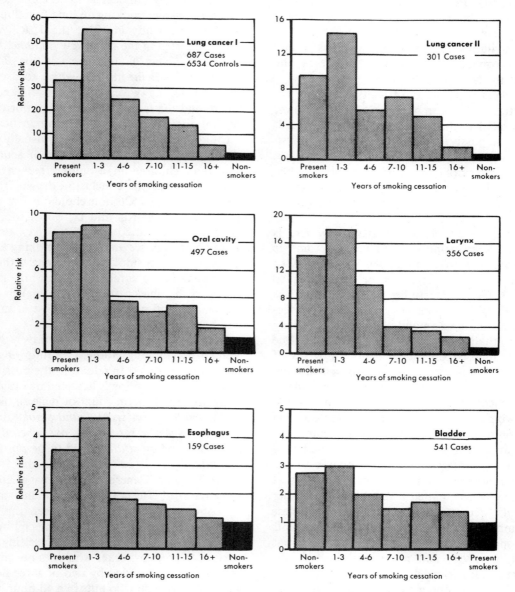

FIG. 7-2 Relative risk of cancer for male exsmokers. In all graphs nonsmokers are assigned relative of one. Lung cancer I — giant cell/large cell, small cell/oat cell, squamous cell/epidermoid, spindle cell, clear cell, large cell undifferentiated; lung cancer II — adenocarcinoma, terminal bronchiolar carcinoma, alveolar cell, bronchial adenoma, acinar, papillary, bronchiolar-alveolar cell. (Modified from Wynder, E.: Your Patient and Cancer, August 1981.)

than adults. People with heart or respiratory diseases or those who wear contact lenses may suffer acute irritations. Cigar smoke is even more irritating than that of cigarettes; cigars can be equated to unfiltered cigarettes at the top of the tar and nicotine range.

Smokers often have difficulty accepting the objections of nonsmokers to their cigarettes, believing that the irritations are exaggerated. Yet, what passive smokers feel are actual physical sensations of discomfort. It is ironic that a person who smokes in an office or other public place could be a considerate individual and yet still cause friends and coworkers to suffer needlessly.

The question of cancer risk, however, is beyond experiencing mild, flulike symptoms. Is secondhand smoke more than irritating? Can it, in fact, be dangerous or hazardous to health? Two 1981 studies presented evidence confirming that nonsmokers exposed to secondhand smoke do stand a greater risk of lung cancer than nonsmokers not exposed. The studies focused on the nonsmoking wives of smokers and nonsmokers and showed that the wives of heavy smokers ran a greater risk of lung cancer than did the wives of nonsmokers. The woman's risk of lung cancer increased in relation to how heavily her husband smoked.

In another study 51 women who had lung cancer were interviewed and compared to 163 other noncancerous hospital patients. Forty of the lung cancer patients and 149 of the other patients were nonsmokers, but among these nonsmokers, more of the lung cancer patients had spouses who smoked. The sample was small, however, and more investigation was recommended to reach a valid conclusion.

A discussion about the risks of cancer from secondhand smoke has been ongoing in the British medical journal *Lancet*. P. N. Lee stated in 1982 that no valid evidence existed that healthy adult nonsmokers are harmed by other's smoke, but C. Rossiter wrote a letter dissenting. Rossiter pointed out that four separate studies have indicated significant adverse effects of passive smoking on lung function: the G. H. Miller study in 1978; the J. R. White study, reported in the 1980 *New England Journal of Medicine*; T. Hirayama in the *British Journal of Medicine* in 1981, which focused on the nonsmoking wives of heavy smokers in Japan; and the L. Garfinkle study reported by the *National Journal of the Cancer Institute*.

Children subjected to smokers, usually their parents, had a greater prevalence of acute illness than children in a smoke-free environment. This was the conclusion drawn from a sample study of 2626 households in five cities done by P. Camaron and D. Robertson. The same study indicated that there may also be more acute illnesses among nonsmoking adults in a home with a smoker than in one without a smoker. Other research shows that children in homes with tobacco smoke have higher heart rates and blood pressures than those in smoke-free homes.

Even an unborn child can be adversely affected by a smoking mother (see following section on pregnancy). In addition, the possibility of a healthy conception is hindered by the genetically abnormal sperm count of male smokers.

The evidence on secondhand smoke at this point is suggestive rather than overwhelming or conclusive. More studies need to be done and undoubtedly will be. At present the United States Surgeon General reports that there are some harmful effects from secondhand smoke.

People studied so far have been the nonsmoking spouses of smokers or the children of parents who smoke in a domestic setting. But what of the office worker who does not smoke, yet may be surrounded by two or three people who do? A person who puts in a 40-hour week, 50 weeks a year in a moderate-sized office space where just one other person smokes is breathing air polluted up to three times above national standards.

Americans spend roughly 90% of their time indoors, and many people work in offices located within buildings that have nonopening windows. Smoke may pollute these contained buildings ventilated by recirculated air as the air becomes filled with higher than normal levels of carbon monoxide. Controlling pollution from tobacco smoke is ineffective primarily because the high costs of doing this defeat efforts to conserve energy inside buildings.

A 1980 study by the National Ambient Air Quality Standards of the public's exposure to tobacco particles—not gases—in indoor air found levels high enough to be in violation of national standards. Unfortunately, it only takes a little cigarette smoke to raise the pollution level of an enclosed space quickly.

In a study of 10,000 nonsmoking office workers, over half said that it was difficult working next to smokers. Another 36% reported that they had to move away from their desks or stations because of irritation from other people's smoke. In 1982 a nonsmoker named Irene Parodi won the first court case relating to secondhand smoke. The U.S. Court of Appeals in San Francisco said she should either have a smoke-free environment in which to work or disability pay because she suffered from the smoke of others. The attorney who won the case said, "The court is essentially recognizing that secondhand smoke can be harmful to one's health." This may be a landmark decision.

Two researchers, J. Ropod and A. Lourey of the Environmental Protection Agency, reported that the emissions from coke ovens are chemically similar to tobacco smoke and produce higher rates of "many forms of cancer in coke-oven workers." They also stated that some non-smokers have tarry fluid in their lungs "strikingly similar to that found in smokers." Based on this and other evidence reviewed, they concluded that indoor pollution and the health problems it causes deserve more attention and research. They are not alone in their conclusions. The World Health Organization recommends intensified efforts to prohibit smoking in public areas and continued study of the effects of secondhand smoke.

The issue of secondhand smoke will remain controversial until more comprehensive and conclusive studies are completed.

Smokers as employees

Several large American corporations have become increasingly concerned about the cost of employees who smoke. When the Dow Chemical Company discovered that smoking workers were absent 5.1 days per year more than nonsmokers—costing the company an estimated $500,000 every year—they introduced financial rewards for employees who quit smoking. Merle Norman Cosmetics Corporation, which requires its 850 employees not to smoke, returns the annual savings of $33,000 a year from loss of working time to its employees in cash bonuses.

IBM currently requires that nonsmokers and smokers have separate offices or separate sections in larger work areas. In a 1981 survey of 223 Seattle-area managers, 119 said they would choose nonsmokers over smokers if both were qualified. Asked to imagine a situation in which they had the power to ban smoking on company premises, a substantial 68% said they would rule in favor of no smoking on the job site. After all, with nonsmoking employees, there is a decrease in absenteeism, as well as a decrease in maintenance costs because cigarette smoke dirties walls, carpets, and drapes.

The added risk of synergism

These managers oversee people who work in offices, which are relatively clean environments, but many smokers work around chemical substances that are themselves toxic. Some of these chemicals interact synergistically with the toxins found in tobacco smoke. This means that the effect of the two chemicals or chemical systems added together is greater than either of them working alone—something like one and one equaling four. The risk of developing cancer from a synergistic combination is often far greater than exposure to cigarette smoke alone.

The 1979 Surgeon General's report indicated several ways in which cigarette smoke can interact with the workplace environment to increase health risks. Workers are doubly exposed to toxic elements; the elements in cigarette smoke can increase the toxicity of workplace chemicals; and the workplace environment can increase the absorption of the toxic elements in cigarette smoke.

The best-publicized example of this negative synergistic action is asbestos and cigarette smoking. Asbestos workers who smoke have five times the lung cancer risk of smokers who are not exposed to asbestos at work. Asbestos workers who smoke cigarettes have over 50 times the risk of lung cancer of individuals who neither smoke nor work with asbestos.

Occupational risks and smoking are also linked to bladder cancer. Overall, smokers appear to develop bladder cancer at about twice the rate of nonsmokers. If on-the-job exposure to beta-naphthylamine and other specific aromatic amines is added to this, the risk of bladder cancer multiplies. People in occupations that expose them to these substances include rubber workers, painters, textile dryers, and workers in the manufacture and use of dyes. Synergism also occurs in uranium miners who smoke and when smoking and exposure to sulfur dioxide and arsenic are combined. Much of this information is just beginning to be studied.

The relationship between occupational exposure and smoking has particular significance for black men. The adjusted cancer death rates for nonwhites in the United States rose 63.2% in the years from 1950 to 1977, whereas the increase for whites was only 20.2%. The rate fell slightly for women of all races. Cooper and Miller, who analyzed the data, believed that the increase was caused mainly by lung cancer deaths. Rather than crediting the rise in lung cancer among blacks to any differences in their smoking habits, Cooper and Miller thought that larger percentages of blacks than whites are in

occupations exposing them to chemicals, dusts, fumes, and other toxic airborne particles.

To reduce the incidence of lung cancer and reverse this growing trend, blacks — and all industrial workers — must have improved conditions on the job site and *must* reduce their smoking. Continued efforts to clean up the workplace are needed. Some clinicians have also proposed establishing industry-based smoking clinics to help smokers exposed to cancer-causing substances at work quit smoking. Such clinics would probably increase the economic efficiency of many industries as well as promoting the health of individuals on the job.

The combination of smoking and other chemicals leading to increased risk of cancer is not limited to industrial sites. The most common tobacco synergism takes place in your local tavern or almost anyone's living room whenever a smoker takes an alcoholic drink. Alcohol acts as a cocarcinogen, a substance that may assist in causing cancer, and is potent with certain carcinogens. Mixed with tobacco smoke, which is itself a carcinogen, alcohol — especially high-proof alcohol — acts synergistically to sharply increase the risk of cancer in the oral cavity: mouth, cheeks, palate, and larynx (voice box). The same synergism increases the risks of cancer of the esophagus, which has its own high mortality rate. The combination of excessive drinking and smoking leads to a greater risk of developing these cancers than either cigarette smoking or alcohol consumption alone. Roughly 75% of all oral cancers in males are estimated to result from the alcohol/tobacco synergism. As women's smoking and drinking habits become more like men's, their risk increases likewise.

Chewing tobacco and smoking are synergistic, too; their use together increases the risk of oral cancer 10 times. Of all oral cavity cancers, 70% can be traced to chewing or smoking tobacco or doing both.

Drinking and smoking are so linked in our social behavior that it is difficult for some people to imagine doing one without the other. Ex-smokers will sometimes resume smoking when drinking in a social setting because the behavior pattern is so strong. Yet tobacco and alcohol together represent one of the strongest combinations most widely known to increase cancer risk.

At first people suspected that smoking might be hazardous; studies were then done, and now we know that it is dangerous to smoke. We discover new information all the time that details the hazards of smoking and why everyone should quit. Perhaps the least important is that the addiction costs from $250 to $600 per year to maintain, not counting any related medical expense or cleaning bills. But the fact remains that millions of people still smoke, although millions have also quit. This chapter discusses how the cigarette poisons, as well as the nature of the smoking addiction and the possible courses to take in quitting. But first we should look at the history of how this national addiction began and what the current status of tobacco use is in the United States, including the increasing roles played by women and the new "safer" cigarettes.*

HISTORY AND CURRENT USE

Before the 1940s, lung cancer was believed to be hereditary. In the first decade of this century it was a rarity; worldwide, there were 374 reported cases in 1912. About the same year, a new, milder tobacco was developed in Virginia. Previously, cigarettes could not be deeply inhaled without irritation or choking. Camel cigarettes was the first blend of these lighter Burley and Turkish tobaccos. They were introduced in 1913 and within months had a national market with the slogan, "Have a Camel, They Satisfy." Lucky Strike followed in 1916 with "It's Toasted," and Chesterfield was introduced for

*No cigarette is safe—at best there is a 15% to 20% improvement over conventional cigarettes.

"People with Discriminating Taste" in 1919.

In the 10 years between 1910 and 1920 annual cigarette consumption in America skyrocketed from 4 to 25 billion, and an ever-increasing death rate accompanied this jump in cigarette smoking. In the 2 years between 1919 and 1921 there was an 800% increase in lung cancer nationwide.

By 1919 young New York women were seen smoking at dinner parties. That same year the first advertisement appeared showing a woman smoking. In 1922 New York women were smoking openly on the streets. By 1923 a Milwaukee survey reported that more than 51% of males over age 18 smoked cigarettes.

During World War II over 25% of all cigarettes produced in the United States were distributed to overseas armed forces. By 1948 over 60% of adult males smoked cigarettes. A 1947 survey of Columbus, Ohio—a typical midwestern city—revealed that about 28% of white women and 36% of black women also smoked cigarettes. Women were beginning to catch up.

By 1950 there were 18,300 lung cancer deaths in the United States in 1 year. After an initial 20-year latency period—the approximate time it takes for cancers to develop—the results of the increase in smoking was starting to show up. By 1977 this figure had risen to 75,000 lung cancer deaths, and the American Cancer Society estimated that in 1983, 117,000 Americans would die of lung cancer alone (83,000 men; 34,000 women). This is a 650% increase in the deaths from this cancer over a 30-year span. These deaths occur despite new diagnostic treatments and social campaigns against a disease that would not appear in 90% of those afflicted if they did not smoke or if they quit smoking.

According to the 1981 report of the Federal Trade Commission on cigarette advertising practices, fewer than 3% of adult smokers ever read the health warning on every pack. Forty percent did not know smoking causes most cases of lung cancer; 50% did not know smoking causes most cases of emphysema; and 50%

did not know smoking causes many heart attacks. From this information, it seems that people simply do not think that the dire outcomes of smoking could happen to them personally, especially if they feel in good health.

Since the Surgeon General's report in 1964 about the harmful effects of smoking cigarettes, smoking rates in the United States have dropped 9%, from 42% in 1965 to 32% in 1980. However, because of population increases and the regular influx of new, young smokers, we have about the same number of smokers in 1982 as we had 20 years ago — 54 to 55 million. And the actual number of cigarettes smoked has increased — currently 600 billion per year. Another discouraging fact is that there has been a substantial increase in the use of chewing tobacco and snuff, particularly among young people. Both of these forms of tobacco carry serious health risks, as we will discuss shortly. Filter-tipped cigarettes, introduced in the early 1950s, went from 1% of the market to 90% by 1981; most smokers are at least smoking filtered cigarettes.

According to the August 1981 Gallup Poll, the number of smokers in the United States in 1981 was 35%, the lowest level recorded in 37 years of regular surveys. The decline since 1972 was greatest among Americans in the 18- to 29-year-old age-group. Sixty-six percent of those who still smoke said they would like to stop. No less than 84% of smokers had given up smoking for at least 1 day, and those who quit for 1 year totaled 13%. More people favored stronger measures against smoking than ever before, up to a complete ban on cigarette advertising, which was supported by 43% of those interviewed. Forty-six percent of the people interviewed thought federal and state taxes on cigarettes should be increased, compared to 38% in 1977.

These figures seem to indicate a trend: smoking is not taken for granted as it was during the 1950s and 1960s. Many people seem to be aware that smoking can hurt them, and many have tried to quit. Since 1965, when 53% of American males were reported to be smokers, the rate has declined to 37% today, and teenage smoking since 1979 also appears to be declining. But there is a disturbing trend among young women. In the past 25 years, age-adjusted death rates from lung cancer among women have increased by nearly 500%. The upturn of women who began smoking during the Second World War has culminated in 29% of women who now smoke. The percentage is increasing, whereas for men smoking has decreased and is now about 37%. More women under age 25 smoke than men.

Women have come a long way

From the mid-1950s to the mid-1970s, adolescent girls were less likely to smoke than boys, or else they started at a later age. Then a 1979 survey indicated that a higher percentage of girls in their teens smoked — 24% compared to the previous 20%. Many of those surveyed said that their physicians had never warned them about the hazards of smoking. These young women will not feel the effects of their smoking for many years, but smoking-related diseases among women are becoming epidemic.

One in every four people who die from lung cancer today is a woman. In 1950 only 9% of lung cancer deaths were in women. In 1983 30% of lung cancer deaths will be in women. Cancer Society epidemiologists estimate that in 1983 34,000 women will die of lung cancer, while some 37,200 will die of breast cancer. It is expected that by 1985 lung cancer will pass up breast cancer as the leading cause of death and the number one cancer killer among women (see Fig. 7-3).

Women were slower to take up smoking than men, and even when a woman did smoke, she smoked less. Now that more women smoke more cigarettes, the rates of lung cancer, coronary heart disease, and chronic lung diseases such as emphysema, bronchitis and asthma, as well as other cancers, have all increased. Women born between 1921 and 1940 are currently at high risk. Unless they quit smoking in large numbers, these women aged 43 to 62 will soon

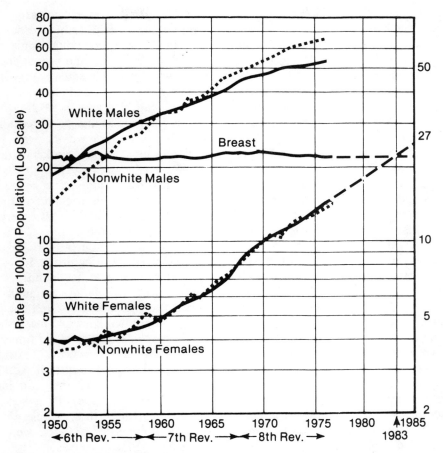

FIG. 7-3 Age-adjusted death rates for malignant neoplasm of trachea, bronchus, and lung, by color and sex compared to rates for malignant breast neoplasm, United States, 1950-1977; projection for white females to 1985. (From The health consequences of smoking for women, a report of the Surgeon General, U.S. Department of Health and Human Services/Public Health Service.)

pass up women who began smoking in the 1920s in (1) total number of years as a smoker, (2) total number of years smoking unfiltered cigarettes, and (3) total number of cigarettes smoked. Even if every woman in the United States stopped smoking today, lung cancer rates would still continue to climb for several years because of the long latent period (measured in years) associated with lung cancer.

The more cigarettes smoked, the longer women continue smoking, the deeper they in-

hale, and the higher the tar and nicotine level of the cigarettes—all of these increase the chances of women getting lung cancer, just as they do with men. According to the U.S. Department of Health and Human Services, "Lung cancer is now an equal opportunity tragedy." Unfortunately, women are not quitting at the same rate as men. While the rate for male smokers dropped 13%, the number of female smokers stayed roughly the same, dropping only 1% (from 33% to 32%) up to 1978. The number of women smoking continues to drop, but more slowly than the number of men who stop. One can speculate about this difference and what causes it.

The 1980 Surgeon General's report on smoking, which focused on the health consequences of smoking in women, stated that women as a group have a more difficult time quitting than men do. But there is more to the situation. Women may not be well informed about the dangers of smoking because in part women's magazines have been remiss in warning them. A study of the hazards of tobacco as dealt with in women's magazines done by E. Whelan, M. Sheridan, B. Mosher, and K. Meister reveals that magazines accepting cigarette advertising many tend to downplay any mention of the dangers of cigarettes. One magazine had had no articles on smoking in the entire 12-year period surveyed (1967 to 1979). Information about smoking had been *edited out* of articles submitted to some women's magazines that accepted tobacco advertising, despite the policy of women's magazines to offer regular columns and special features on the latest health findings and how they relate to women. Middle-class respondents to one survey indicated that they considered "magazines to be a source of health information second in reliability only to their doctor's advice."

In 1980 the American Council on Science and Health (ACSH) wrote several women's magazines asking them to participate in their antismoking campaign by publishing an appropriate article of some kind in their July issue. Of the magazines contacted — *Cosmopolitan, Family Circle, Glamour, Harper's Bazaar, Ladies' Home Journal, McCall's, Mademoiselle, Ms., Seventeen, Vogue, Women's Day,* and *Working Women* — only *one* responded positively. *Seventeen* ran an article called "Up in Smoke" by a young woman who had decided to quit and succeeded.

Women received little or no information about the dangers that accompany smoking.

They did get, however, increasing encouragement to smoke with seductive advertisements that emphasize a smoking woman's independence, attractiveness, and overall liberated flair. Small wonder that women continue the dread habit that contributed to one quarter of women's cancer deaths in 1979.

This figure is bound to increase in the next years because more women who smoke also work. As more female workers enter the paid labor force, more of them are exposed to pollutants, dust, fumes, and chemicals on the job. If these women also smoke, they increase their risks of cancer through synergism in the same way that men do.

Half a million women work in the plastics and rubber manufacturing industries, and 219,000 women who are laundry workers are exposed to a variety of contaminants in the clothes they wash. Thirty-five thousand female meat wrappers work around plastic heating and sealing machines that give off fumes of hydrochloric acid and phosgene. Textile workers, cosmetologists, and industrial workers are all exposed to substances that can increase the risks of cancer, especially when they also smoke. Women artists, jewelers, and crafts workers are exposed to carcinogenic or cocarcinogenic chemicals as well.

A further danger occurs for women who use oral contraceptives: they face special health risks that involve cardiovascular disease. All these factors — smoking, increasing occupational exposure to physical or chemical agents, and use of oral contraceptives — can combine and possibly greatly multiply the health risks for women. These risks in turn affect the unborn, the newborn, and the growing children of smoking mothers.

Pregnancy, children, and smoking

Pregnant women who smoke carry babies that differ from the babies of women who do not smoke. Because the mother smokes, the fetus grows in a different environment. Many of the chemicals in cigarettes, such as nicotine and cyanide, reach the developing baby directly through the placenta. Studies have shown that smoking by the expecting mother leads to increased spontaneous abortion and premature births, vaginal bleeding, a higher incidence of birth defects, and a lower birth weight, no matter how much the mother eats.

Dr. Arthur Holleb of the *CA—A Cancer Journal for Clinicians* states that "the hazards of smoking while pregnant cannot be emphasized enough." Spontaneous abortion is 30% to 70% higher in pregnant smokers than in nonsmokers, and this risk increases with the number of cigarettes smoked. The higher death rate for fetuses of smoking women is caused by complications of pregnancy rather than fetal abnormality. The Surgeon General has found that smoking a low-tar and low-nicotine cigarette *does not* significantly reduce the hazards to the fetus.

These hazards extend into the life of a new baby. Mothers who smoke lose more newborn infants as a result of "respiratory difficulty" and "immaturity" than do nonsmoking mothers, according to the 1980 Surgeon General's report. An infant also has a much higher chance of developing sudden infant death syndrome (SIDS) if the mother smokes during the pregnancy. Although no one seems to know exactly what causes these "crib deaths," as they are called, women who smoke during pregnancy and after increase the risk of SIDS; the more she smokes, the greater the risk. The 4- to 6-day-old babies of smokers also tend more toward irritability and show less interest than the newborns of nonsmokers.

The children of smokers have been followed in studies done over several years. One such study of several thousand children was done from 1 month to 5 years after they were born. The children of mothers who smoked had death rates almost triple those of nonsmoking mothers, about 11:1000 compared to 4:1000. In Sweden a study showed that the children of smokers were hospitalized more often, stayed in the hospital longer, and had more visits to their physicians. These children were hospitalized more often for acute respiratory illnesses, bronchitis, and pneumonia. The same study found that light smokers who quit during the last 3 months of pregnancy had children with the same lower death rate as the children of the nonsmokers.

The children of nonsmoking mothers scored higher in psychologic tests and behavior ratings and in school placement, according to one British study involving several thousand children. In contrast, the children of women who smoked during pregnancy were slightly shorter in height than the children of nonsmokers and were 3 to 5 months retarded in reading, mathematics, and overall ability. The old saying, "Don't smoke—it will stunt your growth," may turn out to be true. These problems were found to be dose related, that is, directly related to the number of cigarettes the mothers smoked. There is also a strong relationship between heavy maternal smoking—more than a pack a day—and hyperkinetic, or hyperactive, children.

The children of parents who smoke are more likely to suffer from respiratory diseases and allergies than the children of nonsmokers. These illnesses also seem to be dose related; when only one parent smokes, the chances of getting these illnesses are less than when both parents smoke. When one parent smoked, the children had more respiratory disease than children in a smoke-free house.

The facts seem inescapable. Smoking tobacco not only hurts the individual, it hurts those who are closest to the smoker—the as-yet unborn, the newborn, and the growing child.

OTHER FORMS OF TOBACCO

People sometimes turn away from smoking cigarettes and use other forms of tobacco as a means of reducing the health risks to themselves and others. Does this strategy for tobacco use work?

Cigars and pipes

Many people assume that there is less risk of lung cancer associated with pipe or cigar smoking because the smokers do not usually inhale as much smoke as cigarette smokers do. As far as inhalation goes, this is correct. Cancers are nonetheless associated with these alternatives to cigarettes: there is increased danger of cancer of the mouth, esophagus, and parts of the larynx, and pipe smokers have more cancer of the lip.

According to the Department of Health, Education and Welfare in 1979, cigar smoke has concentrations of tumor-causing agents equal to or in excess of those found in cigarette tar. Further, cigar and pipe smokers may run a higher risk of lung cancer—even though they inhale less—because the smoke from cigars and pipes is much more alkaline than cigarette smoke. This alkaline smoke allows nicotine to be absorbed directly into the bloodstream more easily from the mouth; thus *nicotine can be absorbed* while the pipe or cigar smoke is just held in the mouth, *without any inhalation into the lungs.*

People who have only smoked pipes rarely inhale the smoke, but people who smoke both cigarettes and a pipe or who have switched from cigarettes to pipe smoking often inhale the pipe smoke deeply and are at proportionally greater risk. The only significant difference between cigarette, pipe, and cigar smoke is the proportion and amount of smoke material inhaled and the length of time a person smokes. Smoking tobacco in any form has its attendant dangers.

Chewing tobacco and snuff

Chewing tobacco and snuff-dipping are two nonsmoking uses of tobacco. People who chew tobacco place a golf-ball-sized "chaw" or wad of tobacco in the pouch of their cheek and suck on it. Snuff, which is a powdered, flavored tobacco, is "dipped" by placing a pinch of it between the lower lip and the teeth or between the gum and cheek and then sucking on the "quid" or liquid that results.

Although people may turn to these tobacco alternatives because they seem to present no risk to health, this is *not* the case. A 1981 study by the University of North Carolina and National Cancer Institute showed that white women in the South who habitually dipped snuff had a higher death rate from cancers of the mouth and throat. In countries where people commonly use chewing tobacco and snuff, such as India, China, and Ceylon, death rates from mouth and throat cancers are among the highest in the world.

People who chew or dip tobacco have more cancers of the mouth and throat simply because they put the tumor-causing agents in direct contact with those areas of their bodies. The most important of these agents seem to be the tobacco-specific nitrosamines that are formed during tobacco curing and fermentation. They have been found in both chewing tobacco and snuff.

Smokeless forms of tobacco still contain nicotine and are therefore habit forming, addicting, and disease inducing, especially with regard to cardiovascular disease and oral cancer. In addition, the American Cancer Society points out that chewing or dipping tobacco is much more destructive to the mouth than smoking cigarettes and leads to such dental problems as receding gums, tooth decay, bone destruction, and the growth of leukoplakia—a white premalignant skin or membrane change. More than 1 in 20 or 5% of cases of leukoplakia change into cancer.

People who use snuff nasally can develop lesions in the nose and other problems. Use of any smokeless tobacco—and tobacco in any form—damages the senses of taste and smell, and a side effect is that users increase their intake of salt and sugar to give things more taste. Increasing sugar and salt use over an extended period can in turn produce or encourage additional health problems—becoming overweight or developing hypertension or high blood pressure.

In spite of the negative effects of smokeless

tobacco, sales have increased 12% per year each year since 1974. In 1983 data published by the USDA indicate that 11 million Americans use smokeless tobacco annually. Use is increasing most rapidly among male high school and college students, particularly athletes. Televised advertisements for smokeless tobacco products featuring professional athletes were aired during the 1980 Olympics at Lake Placid, New York. Not surprisingly, one of the sponsors of the Olympic games was a manufacturer of the product. Sports celebrities and country rock stars are well paid to do advertisements for smokeless tobacco products, with the young as the target audience.

Chewing tobacco is portrayed as being a "with it" thing to do because you do not get hooked on smoking. The spitting that goes along with chewing is pictured as fun, not a disgusting and unhealthy habit, and, of course, the bad breath and discolored teeth are not mentioned at all.

Tobacco companies give out free samples of smokeless tobacco products at colleges to get young people started, the same technique used to start people smoking cigarettes. In spite of the health dangers inherent in these smokeless products, *no* warnings are required on packages or advertisements for them.

Publishers and broadcasters as yet have taken no position to protect young people from the promotion campaigns of the tobacco companies. These campaigns are seductive and effective; when a male sports celebrity gives a testimonial for a smokeless tobacco product, no one points out that he is pushing a damaging and addictive drug, which is exactly what he is doing. Difficult as it may be to take an ethical stand that goes against commercial gain, it needs to be done, and the publishers of magazines, the owners of media outlets, and responsible journalists can do it.

Tobacco is tobacco. Whether smoked, sniffed, or chewed, the negative effects of it remain because of the nicotine in tobacco and the tar that results from smoking. In addition, multiple tobacco use (e.g., dipping, chewing, and smoking) is a likely contributor to an increased cancer risk. The question becomes: if the nicotine and tars are reduced, can tobacco be safe? Thus far the answer is NO.

LOW-TAR CIGARETTES

With an addiction that is pleasurable but dangerous, people would rather find a way to make it safe than give it up. This has been the approach of the industry, which survives on tobacco sales; the government, which gets millions from cigarette taxes; and the consumer, who would rather do anything than kick the habit.

Reports started cropping up in the popular press during the 1950s linking smoking to lung cancer. At that time, only 1.5% of all cigarettes sold were filter-tipped, but as the news of the health dangers from smoking spread, people quickly switched to filtered cigarettes. Over 20 years later, in 1980 over 90% of all cigarettes sold were filter-tipped. (See Fig. 7-4 for cancer risks of filtered and unfiltered cigarettes.)

The typical cigarette Americans smoked in the 1940s, such as the one always shown hanging casually from Bogart's lips, contained 40 mg of tar. Roughly one third of the brands today have 10 mg of tar or less, and some have correspondingly lower levels of nicotine as well. There has also been a reduction in some other health threatening elements — benzo(a)pyrene and polynuclear aromatic hydrocarbons. One might think from these facts that the tumor-initiating activity of cigarette tars would be decreased, making low-tar cigarettes safer to smoke.

The tobacco industry certainly encourages this view: it spent $420 million in 1978, or half its annual advertising budget, to promote low-tar brands. Even in the beginning, cigarette advertising was "health conscious." As early as 1954, one cigarette advertising slogan claimed

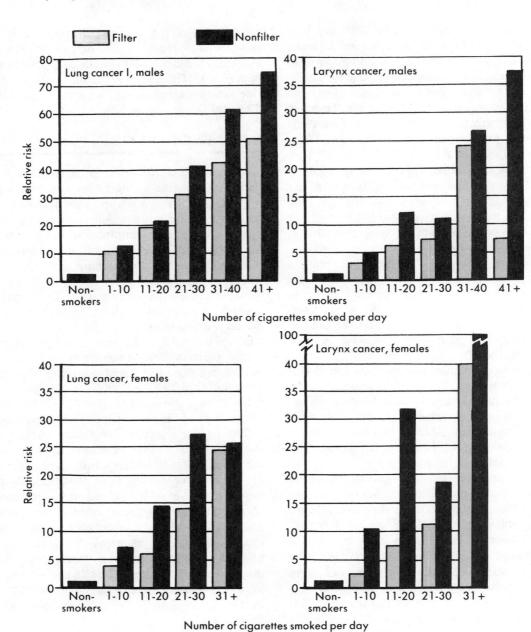

FIG. 7-4 How filtered cigarettes affect risk of cancer. Duration of smoking: 10 years or longer. Lung cancer I—giant cell/large cell, small cell/oat cell, squamous cell/epidermoid, spindle cell, clear cell, large cell undifferentiated. (Modified from Wynder, E.: Your Patient and Cancer, August 1981.)

its filters gave "the greatest health protection in cigarette history." Another brand advertised the "miracle of the Modern Miracle Tip," even though the tar of the cigarette was up to 40% and nicotine was up 70% from the levels that existed before the filter was introduced on the market. Today, brands like Cambridge, Carlton, and Now *all* claim their product has the lowest tar content of any sold.

What is the truth of the matter? Is a low-tar low-nicotine cigarette safe? Does the tar/nicotine dosage on the package mean anything? What have scientific studies shown?

At present the data available are limited because people have been smoking the low-tar low-nicotine cigarettes for too short a time to assess the health risks completely and accurately. More in-depth and long-term studies need to be done. The American Cancer Society has found some decrease in mortality rates in some cancer sites with low-tar low-nicotine cigarettes (defined as less than 17.6 mg tar and 1.2 mg nicotine). On the other hand, a report from a Study Committee of the National Academy of Sciences stated, "Evidence of health benefits from switching to a reduced tar and nicotine cigarette is doubtful." They also said that the amount of tar and nicotine printed on the packs *does not* represent the smoker's actual exposure. According to Kozlowski, in an 18-hour waking day, a two-pack-a-day smoker spends 3 to 4 hours with a cigarette in mouth, hand, or ash tray, takes about 400 puffs, and inhales up to 1000 mg of tar.

The 1981 Surgeon General's report entitled *The Changing Cigarette* concluded unequivocally, *"There is no safe cigarette and no safe level of consumption."* There was a partial concession that low-tar low-nicotine cigarettes can reduce risks "to some extent . . . provided there is no compensatory increase in the amount smoked. However, the benefits are minimal in comparison with giving up cigarettes entirely."

What does the average smoker make of all

this information or lack thereof? In a survey reviewed in the 1981 Surgeon General's report, the public was queried about the health hazards of cigarettes lower in tar and nicotine. One-third believed that there was *no* increase in health hazards from smoking low-tar low-nicotine cigarettes over nonsmoking. Another third did not know if smoking cigarettes lower in tar and nicotine was as safe as not smoking. The conclusion was that the general public is not worried about any health hazards from smoking low-tar low-nicotine cigarettes, and the report concludes, "Many smokers may *falsely* believe that smoking is not dangerous to them if they smoke low tar and nicotine cigarettes."

This lack of concern may be connected to the increase in the average number of cigarettes smoked. In 1954 the average number smoked was 22 per day or 8030 per year. In 1978 the average was up to 30 a day or 10,950 per year. This increase may be related to the decrease in tar and nicotine in cigarettes.

One of the reasons smoking a low-tar low-nicotine cigarette can be as dangerous as smoking any other cigarette is that smokers engage in what is called *compensatory smoking*. Smokers who switch to a cigarette lower in tar and nicotine often unconsciously adjust their smoking patterns so that they get the same amount of nicotine they are used to; they either puff more often and inhale more deeply or smoke more cigarettes each day.

A study done by the American Cancer Society concluded that the tar and nicotine rating was not as important as the number of cigarettes smoked. An experiment done at Johns Hopkins University had volunteer smokers puff on cigarettes using special holders. The cigarettes were in four different strengths of tar and nicotine. The special holders blocked out varying amounts of cigarette smoke: all the smoke, 75%, 50%, or no smoke blockage. The results were that smokers always puffed more when more smoke was blocked out.

This experiment shows that smokers adjust

their patterns of smoking to regulate their intake. When people smoke they get a rush of nicotine to the brain about 7 seconds after they inhale. The smoker's body learns how to concentrate the cigarette's nicotine in the brain for this "7-second hit," which produces a feeling of pleasure. When the cigarette offers less than the habitual amount of nicotine, the smoker changes something to compensate. The process of maintaining a certain level of nicotine in the blood is called *self-titration*.

In a study done at the Addiction Research Foundation of Toronto, the subjects were people who smoked cigarettes advertised as being ultra-low tar. The actual tar and nicotine level of the cigarette was not low, however; it merely had a filter with "microscopic ventilation holes." At least half the people in the group reported that they blocked the ventilation holes when they smoked; some even carried a roll of tape around with them to block the holes before they lit up. The smokers did not realize that it was the holes that made the cigarette safer; they thought that the tobacco itself was a "special mild variety." In another experiment, smokers were able to make a low-tar cigarette in the 11-to 16-mg range deliver as much tar and nicotine as cigarettes in the 31- to 35-mg range just by changing their smoking patterns.

Someone pulling deeper and harder on a low-tar cigarette to get more nicotine also gets a lot more of the other toxic particles and gases than with a normal smoking pattern. Additionally, low-tar low-nicotine cigarettes have a variety of unregulated additives to enhance the flavor. This "product modification" may cause added risks to those caused by nicotine. So much is yet unknown that calling a cigarette low tar or "lower yield" does not tell the whole story. The number of cigarettes smoked, the way they are smoked, and the tobacco additives can all increase the health risk of cigarettes that many people mistakenly consider safe. There is also the sad possibility that in tasting smoother and being easier to smoke, low-tar cigarettes encourage youngsters to experiment with smoking and then discourage their efforts to quit because the cigarettes are widely advertised as safe.

Our approach is straightforward. The only safe cigarette is a dead cigarette with a cement filter. There is no cigarette that is healthy. Smoking any cigarette is hazardous to your health — seriously hazardous.

If a person does no compensatory smoking — does not inhale more often or more deeply and does not smoke more cigarettes per day — then low-tar low-nicotine cigarettes are *slightly* better than high-tar cigarettes. But nothing compares in health benefits to not smoking at all. The most important thing you can do to prevent cancer and serious respiratory disease deserves to be repeated: either do not start smoking or quit completely.

Finally, if you feel that you must smoke, then do the following: smoke a low-tar filtered cigarette, smoke only half of each one, and do not inhale. Then cut down on your smoking and keep trying to quit. Cigarettes are coffin nails; whether filtered, low tar, with special papers, or whatever, those "little white sticks" are killers.

ANATOMY OF A KILLER

This title might sound more like a mystery story than a description of what makes up a cigarette, but it fits. That cigarettes kill is known, but cigarettes are still a mystery in spite of being intensively studied. A burning cigarette releases approximately 6800 different chemicals, and the effects of their interactions on each other and on our bodies are not fully known and may never be. The additives put into cigarettes by their manufacturers are also a mystery, kept secret and not reviewed or regulated by any impartial agency outside of the industry itself.

What we do know about cigarettes is that they are tobacco and other unknown products wrapped in paper and rolled into a cylindrical shape. Most of the time a filter is placed on one end. The tobacco itself comes in a thousand or so varieties. Depending on the tobacco leaf and how it is cured, the nicotine content of tobacco can vary from 0.2% to 4.75% of the tobacco. Even growing methods can affect this percentage. For example, using high levels of nitrogen fertilizer can increase the nicotine and nitrate levels of the tobacco.

The pesticides currently registered for use on tobacco leaves have been tested as contributors to the carcinogenic activity of tobacco smoke. When used as directed, they are found to cause no major change in the human body, which is somewhat reassuring. However, sometimes a pesticide is used that has not yet been tested, as happened once when blue mold was found on tobacco leaves. No one knows whether the new pesticide used then added to the health hazard of smoking or not.

The next step in making cigarettes is the manufacturing process, which introduces several new chemicals and mechanical factors. Reconstituted tobacco sheet is used, and it contains tobacco stem as well as leaf (stem, incidentally, has a lower nicotine content than leaf). The tobacco is also expanded or "puffed" so that less is required to make a cigarette, which also means less tobacco. The way this is done—how the tobacco is shredded—affects how it burns and even the chemical composition of the cigarette. To complicate the issue even more, cellulose-based substitutes for tobacco are used as well. These cause substantial differences in total yield of chemicals and in the chemical composition of the smoke.

When tobacco is smoked in a cigarette, tar results. Most of us think of tar as the smelly, black, sticky stuff used for fixing roads or putting on roofs. Cigarette tar is not much different. It is all the physical matter without the moisture that results from burning tobacco, and it consists of approximately 5000 organic and inorganic chemicals.

The particles that make up the tar are seen as the main contributors to cancer, heart disease, and chronic lung disease. Some of these chemical particles are known tumor initiators or carcinogens, others are cocarcinogens, and some are both. Many known poisonous substances are in cigarette smoke: nicotine, carbon monoxide, nitrosamines, nitrogen oxides, and polycyclic aromatic hydrocarbons—and there may be even more (see Fig. 7-5).

Nicotine is the single most active, fast-acting agent in tobacco smoke. It is also an extremely toxic chemical poison that can kill as effectively as cyanide at a dosage of approximately 60 milligrams. Among other things, nicotine narrows blood vessels, causing high blood pressure and an increased heart rate in smokers, as well as in those nonsmokers nearby and in the unborn young of smokers.

In addition to being poisonous itself, tobacco aids the formation of *tobacco-specific nitrosamines*, which are themselves powerful carcinogenic substances. Called *TSNAs*, they are formed in the curing and fermenting process as well as when the cigarette burns. TSNAs induce cancer in the lungs and tracheas of hamsters and are believed to contribute to cancer of the human trachea. As cancer-causing agents, they affect other organs of the body as well.

No one seems entirely sure, which is another mystery, but the cancer-causing potency of cigarette smoke is believed to depend on how much nicotine is in the tar. The activity that actually causes cancer could occur when the nicotine combines with other unknown cancer-producing chemicals or it could be the result of nicotine converting to nitrosamines (TSNAs).

A secondary, yet important, effect of tobacco smoke is that it contains oxidants that reduce the cleansing activities of the lungs. Many gas components in cigarette smoke are also *cilia toxic,* damaging the cilia, or cleansing brushes, of our lungs, as well as inhibiting cilia movement and mucous flow. Both the cilia and mucous flow help maintain disease resistance, thus damaging them would tend to reduce a

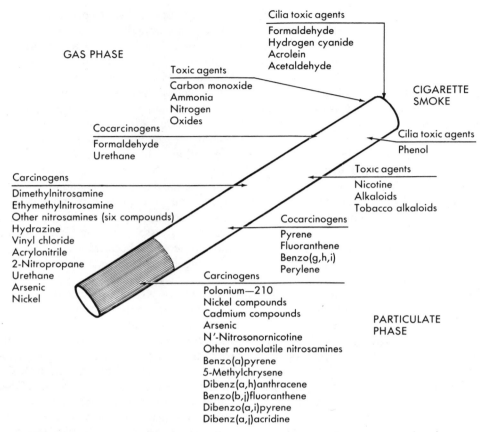

GAS PHASE

Cilia toxic agents
Formaldehyde
Hydrogen cyanide
Acrolein
Acetaldehyde

Toxic agents
Carbon monoxide
Ammonia
Nitrogen
Oxides

CIGARETTE
SMOKE

Cocarcinogens
Formaldehyde
Urethane

Cilia toxic agents
Phenol

Carcinogens
Dimethylnitrosamine
Ethymethylnitrosamine
Other nitrosamines (six compounds)
Hydrazine
Vinyl chloride
Acrylonitrile
2-Nitropropane
Urethane
Arsenic
Nickel

Toxic agents
Nicotine
Alkaloids
Tobacco alkaloids

Cocarcinogens
Pyrene
Fluoranthene
Benzo(g,h,i)
Perylene

Carcinogens
Polonium—210
Nickel compounds
Cadmium compounds
Arsenic
N′-Nitrosonornicotine
Other nonvolatile nitrosamines
Benzo(a)pyrene
5-Methylchrysene
Dibenz(a,h)anthracene
Benzo(b,j)fluoranthene
Dibenzo(a,i)pyrene
Dibenz(a,j)acridine

PARTICULATE
PHASE

FIG. 7-5   The chemical anatomy of a cigarette: toxic gas and particulate phases of cigarette smoke.

smoker's resistance to germs, leaving him generally more vulnerable to illness, especially infections (bronchitis and pneumonia).

Another potential risk factor is the alpha-radiation from polonium-210 in tobacco-related cancer. This risk factor merits further research, but underground miners who are or have been exposed to radiation should be cautioned not to smoke.

Other elements that alter the composition of cigarette smoke are the type of filter and the cigarette paper used. Of the two types of filters currently in use, regular and perforated, the

regular filter does lower the tar and nicotine levels but it delivers *more* carbon monoxide than unfiltered cigarettes of the same tar content. With perforated filters, the carbon monoxide content is slightly less but still much higher relative to the nicotine and tar. A highly porous cigarette paper can reduce the tar intake because more air comes through the paper and mouthpiece so less comes directly through the burning coal of the cigarette. The paper can alter the temperature of the burn, as well as the combustion process and the way the cigarette burns.

The only conclusion to draw from all of this

information is that taking cured, fermented, and processed tobacco, wrapping it in paper with a filter at one end, then lighting a match to it and inhaling the smoke that comes from the burning product results in a "miniature chemical factory which produces numerous toxic substances," as stated by J. Holbrook in the 1981 Surgeon General's report.

Additives

Into this already complex situation we must now inject a relatively new factor—additives. Although moisturizers and flavoring agents have long been used in cigarettes, the recent use of reconstituted tobacco "sheet" makes it easier to add more substances to cigarettes. These additives can be used to get a faster or slower burn rate, to replace tobacco, to flavor or extend the tobacco, or to bind or humidify it.

In 1972 R. J. Reynolds published a list of 1500 "tobacco flavorings," although the company was not required by law to do this. Since tobacco is not classified as either a food or a drug, it does not come under the laws governing such products. Cigarette manufacturers are not required to report the additives they use or to test them first. Yet, it is believed that more than 300 substances are added to cigarettes, possibly including shellac, caramel, and eugenol, according to the *Journal of the Addiction Research Foundation.*

Since no one except the cigarette manufacturer knows what is being added to cigarettes, the substances are not examined for carcinogenic or other effects. Additives undoubtedly alter the cigarette by their presence, but again, since they are secret, "It is not known what effect tobacco additives may have on chemical composition and biological activity of smoke" and "their presence represents an essentially unmeasured risk for the active smoker, passive smoker and fetus," according to the 1981 Surgeon General's report.

The making of cigarettes lower in tar and nicotine almost certainly involves using various additives for both processing and flavor. The use of additives themselves might introduce increased, as well as new and different, health risks into cigarettes.

Because of the many chemicals in smoke and the constantly changing chemical composition of cigarettes, with their many additives, as well as the use of different growing, curing, processing, and filtering methods, the exact composition of smoke will probably never be fully known. For this reason, the stated tar yield of cigarettes cannot be used as a precise measure of the health risks from smoke exposure nor as an indication of relative safety compared to cigarettes higher in tar.

Testing

The tar and nicotine ratings on cigarette packages come from studies done by the Tobacco Testing Laboratory of the Federal Trade Commission (FTC). This laboratory has been in operation for 16 years and is responsible for determining the levels of carbon monoxide, nicotine, and tar in each of the 208 brands of cigarettes made in the United States (H. Pillsbury, director of the FTC laboratory, quit smoking shortly after the facility was opened). It was the report of this laboratory that encouraged Congress to pass the Federal Cigarette Labeling Advertising Act, which authorized the FTC to determine the nicotine and tar figures and required that these figures be included in advertisements.

To test cigarettes, all 208 brands are bought in 50 locations throughout the country. From an initial 416,000 cigarettes bought, 200 of each brand are chosen at random. Each cigarette is then put on a smoking machine, a mechanical pump, that is equipped with various devices to filter out the tar and nicotine in the "inhaled" smoke. Presumably, this is what the lungs do with the cigarette smoke inhaled by the smoker. A smoking-machine puff lasts 2 seconds, and the machine puffs once a minute until the cigarette, 23 mm long, is used up.

The amount of tar and nicotine is measured, and the figures per cigarette are calculated and printed on the cigarette packages. There is tremendous competition between the various companies over which one can produce the lowest-tar cigarette. In December 1981 R.J. Reynolds and Phillip Morris accused Brown and Williamson Tobacco Corporation of fraud. They said this corporation had used a filter on their low-tar cigarette Barclay that "fooled" the testing machine by causing more air to be blown into the machine than usual. The air diluted the cigarette smoke and may have led to a misleading report. In addition, the four grooves that added air to the machine's inhale mechanism had a tendency to collapse or become blocked when smoked by a person.

What all this testing amounts to may not be much. We know the quantity of nicotine and tar the smoking machine gets per cigarette, but our concern is with humans who smoke, and humans do not follow the same smoking pattern that the machine does. For example, four of the most popular king-size low-tar filter cigarettes, representing 35% of all sales, were machine tested. After 8.7 puffs, they measured out to have 1.2 mg of nicotine and 18.6 mg of tar. But human smokers take an average of 9.8 puffs per cigarette and commonly up to 14 or more puffs on a king-size cigarette. Using the 14-puff figure, the same cigarette testing would yield 58% or *more* tar and nicotine than the package rating. According to L. T. Kozlowski, a cigarette advertised as being in the 1- to 5-mg range can turn into a 15- to 20-mg tar cigarette if a smoker takes more and deeper puffs than the machine allows for or even partially blocks the ventilating holes or channels that are to be found in many cigarette filters. As the 1981 Surgeon General's report concluded, these "published machine-smoked tar and nicotine levels imply an estimate of relative risk which fails to account for actual individual smoke exposure and for all the smoke constituents," and "the 'tar' and nicotine yields obtained by present testing methods do not correspond to the dosages that the individual smokers receive; in some cases, they may seriously underestimate these dosages."

What the testing does reveal is exactly how much tar and nicotine a smoking machine is exposed to, but the incidence of lung cancer among smoking machines is not a problem. The tar and nicotine levels may be less than useless for the smokers who suffer and die from lung cancer because the figures can be misleading and are widely exploited. These levels are heavily advertised, and smokers take the figures seriously, thinking the lower tar and nicotine figures guarantee a "safer" cigarette.

Despite the tobacco industry capitalizing on the testing reports of the government laboratory, they also maintain their own laboratory. The Tobacco Institute, the public relations arm of the tobacco industry, operates a smoke testing laboratory in Bethesda, Maryland "to keep the FTC honest," according to an Institute spokesperson. There is a lot at stake in these figures because of what the tobacco industry represents.

TOBACCO IS BIG BUSINESS

The tobacco industry as a whole has an annual advertising budget of more than $1 billion ($1.24 billion in 1980) and retail sales of $17 billion. The worldwide industry spends more than $2 billion annually on advertising, according to the United Nations Conference on Trade and Development. Tobacco is America's fifth largest cash crop, and hundreds of thousands of people are directly employed in the tobacco industry. No wonder the industry's very subtle yet effective lobby, the Tobacco Institute, still claims that a cause-and-effect relationship between cigarettes and lung cancer, emphysema, and heart disease has not been established. Although the latest Surgeon General's report is very conclusive and specific on these points, billions of dollars in profit ride on the industry's attempt to deny this fact.

The 1981 Surgeon General's report states that "current . . . advertising conveys the implicit message that substantial reductions in machine-measured tar and nicotine levels may be equated with substantial reductions in risks for smokers." The "substantial reduction in risk" is *not* a fact and could be a fantasy, but the industry has a huge stake in promoting the idea of a safe cigarette, even though no such thing exists. By 1978, $420 million—half the annual budget for cigarette advertising—went to promote sales of "low-tar" cigarettes. One company, Brown and Williamson, spent roughly $150 million in 1980 on advertising and promoting one new product —the "ultra light" cigarette, Barclay. Part of the promotion campaign was to give away free cartons of the cigarettes.

While the six major cigarette companies spent over $1 billion to advertise their product in 1980, the American Cancer Society, the American Heart Association, and the American Lung Association combined spent only $10 million, or 1% of the industry advertising budget, on smoking-prevention programs; and under the current administration, the United States Government Office on Smoking and Health is facing a 50% cut.

A total ban on cigarette advertising has been adopted in Norway, Sweden, Finland, Iceland, and Italy. The United States banned cigarette advertising from television in 1971, which only sent the tobacco advertising dollars elsewhere, mostly to the print media. The tobacco industry outspends all other national advertisers in newspapers, and the eight leading cigarette companies spent $386 million in 1981 on magazine advertising. Magazine ads for cigarettes are large and glossy, colorful and seductive; they associate smoking with having fun and being mature, attractive, and worldly. The models who smoke in the ads all look vibrantly healthy and energetic.

These advertisements attract more than just their readers; magazine publishers love the money that comes with them. According to the editor of *Good Housekeeping*, the money from cigarette advertising helped several magazines survive the 1973 recession. In an average year, *TV Guide* carried $26.9 million worth of cigarette advertising; *Time*, $40.4 million; *Playboy*, $9.4 million; *U.S. News and World Reports,* $11.2 million; *Newsweek*, $20.8 million; *Family Circle,* $12.9 million; *Woman's Day,* $12.8 million; *Better Homes and Garden,* $11.4 million; *Sports Illustrated,* $20.8 million; *People,* $15.4 million.* In some Sunday supplements 80% of the advertising is for cigarettes, according to *Mother Jones* magazine.

Redbook receives $8.7 million of ad revenue from cigarettes; *Ms.*, $573,000; *Cosmopolitan*, $5.2 million; *McCalls*, $9.4 million; *Glamour* and *House and Garden*, $2.5 million each. Between 1971 and 1981 *Cosmopolitan* published 155 articles on dieting but only eight on smoking. *Ms.* has no articles on the hazards of smoking, which is bizarre for a magazine that covers women's health issues and is aware that soon smoking will be the number one cancer killer of women. *Harper's Bazaar* receives $597,000 yearly from cigarette ad revenues. A recent article on health hazards in the office had three uncomplimentary paragraphs on smoking reduced to one. The magazine's health editor states, "We do have to consider the advertisers but we've still managed not to quench the story."

Many advertisers cancel ads when the newspapers report negatively on cigarettes. Tobacco companies require their ads not be run near obituaries or antismoking stories. When these guidelines are not observed, the tobacco companies ask for a free ad or an adjustment in cost. Tobacco companies are not accused of heavy-handed pressure techniques in dealing

---

*Hutchings, R.: A review of the nature and extent of cigarette advertising in the U.S., Proceedings of the National Conference on Smoking or Health, November, 1981, p. 255.

with editors and publishers, but the smaller and weaker publications especially may employ self-censorship on the smoking issue. On the other hand, the industry does place its ads in parts of magazines and newspapers that have less reporting and publicity critical of cigarettes.

Magazines that carried cigarette advertising did not, over a 7-year period, publish any articles that related the dangers of smoking, according to a study in the *Columbia General Review*. For example, two articles appeared in women's magazines focusing on preventive health care: "The ABCs of Preventive Medicine" and "Seventy-Six Ways to Save Your Life." Neither mentioned smoking at all. Magazines such as *Time, Newsweek,* and *U.S. News and World Report* have had articles on the causes of cancer, but none made a strong case against smoking, although smoking is now firmly established as a known cause of cancer.

The magazines that do run articles on the health hazards of smoking are usually the same ones that have a policy of not accepting cigarette advertising: *Good Housekeeping, Science Digest, Consumer Reports, The New Yorker, Reader's Digest, Hustler,* and *Washington Monthly.*

The clearest example of how the tobacco industry uses its advertising money to influence editorial content occurred with *Mother Jones*, a celebrated muckraking journal. When *Mother Jones* ran an article on smoking and health in its April 1978 issue, $18,000 worth of cigarette advertising was immediately withdrawn. In January 1979 another article relating to tobacco and health appeared. Within 2 weeks two other tobacco companies canceled their ads, and *Mother Jones* was told it "would never get any more cigarette advertising."

The *Mother Jones* example illustrates a covert form of suppression. In a more obvious maneuver Phillip Morris took legal steps to prevent a film entitled "Death in the West" from being distributed, even though two of its executives star in the documentary. One executive

chain-smokes whenever he is on camera. The other, a medical doctor who does not "care to smoke" rejects the idea that smoking is harmful and contends that too much of anything can be bad for you, including applesauce.

The film is a half-hour documentary produced by Thames Television, a British company. It was shown to 12 million British viewers before it was suppressed by the Phillip Morris Tobacco Company. Several years later a professor at the University of California at San Francisco obtained a copy of the film, which was loaned to a local television station that has aired it several times on prime time, local and national.*

The film opens with the "Marlboro man" theme music and one of the TV ads that are now illegal. Then five or six real-life cowboys, all suffering serious illnesses from the effects of smoking, come on camera one at a time. John Holmes is shown riding on his New Mexico ranch with an oxygen tank strapped to his saddle and tubes running to his nose; he started smoking at age 17. He explained, "It was the only thing to do. I thought it was going to give me stature, make me a man." After each cowboy appears, his physician comes on and makes a statement: "Ninety-nine out of a hundred cowboys I see would not have cancer if they had not been smokers." Between these sequences are more romantic commercials and interviews with the two Phillip Morris executives, who try very hard to defend their products and thus their livelihood.

Airplane accidents, environmental dangers, and war frequently appear on the front pages of our newspapers. Yet it is very difficult to find the same attention paid to a habit that kills more than 110,000 people each year, every single year—a million people a decade go up in smoke!

---

*The film is now used as part of a smoker's education program in elementary, high, and prep schools in California. The program was developed by Stanton Glantz, in cooperation with California Nonsmokers Rights Foundation, with curriculum developed in cooperation with Herb Thier and Alan Schnur, Laurence Hall of Science, University of California at Berkeley.

Fortunately for all of us, the news is out, and Americans have become much more aware of the dangers associated with smoking. As this happens and the number of smokers continues to decline, the tobacco industry will face decreasing sales. For example, the industry growth in 1980 was only 1% despite the $1 billion spent on advertising.

The big international tobacco companies such as Phillip Morris (Marlboro) approach declining sales by seeking new markets in the Third World. Phillip Morris sells its products in more than 160 countries, and sales have increased there 18% in the last decade. Advertisements present smoking as an adult, healthy, and macho or sexy activity, and Third World consumption of cigarettes is now growing at 5% a year. Most Third World governments are too short of funds to give up the revenues they get from tobacco taxes or to fund effective antismoking campaigns. They are also, unfortunately, the countries that can least afford the heavy health care costs of smoking-related diseases.

The U.S. Government and tobacco

No means currently exist to restrain the giants of the tobacco industry from seeking markets in the Third World. The industry is as unregulated abroad as it is in this country. The one exception to this is the requirement by the Federal Trade Commission that a warning be put on cigarette packages and advertising that tobacco is hazardous to your health. Other than this, cigarette companies are not required to list the ingredients in cigarettes—as a food manufacturer must on a soup can or a drug manufacturer must on a drug label—since tobacco is considered neither a food nor a drug. As already mentioned, of the hundreds of potential cigarette additives, none must be disclosed or tested for safety before use. The tobacco industry is the only industry that stands outside the scrutiny for safety of the Food and Drug Administration.

You might wonder how the tobacco industry achieved the special status that it has, and one factor is probably the TPPAC—the Tobacco People's Public Affairs Committee. TPPAC is the political action group of the industry's lobby, the Tobacco Institute, and it has made financial gifts to members of both houses of Congress, according to an article in *Mother Jones* magazine. These gifts must certainly help increase the immense lobbying power of the Tobacco Institute.

In addition to the Tobacco Institute in Washington, the government itself has an ambiguous relationship with the tobacco industry. For example, if everyone in the United States should suddenly quit smoking, the federal government would lose $500 million—half a *billion* dollars—in tax revenue each year. Yet, several government agencies exist just to reduce the number of cigarettes smoked. A lot of the antismoking literature in use has been developed by the National Cancer Institute or the Office on Smoking and Health of the Public Health Service, although the total antismoking budget was still well under $1 million.

The government has also funded the search for a "safe" cigarette, spending $40 million on this project during the past 10 years. This is the only time the government has financed research to develop a safe consumer product, even though many other industries would probably appreciate this kind of help.

Critics of the government believe that it can play a much stronger role in the regulation of the tobacco industry. Suggestions include instituting safeguards on the use of additives, studying them, and disclosing the health effects of their use; pushing for more effective cigarette labeling, including the warning that tobacco is addictive; working toward a total ban on cigarette advertising; and promoting a stiff tobacco excise tax to reduce cigarette consumption. Part of the monies from this tax could be used to research either alternate healthy uses for tobacco or programs to retrain tobacco workers for other livelihoods; if Americans are to be healthy, the cigarette industry has to die. This, however, is not something that will happen quickly or easily. At present, we still have 55 million people in the United States who are addicted to a substance that endangers their health and shortens their lives.

ADDICTION AND CURE

Twenty-five years ago, smoking was thought of as a social habit; today it is recognized as an addiction. This puts smoking in the same category in some respects as alcoholism and other drug addictions. In fact, former drug addicts and exalcoholics who smoke state that it is more difficult to give up tobacco than heroin or liquor. Research shows that 10% of alcoholics will quit drinking, whereas only 7% of smokers will stop smoking.

The addiction to tobacco, specifically to nicotine, is socially encouraged and reinforced, something that is not true of heroin addiction, but the same for alcohol addiction. Smokers are surrounded by billboards and ads showing attractive, healthy people smoking, but these are social and psychologic inducements. The real problem is physical dependence—the biologic hook of nicotine and tar. Fig. 7-6 depicts the tar and tobacco content of the average cigarette.

Nicotine is similar to certain amphetamines that are central nervous system stimulants and are considered more addictive than the opiates, including heroin. Cigarettes do not make you feel intoxicated, as do alcohol or other drugs, so the addiction may not seem so intense, but it still exists, as any honest smoker can tell you. The American Psychiatric Association, in their most recent diagnostic manual, termed tobacco dependence from cigarette smoking "an organic mental disorder and an addiction." The psychiatrists labeled tobacco an addictive substance because it meets all the major criteria, including having a withdrawal syndrome. Withdrawal from tobacco is characterized by the following:

1. A craving for tobacco
2. Insomnia
3. Increased appetite
4. Difficulty concentrating
5. Restlessness
6. Irritability
7. Drowsiness
8. Anxiety
9. Headache
10. Gastrointestinal disturbances

The craving becomes noticeable within 2 hours of smoking the last cigarette and usually reaches a peak within 24 to 96 hours. Then the intensity of the craving gradually declines over a period of days to 4 weeks. Exsmokers will still experience an occasional intense longing for a cigarette months after they have quit, usually in a situation or atmosphere in which they once smoked habitually: at a party, after dinner, to relieve stress, to break up a dull routine. According to statistics, more than half the people who quit smoking will relapse within 6 months, probably giving in at just such a moment. But after not smoking for a year, most smokers never smoke again.

In labeling smoking an addiction, the psychiatrists hoped to help people who wanted to quit. The thinking was that if the smoker who wants to quit understands the actual addictive nature of nicotine, the tactics for quitting can be more realistic and effective.

People who smoke associate smoking with relaxation or else they smoke to reduce tension in stressful situations. Although the association between smoking and taking a break is strong, nicotine is not a depressant that helps one relax; as a drug, it is a stimulant. Most smokers who try to quit without understanding the normal withdrawal symptoms feel very anxious, which is a direct result of the physical withdrawal from nicotine. But the smoker who does not know this only thinks, "I get very nervous when I don't smoke," and lights up to keep calm. The anxiety would pass, along with all the other withdrawal symptoms, given some time. The

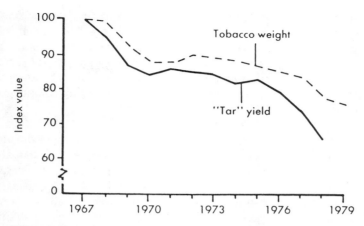

FIG. 7-6 Index of average "tar" and tobacco per cigarette, annually, 1967-1979. Base year 1967—100; 1979 estimated. (Modified from U.S. Department of Agriculture.)

uneducated quitter will often not be able to wait this out, however, not knowing the symptoms will pass quite soon.

M. Russell, director of the Addiction Research Unit in London, says that people do not "recognize the extent to which smoking for most smokers is really a very finely adjusted drug-taking activity. Smokers modify their self-dosage by the size of the puffs, the depth of inhalation, and the number of cigarettes they smoke." The smoker goes for a certain nicotine blood level just like a junkie goes for a fix.

Cure: quitters are winners

Thirty million people have kicked the smoking habit or addiction. About 95% of these exsmokers quit on their own with no apparent outside assistance. The motivating factors for most quitters were positive: they were interested in health and greater mastery over their lives and wanted more energy and endurance to live stronger lives longer or to have a more vigorous sex life. Smokers are more likely to quit at a time when they have symptoms such as shortness of breath, cough, or sore throat or have fear of heart or lung damage.

Exsmokers get the rewards that they seek.

After a time, smokers who have quit say they feel "more alive," which is an accurate description of what happens to them. As soon as smokers quit, various parts and processes in their bodies begin working to clear away the effects of smoking. Precancerous cells lining the lungs start to return to normal; the lung cilia begin sweeping out impurities; and the levels of carbon monoxide and nicotine in the system decrease rapidly.

Exsmokers commonly report that physical symptoms that have bothered them for years seem to disappear overnight; other symptoms disappear more gradually. Among the disappearing symptoms are smoker's "hangover" and chronic fatigue, shortness of breath, heavy morning phlegm, as well as more subtle discomforts like feeling headachy, not enjoying food, and feeling guilt about needing a cigarette. Along with the bad health effects of the habit, the exsmoker gives up yellow, nicotine-stained fingers and teeth, burned holes in clothes and furniture, and worry about fires. Fires caused by lit cigarettes account for 40% of all fatal fires in the United States, and they burn up as much as $300 million of property a year.

Exsmokers are also proud of the example

they set for their children. Children do not like being exposed to secondhand smoke. Of more than 2000 children between the ages of 7 and 15 interviewed, 80% indicated a strong dislike for their parents' smoking habits, mentioning they experienced coughing and eye irritation from the smoke. The comments included, "It's bad for them," "They might get cancer," "They have bad breath," and "I don't like the smell." Sixty-seven percent of the children interviewed said they would respect their parents more if they did not smoke.

As a group, physicians have quit smoking in great numbers: going from 38% smokers to 8%. Former Secretary of the Department of Health, Education and Welfare, Joseph Califano, Jr. turned his back on a three-pack-a-day habit in 1975. He labeled smoking "slow-motion suicide." Obviously, these professional people were impressed by the facts; the known dangers may have been a motivating factor. The health risks became very personal, not just empty statistics, because those who quit saw the physical effects smoking had on health.

Many people, however, start tuning out danger warnings beyond a certain point. The health risks do not seem to relate to them, and they just do not want to hear any more about them. It is difficult to motivate people to do anything with a warning about the increasing threat of getting cancer X number of years down the pike. The statistics have no impact or personal meaning, especially for young people, who often tend to think of themselves as somehow immortal.

All in all, positive incentives seem to work better than warnings or threats in helping people to stop smoking. If there are warnings of health dangers, they have to be personal and as immediate as possible. Another thing is that people who thought they would be successful in quitting were successful. Their positive attitude and motivation seemed to work together for them. This is important information because research shows that 80% of all smokers would like to quit. Nicotine gum has been used in

Europe and Canada for smokers who wish to go "cold turkey" to stop. It is being tried experimentally in the United States and may be an aid to reduce symptoms during quitting. Nicotine gum may prove to be an acceptable source of nicotine for aiding smoking cessation.

Becoming a quitter

One way to accomplish something difficult is to find someone who has already successfully done it and follow his or her lead. This approach might work well with solving math problems or climbing a rock wall, but with smoking things are more complicated. The situation with giving up smoking can be compared to a popular song by Paul Simon called, "There Must Be Fifty Ways to Leave Your Lover." Studies of successful quitters show that a variety of strategies works and what works for some does not work for others. In spite of the various techniques used, overall patterns did show up.

Most people seemed to feel more comfortable quitting on their own than through a clinic. Most successful quitters chose from a wide variety of strategies the ones that suited them. In general, they found self-reward and "active problem-solving strategies" most helpful in quitting.

There are people who decide one day, after years of smoking, that they will never smoke another cigarette. They put out the half-smoked cigarette they have been looking at with disgust and they never light up another cigarette again. This is called the cold-turkey approach, and although this is not a fairy tale, it might as well be for many smokers. A lot of successful quitters could not have quit with a cold-turkey cure. Instead, they used help—pamphlets, a quitting schedule, audio tapes, or a smoking diary. They also rewarded themselves—had their teeth cleaned, bought new clothes, saved their cigarette money for treats, or went out. They figured out strategies for keeping off the drug—gum, toothpicks, or fiddling with something to keep their hands busy. They made pacts with friends or spouses or bets with friendly enemies. Some attended smoking cessation clinics and went through formal programs.

One important aid toward eventual cessation can be to make a diary of each cigarette smoked. Record each cigarette on the chart, as often as possible, *before* smoking the cigarette. That way, you might think twice before lighting up and will often forego that cigarette. This technique is part of reconditioning or changing smoking behavior. It is a helpful strategy to use before actually quitting.

Those who want to quit on their own should be aware that several national organizations exist whose sole business is to help them. You can contact your local community resources, both public and private, in your area (see the resources list in Appendix B).

The American Cancer Society (ACS), American Heart Association (AHA), American Lung Association (ALA), the National Interagency Council on Smoking and Health, and the Office of Cancer Communications all have excellent booklets that tell you what you need to know in order to quit: how to substitute for your smoking pattern, what to expect after cutting down and quitting, how to control weight, and so on. Many of these pamphlets are designed to guide you through the quitting process day by day, and they contain a variety of tips, approaches, and gimmicks that have been popular and successful with exsmokers. It is a matter of choosing what makes sense to you as an individual. One ACS quitter's guide includes a form to wrap around the cigarette pack and use to record the number of cigarettes smoked daily and when, where, and why. The same pamphlet gives six key reasons why most people smoke compulsively and how to handle each of them. One especially good pamphlet is *Calling It Quits*, published by the National Cancer Institute in Bethesda, Md. 20205. The approach and ideas are upbeat and creative and sure to challenge and inspire the motivated quitter with some practical ammunition for the job.

One of the ways to determine what approach to take as a quitter is figure out when and why you smoke. Then you can choose an appropriate substitute. A smoker's log (Table 7-2) can help you figure this out. If you smoke for the stimulating effects of the drug when you are feeling tired or bored, you can achieve the same results with a brisk walk or jogging in place if you work. (Most employers will actively support their employees who want to quit smoking; it saves money for them in less sick leave and less cleaning and maintenance.) Some people smoke because they have lots of energy. If this applies to you, you can try playing with a paperclip or doodling instead. If smoking is just a habit with no reason and not even much pleasure anymore, you can use the awareness techniques such as the diary and then make a game of eliminating smokes or putting them off by calling a friend or doing something else that is pleasurable instead of lighting up.

The most common reason people give for smoking is stress, and this is especially the case with women. People tend to light up in tense situations to withdraw or pull back from the stress, and of course, everyone has some stress-producing situations in their lives. It may not be possible to do away with stress—although you can usually reduce it—but there are other effective ways of dealing with stress rather than lighting up a cigarette. To begin making a change, a smoker needs new forms of stress management. Some of the things that work are undertaking an exercise program such as walking, jogging, or dancing; learning relaxation, meditation, or self-hypnosis techniques; enrolling in stress reduction or behavior modification classes; or taking up a new sport or hobby such as gardening, bicycling, or tennis. Stress-management alternatives to smoking are as varied as people themselves, and workshops are available, often through local community colleges, in stress management. Each method may work initially: 40% to 80% quit, but tragically the majority relapse. Patients may respond best to direct advice from their physicians on how to quit smoking.

TABLE 7-2   Quitter's log

Day	Time	Desire rating*	Available aids; psychologic support*	Depression/ frustration level*	Success rating†

*0 to 100.
†0%—None; 100%—Must smoke

What keeps most people from quitting?

Stress and fear of gaining weight are the two most common reasons people give for not quitting. If people smoke in response to stress and then know when they quit they will experience the added stress and anxiety caused by withdrawal symptoms, the combination may seem overwhelming. They do not even want to try. Stress reduction and/or nonsmoking means of stress management are the methods these people should use. It is important to start alternative ways of dealing with stress *before* quitting smoking, however. Once stress is reduced or managed by some change in schedule, new habit, or practice, quitting smoking will also be more manageable—not an added burden. Giving up smoking can thus become part of a lifestyle change toward better health, vigor and enjoyment of life.

On the average smokers do tend to weigh less than nonsmokers. This is because it takes slightly longer for a smoker's stomach to digest food than a nonsmoker's stomach and because smoking has an effect on taste, tongue, and mouth. Smokers also have blunted appetites as a result of their smoking habit. It is important for smokers to realize that not all people who quit smoking gain weight. Twenty-five percent stay the same, and another 25% actually lose. One in two smokers who quit have no problem at all with any weight gain. Exsmokers who lose weight attribute their loss to increased energy levels and improved self-image, both positive gains they achieved by giving up smoking. (See Chapter 5 for weight-control diet.)

Tips to help you stop smoking

1. Prepare to quit

- Set a "quit" day about a week ahead and mark it as a "red letter day" on your calendar.
- Keep a daily record of each cigarette smoked.
- Collect all butts in a jar.
- Buy cigarettes one pack at a time.
- Wait a full five minutes after an urge occurs before lighting up.
- Smoke only when a cigarette is strongly craved.
- Stop using all smoking paraphernalia such as cigarette cases, lighters, or holders.
- Figure out the lifetime monetary cost of smoking.
- Read some literature from the American Cancer Society.
- List reasons for quitting and benefits that will accrue.

2. Positive attitude

- When "quit" day arrives, become your own source of positive reinforcement and positive feedback.
- Remember that quitting cigarettes is adding, rather than subtracting something from your life.
- Silently repeat positive statements, such as "I choose not to smoke," "I shall not be a slave to cigarettes."
- Repeat these statements in front of a mirror.
- Post quit smoking signs or slogans in your home and work area.

3. Stimulus control

- Get rid of smoking stimuli at home and at work.
- Change your routine: Go to work a different way; sit in a different place in the cafeteria; choose a "no smoking" section; leave the "scene of an urge."

4. Develop incompatible behavior

- Smokers derive both oral and manual satisfaction from cigarettes. So use coffee stirrers, sugarless gum and mints, pen or pencil, etc., to keep both your mouth and hands occupied. Also keep *yourself* busy — not only your mouth and hands — since smoking serves as an activity to combat boredom and loneliness. Get involved in movies, books, walks, hobbies, arts and crafts.

5. Aversive techniques

- Butt bottle — Keep the jar with the cigarette butts that were collected during the preparation period. Add some water to enhance the unsightliness. Look at the butts when an urge occurs.
- Ex-smoker's ritual — Select a negative consequence of smoking, such as climbing a flight of stairs breathlessly, or being diagnosed as having lung cancer. Imagine this experience for 15 seconds whenever an urge occurs.
- Urge zapper — Wear an elastic band (or rubber band) on your wrist. "Zap" yourself whenever an urge occurs.

—From the Stop Smoking System of the American Health Foundation.

From Powell, D.R., and Bohm, E.: Your Patient and Cancer, March 1983, pp. 110–111.

Continued.

Tips to help you stop smoking—cont'd

6. Stress management

- Deep breathing—Inhale deeply, hold your breath for three seconds, and then exhale slowly through pursed lips. This increases the flow of blood to the heart, reduces tension, and will relax you.
- Mental imagery relaxation—Visualize, as vividly as possible, a very peaceful scene such as walking along a beach or through a forest.
- Emotional release—Tighten the muscles in your body and then release them while groaning or sighing or even shouting.
- Physical activity—Exercise is an excellent way to reduce tension. Walk part of the way to work or during lunch hour.
- Take warm showers or baths.

7. Eating management for urge control

- Don't skip meals. Eating regular meals prevents the blood sugar level from dropping and triggering the desire to smoke for a "lift."
- Don't consume foods containing sugar such as pastries, candy or ice cream. Eliminating sugar prevents the blood sugar fluctuations that lead to increased desire to smoke.
- Don't consume coffee, tea, and cola drinks. Strong associations have been made between these drinks and cigarette smoking. They seem to "go together."
- Don't consume alcohol. Alcohol too has been psychologically connected with cigarettes. It produces a laissez-faire attitude and inhibits motivation towards goals such as quitting smoking.
- Do drink up to 8 glasses of liquids per day. It will help flush out nicotine.
- Do eat three meals per day. This maintains constant blood sugar levels, thus preventing urges to smoke.
- Do drink fruit juices or take a piece of fruit between meals. This also maintains constant blood sugar levels and prevents fatigue.
- Do eat lean meats, fish, poultry, cheese, vegetables, whole grains, and salads.

8. Self-reward

- You may experience a sense of deprivation due to the withdrawal of cigarettes from your life. This can be lessened if you indulge in small daily treats throughout the quitting process—fresh cut flowers, a new book or record album, a phone call to a friend.
- Collect in a bank the monies you would have spent on cigarettes. Watch it accumulate and plan for a weekend vacation or other "splurge of your choice."

9. Self-control technique

- "The urge for a cigarette will go away whether I smoke or do not smoke a cigarette." Repeat this *Ex-Smoker's Inspiration* often.

10. Buddy system

- Some people benefit from quitting smoking in conjunction with a friend.

In those who do gain weight, successful strategies for weight control focus on why people put on weight in the first place. The range of reasons for eating more once a person quits smoking are (1) gaining a sharper sense of taste and more overall appetite, (2) using food as an oral substitute for smoking, (3) eating to counter nervousness or stress, and (4) eating to alleviate feelings of psychologic deprivation. The strategies for satisfying the need for oral stimulation without cigarettes involve substitution, including chewing gum, eating low-calorie foods such as celery or carrots, and chewing on stick cinnamon. If the food makes up for a feeling of psychologic deprivation, exsmokers are advised to add pleasurable new experiences to their lives that are not connected with food. With a better sense of taste and appetite, the exsmoker can change diet patterns to lower-calorie, more healthful eating habits and get a double bonus from quitting. The boxed material outlines what happens when you stop smoking.

What happens after you quit smoking

Smoking

1. Makes you tired
2. Gives you headaches
3. May make you jittery
4. Gives you a foul-tasting mouth
5. Deprives you of wind, energy, and health

12 hours after quitting

1. Carbon monoxide level declines
2. Helps heart and lungs

2 to 3 weeks after quitting

1. Taste improves
2. Decreased smoker's hack
3. Gastrointestinal system normalizes
4. Fewer headaches—mind improves, fewer dizzy spells
5. New energy and increased strength
6. Breathing improves
7. Money saved ($1/pack/day equals $350 saved/year)
8. Cleaner home and office

No smoking

1. Less job absenteeism
   a. 1/5 of sick days (of smokers) related to smoking
   b. 1/10 of sick days in bed (of smokers) related to smoking
2. More productive days
3. Improved life span

Symptoms during recovery (temporary)

1. Fluid retention; possible weight gain
2. Sore gums, tongue
3. Mental tension
4. Possible fatigue

To alleviate symptoms after quitting

1. Find other diversions
2. Get enough rest for optimum physical and mental alertness
3. Eat five or six small meals a day instead of two or three big ones
4. Eat foods high in protein for more energy
5. Drink a lot of the *right* fluids: water to increase circulation and stimulate digestion, milk to soothe nerves and avoid fatigue, citrus or tomato juice to give quick energy boost
6. Begin a habit of regular exercise

Giving up on quitting

For most smokers, quitting is a process, not a single event. A single, double, or triple slip is not evidence of failure. In fact, the more times you try to quit, the more likely you are to succeed ultimately. Most successful quitters have a history of previous attempts at quitting that last anywhere from a day to several months and longer, so a relapse should not be regarded as a sign of failure. Rather, it is a predictable response to a stressful situation. Each attempt at quitting is a small gain on the road to quitting entirely—a practice session that gradually develops a person's ability to handle stress without a cigarette.

People who have already quit several times will often get tired of having to face the initial withdrawal symptoms from nicotine one more time. Desire to avoid this discomfort motivates them to stay off cigarettes once they have quit, since they do not want to go through the process of quitting again. There are two hard tasks to giving up smoking: sticking through the initial withdrawal and then staying away from smoking.

What seems difficult for exsmokers is to maintain the new nonsmoking behavior, especially in a variety of situations that formerly stimulated them to smoke. This is true for people in formal programs as well as people who quit on their own. Many exsmokers are not prepared for the stage that occurs soon after quitting. As the lungs clear, there may be increased coughing; as the body works to expel impurities, it can retain fluids, causing a feeling of being fatter and heavier. Then there is the edginess from the stress of withdrawal. The former smoker may well wonder, "If this is good for me, then why do I feel so bad?"

Some kind of follow-up is needed to show exsmokers how their health is improving and the health risk is actually being reduced. Exsmokers already on an exercise program usually notice a change in their wind and endurance without any outside help, but others need some

obvious feedback to prove that the changes toward increased health they wanted are actually taking place. People who want to quit and those who want to maintain their new nonsmoking habit can use all the help they can get. Fortunately, there are many resources available.

Resources

The most valuable resource any potential exsmoker has is his or her family physician. Physicians are highly respected and can give good advice on the effects of smoking, a person's health, and safe, manageable techniques for quitting. Realizing the impact physicians have on their patients, the National Cancer Institute has created a "Helping Smokers Quit" kit. The kit contains posters, handouts, and instructions for using the simple four-step process that only requires one office visit (see Resources list in Appendix B). One kit, which is free, has enough materials for 50 patients, and the materials are geared for all levels of smokers, from those who strongly want to quit to smokers who have not yet considered quitting.

For the smoker who wants company, a variety of clinics and group programs exist. Group settings can be helpful because the potential quitter finds support and can share the discomforts of withdrawal with others who have committed themselves to going through the same process. The group approach ranges from very structured ways of changing smoking behavior to simple group discussions held in a supportive atmosphere. The American Health Foundation is an example of a structured approach with a 5-day program based on the idea that people can quit if they know how to do it. Participants learn how to prevent the urge to smoke or get rid of the urge when it does occur. Private clinics also offer smoking cessation programs; check in your local area. There is a wide variety of commercial programs, as well as clinics sponsored by public agencies; commercially available products such as filters and excellent tapes can also help some people. A host of written material is available from a variety of government agencies and private research organizations. The Resources list in Appendix B gives some of the options, and a call to the local office of the American Heart Association, American Lung Association, National Cancer Institute, or the American Cancer Society will give you many more.

Remember that the overriding factor for success is simply having the desire to stop. Successful quitters have some or all of the following characteristics:

1. They are strongly motivated and committed to making a change.
2. They use various behavioral techniques to change their behavior, including rewards and positive reinforcement.
3. They have social support or else they find it.
4. They have made other successful attempts to stop.
5. They use substitutes to alleviate cravings.
6. They believe that they will be able to quit.

But anyone who has successfully quit can attest to one thing: the simplest way to control smoking is not to start in the first place.

PREVENTION

No one in our society knows exactly how and when they become an adult. Unlike many simpler, primitive ones, our society offers no special test or ceremony to mark the passage from childhood or adolescence to adulthood. But because youngsters are vitally interested in growing up and mastering the skills of adulthood, they are constantly on the lookout for signposts to maturity. The two most obvious marks of adulthood in our society are drinking alcoholic beverages and smoking cigarettes, both legally restricted according to age.

Boys, and more recently girls, drink and smoke as a way of showing that they are mature and worldly, not realizing that smoking also shows that they are misguided and foolish. Their healthy and natural desire to prove their maturity is a motivation played on and encouraged by an expensive, very sophisticated, and attractive tobacco advertising campaign. Using natural psychology and clever advertising, tobacco advertisements work to get people hooked while they are still young and somewhat less discriminating. The ads also give young people the impression that it is safe to smoke with the new low-tar cigarettes.

Statistics show that 85% of teenagers who smoke more than *one* cigarette become regular smokers. With the milder low-tar cigarettes that do not make a person gag or cough when first smoked, new smokers—usually teenagers—find it even easier to get started on a smoking habit. Every 2 minutes, five teenagers start smoking, shortening their potential lifespan by 5½ minutes for every cigarette they smoke. Each year 1 million adolescents stop smoking, but 1.5 million youngsters start smoking.

People begin to smoke for a variety of reasons: as stated, smoking is a way of expressing one's independence or of gaining a false sense of maturity; smoking makes a person feel accepted by others who smoke; smoking is pleasurable and stimulating; it is psychologically enjoyable as an oral gratification; and a cigarette is always something handy to manipulate when nervous.

The most effective prevention approach is motivating teenagers and younger children to reject trying that first cigarette. Parents can play an important part in the prevention process if they themselves do not smoke or if they have quit. When parents do smoke, there is twice the chance that their high-school-aged children will also smoke. Parents can also express and support an approach to health that includes taking responsibility for one's health through life style choices. They can encourage their youngsters to realize that in order to remain healthy or become strong, their bodies need proper consideration and care. An active interest in any kind of physical prowess, endurance, or sports by the parents of young people also encourages this view.

Outside the influence of the home, parents can approach public school officials and ask them to present smoking-prevention programs or materials to the school children. Parent organizations can be especially effective in this area.

There are basically two types of school programs: the traditional health education type—smoking is bad for you, and the type that deals with the social and psychologic reasons for taking up smoking. Warnings about the dangers of smoking seem to have little positive impact, according to research studies. The second approach is more effective with adolescents: showing them how to resist the social pressures to smoke. One program uses videotapes of social situations in which teenagers might feel pressured into smoking. After 10 weeks 10% of the viewers became smokers, compared to 18.3% in the control group that did not take part in the program. This type of social awareness program is especially effective when peer counseling is involved; for example, tenth-graders counseled seventh- and eighth-graders in one California program.

One successful Canadian short-course prevention program portrayed adult smoking as a drug addiction as well as being destructive to health. With the knowledge of the mechanisms of drug addiction, the young people started to see smoking as a weakness rather than something associated with strength, independence, and adulthood. The smoking rate in the schools that used this program was 4% over a 2-year period from the beginning of the seventh grade through the end of the eighth grade, compared to a smoking rate of 17.5% in schools without the program. The total teaching time for the program was under 5 hours, and it combined films, slides, lectures, and discussions.

The 1981 report from the United States Public Health Service, *Helping Teenagers Become Nonsmokers,* describes five smoking prevention programs designed for adolescents. Four of the five programs focus on life-skills training, such as resisting peer pressure to smoke, decision-making, interpersonal communications, and environmental awareness. All the programs include the use of films and biofeedback equipment (instruments that measure stress) to emphasize both short-term and long-term effects of smoking.

Courses such as the American Health Foundation's program "Know Your Body" show promise in being able to influence children in how they think about their health and thus can affect their behavior. This is a 3-month program for grade-school and junior-high students. The program's main thrust is to teach resistance to destructive social pressures, to encourage selection of attractive role models, and to discuss nonsmoking techniques for coping with anxiety, especially in social situations. The program also informs about the consequences of smoking. Results show a high level of success: in schools that used the program, only 8% of the students started to smoke, compared to 19% in schools that did not use it.

A bibliography of *Public and Professional Education Materials* is available from the U.S. Department of Health and Human Services. It lists 290 different materials and services on smoking prevention, including (1) brochures for children and adults, (2) comic books, (3) posters for children and adults, (4) video cassettes, (5) film strips, and (6) foreign language cassettes. In addition, the department has a list of organization committees, environmental action groups, and cessation programs that are committed to smoking prevention.

The Office on Smoking and Health is one of the smallest agencies in the Department of Health and Human Services, with an overall annual budget of $2.5 million and a staff of only 19 full-time employees. It does, however, offer an extremely active information program that is dedicated to carrying out the smoking and health agenda described in its recent *Report on Smoking and Health* in this way: "The decision to smoke is a personal decision, but once this is said, it remains unquestionably the responsi-

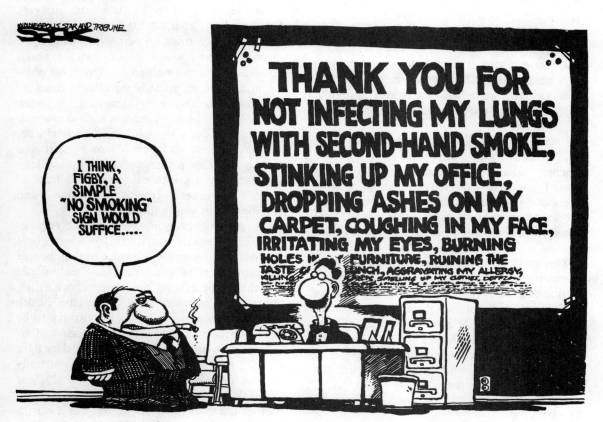

(Reprinted with permission from the Minneapolis Star and Tribune.)

bility of health officials to ensure that smokers and potential smokers are adequately informed of the hazards. This is especially true in a society where hundreds of millions of dollars are spent each year promoting cigarettes . . ."

The Office on Smoking and Health has contracted with several advertising agencies to devise a radio, television, and print campaign addressing three specific objectives:

1. To encourage children and young people, particularly girls, not to take up smoking
2. To encourage women to quit smoking, particularly during pregnancy
3. To encourage less hazardous smoking, that is, the use of low-tar low-nicotine cigarettes

Even without any formal program or back-up, an intelligent, concerned adult (parent, teacher, friend, scout leader, grandparent, coach) can lead a discussion that helps teen-agers and younger children become more critical in their analysis of smoking ads, peer pressure, and the so-called advantages of smoking.

The goal is to eliminate smoking among young people because it is thought to be an addiction of older, cough-ridden people who have no interest in maintaining their looks, health, vigor, or stamina. At present, with 55 million smokers in the United States and glamorous ads in all the print media encouraging people to smoke, this is a dream for the future, but still something to work toward now.

SUMMARY

The 1982 Surgeon General's report on smoking for the first time focused on just one disease — cancer. The evidence, if anything, is more conclusive. To quote the Surgeon General of the United States:

Cigarette smoking, as this report makes clear, is the chief single avoidable cause of death in our society and the most important public health issue of our time.

The Assistant Secretary for Health, Edward Brandt, Jr., states:

Cigarette smoking is the single major cause of cancer mortality in the United States. Tobacco's contribution to *all* cancer deaths is estimated to be 30 percent.

In other words, as a society, we could reduce the incidence of cancer by 30% — one in every three cases — by abandoning tobacco. It is difficult to translate this into personal, manageable terms, however, when we are talking about more than 250 million people. The most obvious and the most socially significant thing an individual can do is to stop smoking. By giving up smoking, a person becomes a good example and role model for children, grandchildren, brothers, sisters, and possibly parents, if it is not too late. One person who gives up smoking can also have a positive impact on at least 10 others — co-workers, friends, associates, and neighbors who would like to quit.

One person who quits can help and encourage other people from starting. Older people can influence younger people; young people can gently remind older people. Children can help their parents quit; parents can advise their children or educate them about the health hazards of smoking. We can all also try to be more honest with our smoking friends and associates who ask half-consciously as they light up, "Do you mind if I smoke?" To say steadily and yet pleasantly, "Yes, actually, I do," or "Yes, I'd appreciate it if you could wait til another time," takes courage, but it is a worthwhile response, especially if you like and respect the person about to smoke. Some people have used signs in their homes or offices requesting people not to smoke. These are less direct but can be effective.

On a societal level, many options are available to counter the tremendous impact of tobacco advertising. We can tax tobacco and use the revenue to study successful smoking cessation techniques. Research can be done on why some people never smoke, and more corporations can be encouraged to offer rewards to employees who quit, as well as to sponsor smoking-cessation clinics for their employees.

Restricting tobacco advertising, as done in several European countries, would probably be the most effective measure of all. A series of clever, colorful antismoking advertisements in all the major magazines would also be effective, but this would be costly. A small step in this direction are the posters one sees in medical offices that announce, "Smoking Is Glamorous," and then show an extremely unglamorous smoker—a more realistic portrait than those painted by the magazine ads.

Health insurance company executives, well aware of the benefits of not smoking, can work out ways to finance or pay people who successfully participate in smoking-cessation clinics. And perhaps one day a person dying of lung cancer can win a liability suit against a tobacco company for damages. If the cigarette companies are held legally responsible for the health

---

Smoking facts

1. Smoking is responsible for 83% of lung cancer deaths among men and 43% among women—greater than 75% overall. Smoking has been implicated in cancers of the mouth, throat, larynx, pancreas, and bladder.
2. Smoking accounts for 30% of all cancer deaths and is a major cause of heart disease.
3. The cancer death rate for male smokers is double that of nonsmokers and 30% higher for female smokers versus nonsmokers.
4. Smoking-related disorders are estimated to cause 325,000 premature deaths each year, with a financial burden of about $27 billion in medical care.
5. From 1976 to 1980 adult male smokers dropped from 41.9% to 36.7% and women smokers dropped from 32% to 28.9%.
6. From 1965 to 1980 the proportion of exsmokers has increased from 20.5% to 24.5% (male) and 8.2% to 15.5% (female).
7. The percentage of high-school seniors who smoke has dropped from 19.4% to 13.5%.
8. There are more than 33 million exsmokers now living in the United States.
9. Ninety-five percent of the successful quitters have done so on their own.
10. The average smoker buys about 11,000 (550 packs) cigarettes per year; the cost: approximately $500 per year.
11. Cessation clinics show a quit rate ranging from 25% to 35%, with several reports among American Cancer Society clinics and others of 50% abstinence 6 months after.
12. There is no such thing as a safe cigarette, but from 1960 to 1972 the average mortality of low-tar and low-nicotine smokers was 16% lower than high-tar high-nicotine smokers.
13. Preliminary research indicates that nonsmokers who are frequently exposed to "second-hand" smoke may have an increased risk of lung cancer.
14. Industrial workers are especially susceptible to lung disease as a result of the combined effects of industrial substances and cigarette smoke; asbestos exposure and cigarette smoking increases individuals cancer risk 60 times.
15. "The chief, single, avoidable cause of death in our society and the most important health issue of our time" is cigarette smoking, according to C. Everett Koop, 1982 U.S. Surgeon General.

Modified from 1983 Cancer facts and figures, American Cancer Society, and Surgeon General's Report on the health consequences of smoking.

damage their products cause (as many other industries are), things would change very quickly indeed.*

These valuable social programs are all possible but not necessarily quick or easy to achieve; they require people to devote a lot of time, energy, and financial output. One way an individual can easily start the ball rolling is' to write or call his or her political representative at the state and federal levels, requesting more public nonsmoking laws, more antismoking literature and advertising, higher taxes on tobacco products, and so on. Employees can request smoking restrictions in their place of work, politely but firmly (see the Resources list in Appendix B). Interestingly, a California appellate court recently ruled that an attorney who was fired for demanding a smoke-free work area can sue his former employer. Individuals who travel by public transport or patronize restaurants can request nonsmoking sections and make a point of expressing their appreciation for these areas, especially to restaurant owners.

_____
*Thanks to Gwenda Blair's article, "Why Dick Can't Stop Smoking," in *Mother Jones* for these ideas.

Parents can ask school principals to institute smoking prevention programs.

The fight against smoking will be long and hard, but there are encouraging signs. According to the Agriculture Department, the annual cigarette consumption by U.S. smokers in 1982 dropped 2% from 1981, down to a per capita intake of 3746 cigarettes. (Compare this to the 4345 average in 1963.) Also, during the 11 days immediately following the Great American Smokeout on Nov. 18, 1982, a Gallup survey reported that 4.5 million smokers quit for that day and 2.3 million were still not smoking the day they were interviewed. It appears that hardcore smokers are testing themselves more than ever.

For the individual who just wants to adopt a life-style that significantly reduces his or her own personal chances of getting cancer, the single most important thing is to refrain from smoking or to stop smoking as soon as possible. There is no way around the evidence. The best way to protect yourself from cancer is to know the facts (see boxed material on p. 197) and to stay away from tobacco or get away from it without delay.

**Thank you
for not smoking.
We'd rather die of
natural causes!**

Anonymous

CHAPTER 8

Environmental and Occupational Risks

"Here you are, lad . . . up you go!"
Stark naked and pitifully thin—the better to negotiate the dark,
narrow passage—the 8-year-old London boy scrambled up the still-warm
chimney, loosening a shower of soot.
"Look alive, mind you," the youngster's master admonished.

PHILLIP POLAKOFF
ERNEST H. ROSENBAUM

Bitter irony; alive, indeed!

Years later, in his young manhood, that London chimneysweep (or someone like him) would die of scrotal cancer in the mid-18th century—the first recorded victim of occupational cancer.

We have dramatized this incident from the factual story that has often been told before: how the English surgeon Sir Percival Pott found cancer of the scrotum among London chimneysweeps in 1775. Often starting as children, they had been exposed in their work to the sooty by-products of coal combustion—substances we now know can cause cancer.

You might reasonably suppose from this that at least we got an early start on protecting workers from cancer-causing agents on the job. Things should be much better after more than 200 years of warning, right?

Wrong! The record is dismal. Coke-oven workers in the steel industry today are still inhaling the very same kinds of substances that caused cancer among the 18th-century chimneysweeps. The death rate from lung cancer among these workers is 10 times as high as that of other steelworkers.

Some 70 years after Pott reported his findings, scrotal cancer was also discovered among copper smelter workers exposed to arsenic. Today, 136 years after the copper-smelting hazard was found, more than a million workers are inhaling the same substance, and they are dying of lung and lymphatic cancer at rates that are from two to eight times the national average.

More than 100 years ago, miners in Central Europe were found to be dying of lung cancer. Fifty years later, scientists identified the cause of the disease as radioactivity in the mines. Despite this, in 1971 thousands of American uranium miners continued to work with radioactive materials—an exposure that tripled their chances of dying from lung cancer.

199

In the late 1890s scientists found that aromatic amines were causing bladder cancer among German dye workers. During the early decades of the 20th century, such amines as benzidine and beta-naphthylamine were banned or taken off the market in the United Kingdom, Italy, Switzerland, Japan, and the Soviet Union. However, there is some uncertainty as to how scrupulously these restrictions have been observed. Less than 10 years ago, according to a report published by the New York Academy of Sciences in 1977, " . . . thousands of American workers were still literally sloshing around in these chemicals." These exposed workers are now developing—and will continue to develop—bladder tumors at an epidemic rate, based on what we know from past experience.

The deadly effects of inhaled or ingested asbestos fibers have been known for at least 80 years. However, it was only a little over 25 years ago that asbestos was identified as a potent cause of lung cancer. Yet, even today, workers are still being exposed in dozens of asbestos factories and in hundreds of asbestos-related trades.

Probably the single largest group to have experienced heavy asbestos exposure within the last 40 years consists of American shipyard workers. Since the latency period for asbestos-linked cancer can range up to 30 or 35 years or even longer, this high-risk population of some 4 million is expected to account for an upsurge in the incidence of lung cancer in the very near future. It may already have begun. In addition, the lungs are not the exclusive target for this potent carcinogen. Asbestos has also been linked with cancer of the stomach, large intestine, larynx, and rectum. It is responsible for virtually all cases of mesothelioma, a rare and always fatal cancer of the lining surrounding the lungs and abdominal cavity.

The long and depressing recital of carcinogens in the workplace over the decades—centuries in the case of the doomed chimney-sweeps—could go on and on. A final example,

however, should suffice to document the sorry record of control or abatement of the hazards.

Vinyl chloride has been a key ingredient in the manufacture of plastics for well over 35 years, but it was not until 1974 that scientists learned that it was a potential and potent cause of liver cancer. How many thousands of workers are exposed to vinyl chloride at their jobs today? How many tens of thousands of people are being exposed because they live near a plant where vinyl chloride is made? How many hundreds of thousands of individuals have been exposed because they have used aerosol sprays in which vinyl chloride was added as a propellant and solvent? What, if any, will be the consequences of these multiple exposures?

The answers are chillingly inadequate: we simply do not know.

KNOWNS AND UNKNOWNS

This thread of uncertainty runs throughout the occupational cancer tragedy—past, present and, unless there are radical changes, future. Scientists have found high cancer rates among various occupational groups, although the specific causes remain a mystery. Workers in the metal fabricating and finishing industries, for example, are known to face significant cancer risks. Four groups—boilermakers, plumbers, structural metal workers, and welders—are susceptible to bladder cancer. Aluminum mill workers and sheet metal workers have high rates of pancreatic cancer. Also, it is not just the coke-oven workers, mentioned earlier, who risk cancer in the steel industry. Studies have shown high rates of bladder, respiratory, and kidney cancer among other steelworkers. In steel finishing operations, lung cancer among workers seems especially prevalent.

Workers in the rubber industry are prone to cancers of the stomach, colon, prostate, respiratory system, and lymph- and blood-forming tissues. The rubber industry uses a vast and ever-changing variety of chemicals, many of them subject to extremely high temperatures. Is this the cancer connection?

What about chemicals in general? Not just in rubber manufacturing, but in industry as a whole, a new and often untested chemical is introduced about every 20 minutes on the average, day after day, year after year. Only a small fraction of the chemical substances now used by industry have been tested and labeled carcinogenic. No one in fact really knows just how many chemicals are in use—let alone their toxicity or carcinogenicity. We do not know what the future will reveal about the effects of such exposures that are taking place right at this moment.

What we can say with some degree of certainty is that occupational cancer poses a problem of staggering proportions. Equally true, we cannot point to any single segment of our society and say: "This is *your* responsibility, what are *you* going to do about it?" This is a problem of total concern—for individuals, for unions, for business and industry, for the scientific and academic communities, and for governments.

In trying to understand and prevent cancer, we are faced with (not yet "dealing with," as we have just seen) a social disease of significant dimensions. To approach rationally the subject of cancer prevention, or at least risk reduction, we first need to clear out some underbrush of fear, misinformation, and despair.

No, everything does not cause cancer. Scientists are simply finding more possible cancer-causing agents and predisposing conditions. This is something like crime statistics, which seem to rise constantly; this may result in part from the improvements being made in detection and reporting. The same is true about cancer, which in a real sense is a crime against your body.

No, there is no magic bullet or space-age pill you can take to prevent cancer—at least not yet.

Yes, there are things you can do for yourself to prevent (or reduce) exposure to known carcinogens. For example, you can stop smoking, cut down the amount of alcohol you drink, avoid too much sun, and when exposed to midday sun, use a sunscreen. These are all within your control, and if not controlled, they are all elements in your life-style and environment that increase the risk of cancer in one form or another.

Yes, there are a number of things that are being done *for* you to prevent cancer.

In the worker's ongoing battle against assault by cancer invaders of the workplace, he or she generally will face an enemy in one or more of four different guises: dusts and fibers, metals, chemicals, and radiation. They may work alone or, probably more often, in concert, often enhancing each other's evil potential—particularly in the presence of cigarette smoke.

DUSTS AND FIBERS

Heading any list of dust/fiber offenders is *asbestos*, which—because of its many applications and widespread use—is a possible exposure hazard for just about everybody. However, the greatest risk is among those who work directly with the raw fiber, such as shipyard workers and longshoremen. Automobile mechanics are also exposed to harmful levels of asbestos dust when grinding brake drums. Floor covering workers are exposed when they sand old asbestos tile floors in preparation for laying new tiles. Office workers may face exposure from old forced air ventilation systems that were lined with asbestos during installation. People who live and work under decaying asbestos ceiling tiles are at risk, too. Even families of workers are exposed to asbestos fibers brought home on clothing or in the hair. (More about this "bystander" effect later.) Clearly, there are virtually no boundaries to potential asbestos exposure.

The cancer rate among asbestos workers is three times the rate of disease among persons not so exposed. About 4 out of 10 workers heavily exposed to asbestos will die of cancer.

Lung cancer related to asbestos usually is the

result of long and continuous exposure. The cancer may not appear until 20 years or more after the exposure began. However, mesothelioma can develop as a result of as little as 2 months of exposure to asbestos.

Curiously, not all persons exposed to asbestos will eventually get cancer. It is still a matter of conjecture why different toxic materials affect people differently. In the case of asbestos, it may cause disease in some people but not in others working right alongside them under virtually identical circumstances. What is known is that the length of exposure to asbestos increases the risk of lung cancer. Equally certain is the vastly increased risk—up to eight times greater—if the person smokes. The figure is 40 to 50 times greater in an asbestos-exposed smoker than in a non-asbestos-exposed non-smoker.

Prevention of asbestos-related cancer (and other diseases from the same source) relies primarily on avoidance of exposure to the fibers. Here are some measures that help to accomplish this:

1. Wearing an approved respirator during all exposures.
2. Wearing protective clothing and hat.
3. Thoroughly vacuuming clothing before removing.
4. Keeping clothing in a well-vacuumed locker.
5. Showering before leaving work.
6. Having separate lockers for work and street clothes.

In addition to these measures, it is important that the employer knows about the OSHA (Occupational Safety and Health Act) asbestos standards and follows the required health-protection rules to the letter. Individual worker's rights are also set forth in the OSHA law passed in 1970, and the worker should know what these rights are and insist on them.

However, it is not only the worksite that is the battleground against occupational cancer. Studies have shown that such substances as as-bestos, arsenic, beryllium, and vinyl chloride are already associated with disease and death among people who have never worked with these substances.

Investigators from Mount Sinai School of Medicine in New York examined 326 relatives of asbestos workers from a single factory who had their first household contact with asbestos 25 to 30 years earlier. X-ray films disclosed evidence of asbestos-related disease in the lungs of 35% of the relatives, including four fatal cases of mesothelioma. Unnecessary cancer death is always tragic, but there is a special poignancy in the deaths of these four victims who never had any direct contact with asbestos. As reported by the New York Academy of Sciences, they included:

1. A 32-year-old woman who, at age 13, lived in the home of her brother-in-law while he worked at the plant for 6 months. Before that, she lived near the plant and often played in the homes of friends whose fathers worked there.
2. A 40-year-old man whose father worked in the asbestos plant for 3 years until the son was 11 years old.
3. The daughter of the plant engineer. She died at age 41.
4. The 42-year-old daughter of a man who had worked in the plant for 5 years. Her contact with asbestos? When she was 10 years old, she took lunch to her father at the plant every day.

These "innocent bystanders" were not asbestos workers. They were victims of a flank attack by this pervasive material. Can their deaths be regarded as occupational? M. Newhouse of the London School of Hygiene and Tropical Medicine has an answer that is hard to dispute: "I really regard these deaths as occupational deaths. If the factory weren't there, they wouldn't have been exposed to asbestos."

Asbestos is an insidious hazard because it is so difficult to remove; 20 years after one plant had closed, asbestos dust was found in the homes of former workers. This raises the grim possibility that unsuspecting occupants of these dwellings could be at risk even after the former asbestos workers and their families had moved.

In view of this chance of lingering hazard, scientists stress that under no circumstances should asbestos workers bring home their dusty work clothes for laundering. Showers and changing facilities should be provided at the worksite, and the work clothes sent out to commercial industrial laundries equipped to handle contaminated clothing. However, even this solution is not adequate. Mesothelioma has occurred among commercial laundry workers who had been handling asbestos-contaminated clothing. As with most industrial contaminants, a better solution is control of the dust at the source.

Using a less hazardous material to replace one known to carry risks is sometimes an effective preventive measure, but this must be done with great care. A good example is *fibrous glass*, which has been showing up in recent years as a substitute for asbestos in many insulating and fireproofing materials. However, since fibrous glass is also made up of tiny fibers, scientists are naturally concerned that inhaling particles of this substitute could also cause cancer.

Investigation of this possible risk has been complicated by a couple of factors. First, the physical characteristics of glass fiber, unlike natural fibers, can and do change continuously according to use. Second, since commercial production of fibrous glass in the United States dates back only to about 1933, not enough time had elapsed until just recently for job-related cancer to begin showing up. In the meantime two possibly related events occurred: (1) various studies showed that fibrous glass causes cancer in experimental animals and (2) a large number of fibrous glass workers were retiring on disability because of chronic bronchitis. In light of these facts the National Institute for Occupational Safety and Health (NIOSH) launched a major study of disease and death in the fibrous glass industry.

NIOSH's study of the causes of death among 1448 workers exposed to low levels of airborne glass fibers showed a high rate of nonmalignant respiratory disease but no excess risk of lung cancer. However, the study did indicate risk of lung cancer among workers involved during the early years of fibrous glass production. At that time a process exposed them to glass particles of very small diameter. Processes used today also produce fibers that are much thinner than in the past, and small-diameter fibers have caused cancer in animals. These relationships are a cause for concern. Until more is known about the risk from fibrous glass, scientists are emphasizing that exposure should be kept to a minimum through good engineering and good work practices.

Workers in two other industrial categories— *wood products* and *textiles*—also face exposure to potentially cancer-causing dusts. A study of nearly 300,000 death records in the state of Washington, conducted by S. Milham of the Washington State Department of Social and Health Services under a NIOSH contract, disclosed an unusually high rate of cancer among workers in the wood products industry. Types of cancer varied with the particular jobs performed. However, cancer of the stomach and of the lymph- and blood-forming tissues was found at high rates among nearly all the occupational groups surveyed. These included carpenters, loggers, professional foresters, pulp and paper mill workers, and plywood mill workers.

Wood products may present a dual risk: dust for the most part but edging into the chemical hazard in some processes. The Washington study indicated that the stomach cancers could have resulted from swallowing wood particles. On the other hand, the cancers of the blood and lymphatic systems might have been caused by the chemical breakdown of wood. This would particularly affect workers at the mills producing pulp, paper, and plywood. Interestingly, the study showed a lesser cancer risk among workers in sawmills, where the wood is simply machined, compared to the higher risks among workers in those occupations where chemicals are involved.

Other types of cancers found in the Washington study and the predominant groups in which they occurred included: prostate (loggers); lungs, pancreas, and rectum (professional foresters whose work exposes them to a variety of environments such as mills, offices, and forests); small intestine (pulp and paper mill workers); and pancreas and testes (sawmill workers and those engaged in other wood-machining operations).

Since all of these groups have one thing in common—they all work with wood—can we conclude that wood is a cancer-causing agent? Studies in England and Sweden reveal some interesting evidence. Cancer of the nasal passages and sinuses was found among English furniture workers. In Sweden researchers found unusually high rates of sinus cancer among woodworkers. According to the Swedish cancer registry, approximately 45% of all recorded cases of nasal sinus cancer in that country occur among woodworkers.

It is noteworthy that the Washington study revealed no nasal sinus cancer among woodworkers in that state. A possible explanation of this somewhat puzzling aspect of the studies here and abroad may be found in the fact that the American workers deal mostly with softwoods, whereas their British and Swedish counterparts work mostly with hardwoods.

Dusts and fibers are also suspected in the higher rates of certain cancers among British textile workers. Cancers of the tongue, mouth, and throat are more common among textile workers than in the general population, with a death rate three times as high. Researchers at the Department of Occupational Health at the University of Manchester (England) have ruled out smoking, drinking, wearing dentures, or chewing regularly on bits of material (apparently a fairly common habit) as possible causes of the cancers.

Thus the prime cancer-causing suspect appears to be dust, particularly that generated in the initial cleaning of the raw fibers. Traditionally, dust and dirt are removed from raw wool and cotton by beating and crushing the unwanted material into fine particles. These are then shaken out and blown or vacuumed away. Obviously, investigators point out, a lot of this dust finds its way into the noses, mouths, and throats of the workers.

Among handlers of wool there may be a dual hazard similar to that mentioned earlier for woodworkers when chemicals are involved. In the British study the cancer incidence and mortality rates appear to be higher among those who work with wool than with cotton. Raw wool often contains residues of sheep dip, a pesticide that contains arsenic.

Whether in woodworking, textile making, or any other activity in which hazardous dusts or fibers can become airborne, the best prevention lies in controlling the offending material at the source. Engineering and design technologies in many cases can enclose, isolate, and mechanize operations. Adequate ventilation of the worksite can prevent dispersion of the dust and fibers into the breathing zone of the workers and the general environment. Respirators to protect individual operators are available, but generally they should be used only to provide an extra margin of safety. They may be used appropriately in emergencies or during maintenance operations in which reliance on mechanical control of the pollution is not feasible. Nevertheless, masks should be required for workers in areas where there are unavoidable dusts, vapors, and mists.

METALS

Occupational diseases associated with metals are among the oldest on record. Slaves toiling in the mines of ancient Greece and Rome were poisoned by such toxic metals as lead and mercury. A number of metals or metallic compounds, including arsenic, cadmium, chromates, iron, and nickel are known to cause cancer in humans and animals. Lead, selenium, titanium, cobalt, and zinc do not cause cancer. Because metals occur naturally in the environment, a worker's on-the-job exposure does not end with the workshift. Outside the office or factory gate, the worker continues to be exposed to metals in the air, in the water, in food; since the body is slow to eliminate many metals, they may accumulate in tissue and produce long-range effects.

As with some woodworkers and textile workers, people who work with metals and metallic compounds also face a double-barreled risk potential. First, they are exposed to the metals and metallic compounds that are the basic ingredients of the products they build or handle. Second, some of the substances used in various processing steps may also be hazardous. For example, in the course of performing their jobs, workers may come in contact with lubricants, chemical fumes, and other agents that might cause cancer.

A study of metal workers in 10 occupational groups in the state of Washington showed high rates of respiratory cancer. The groups included boilermakers, copper smelter workers, machinists, metal molders, plumbers, structural metal workers, sheet metal workers, aluminum mill workers, welders, and tool-and-die makers. As stated earlier, in addition to the lung cancer found in all groups, four worker categories — boilermakers, plumbers, structural metal workers, and welders — also appear to be susceptible to cancer of the bladder. Cancer of the tongue was evident among machinists, plumbers, and structural metal workers. Malignant lymphoma was found to be common among aluminum mill workers and plumbers.

Some reservations have been expressed about the possible metallic cause of the cancers among the aluminum mill workers. The cancers in this group seem to be concentrated among workers in pot rooms where they are exposed to volatiles of coal-tar pitch. Some researchers suggest that these substances, rather than the metal itself, may be responsible for the cancers among the aluminum workers.

For a number of years cancer hazards in the steel industry were throught to be largely confined to coke plants, in particular coke-oven areas. However, a study of workers throughout a large Baltimore steel plant by E. Radford of Johns Hopkins University revealed high rates of cancers of the bladder, kidney, and respiratory system. Although the study did not link the cancers with any specific substances, it suggested that cancer-causing agents may be more widespread in steel manufacturing than was previously thought.

Although perhaps less prone to change than other industries, steelmaking nevertheless is constantly introducing new processes. This may mean that workers are exposed to new substances or combinations of substances that can carry unsuspected health effects. Steel finishing operations, for example, change frequently; it was in this area of the plant that the Baltimore study made the then surprising finding of numerous lung cancers.

A study by the National Cancer Institute found that lung cancer deaths increased steadily with the length of exposure to *arsenic*, ranging from two to five times the expected rate. The same study also showed that the greatest number of deaths occurred among those workers exposed both to arsenic and sulfur dioxide. This suggests that sulfur dioxide may be a cocarcinogen that enhances the cancer-causing properties of the arsenic.

As many as 100,000 workers are exposed to *cadmium*, which studies have shown may be responsible for cancers of the lungs and prostate. A NIOSH study of cadmium workers showed lung cancer rates more than twice as high as the expected rates. Workers exposed to cadmium for 20 years or longer ran an especially significant risk of prostate cancer.

Cadmium is a versatile as well as demonstrably hostile metal with numerous applications in industry. It is used in the electroplating and rubber industries; in nickel-cadmium batteries; in brazing/soldering alloys, pigments, and chemicals; and as a stabilizing agent in plastics.

What about other metals and metallic compounds? *Nickel* is known to cause lung cancer. *Chromium* compounds have been linked with cancers of the nasal and sinus cavities, lungs, and larynx. *Iron oxide* is associated with cancer of the lung and larynx. *Lead*, although it has been recognized as a poison for at least 1000 years, is not believed to be a potent carcinogen in humans. Some studies in which animals were fed large amounts of lead salts showed evidence of kidney tumors. However, a study of more than 7000 smelter and battery plant workers turned up no unusually high numbers of urinary tract cancers.

On the other hand, lead workers are often given drugs known as chelating agents to reduce the levels of lead in their blood. This can give the impression that the workers are exposed to significantly lower levels of lead than is actually the case. This practice, widespread in the industry, is a cause of concern among professionals dealing with workers' health and safety.

Prevention, again, largely focuses on avoiding or minimizing exposure. There are several ways of doing this: using the best available technology, alternative materials, and protective "threshold limit values" (TLVs).

The TLV simply means the highest level of a substance that a person can be exposed to without suffering certain ill effects. However, according to some scientists, there is little evidence that thresholds for carcinogens exist; nobody certainly has ever found one. Although important, TLVs are generally designed to protect workers from short-term effects, such as dizziness or irritation. However, as seen in the case of asbestos, they are far from adequate in protecting workers and their families from carcinogens.

Arsenic is something of a special case when it comes to setting a threshold since it occurs naturally in the environment. This natural level is called the "ambient level," and NIOSH has set the occupational exposure to arsenic at approximately the ambient level found in the United States. Since arsenic can cause cancer in at least three body organs—skin, lungs, and the lymphatic system—it is important that job exposures not add to the body's natural burden of arsenic.

CHEMICALS

Turning to chemicals as possible sources of occupational cancer, we are faced with a bewildering cauldron of substances. No one really knows what the deluge of industrial chemicals introduced over the last few decades is doing to workers' health. We do not even know with any exactness just how many chemicals are in use.

The uncertainty about individual chemicals is complicated by lack of knowledge about how they might work in combination with one another. In our chemical-laden society exposure to combinations of carcinogens is the rule, not the exception. Studies show that some substances acting together produce more tumors in a shorter time than either one acting separately. This synergistic effect is dramatically illustrated in studies showing that cancer rates are far higher among asbestos workers and uranium miners who smoke, for example, than among those who do not. Any listing of all possible chemical risks probably would be out of date by the time you turned this page, but following are some of the most notorious, the longest known or suspected, and the most thoroughly studied substances:

Vinyl chloride leaped into public consciousness as a cause of occupational cancer in January 1974, when the B.F. Goodrich Company announced that three workers at its Louisville, Kentucky, vinyl chloride plant had angiosarcoma, an extremely rare form of liver cancer. The Goodrich disclosure prompted NIOSH to initiate studies of workers at four vinyl chloride plants to get some idea of the extent of the hazard. The plants selected had been polymerizing vinyl chloride for between 20 and 32 years. Because of the long latency period between initial exposure and the appearance of cancer, the researchers focused on those workers who had been working with vinyl chloride for 5 years or more and whose initial exposure to the chemical had begun at least 10 years earlier.

The study found higher than expected rates of death from cancer of the liver—the incidence that triggered the investigation—but also fatal cancers in other organs and systems. These included cancers of the brain and central nervous system, respiratory system, and lymph- and blood-forming tissues. Another finding was that the longer the elapsed time since the first exposure to vinyl chloride, the higher the death rate. Workers who had been exposed for the first time 15 years earlier had higher death rates than those whose initial exposure was 10 years before.

The NIOSH researchers also studied any cancer deaths among former employees of the four plants regardless of whether the victims had been exposed for 5 years or had passed the 10-year latency period. This phase of the study revealed the case of a man who had been exposed to vinyl chloride for about 3 years and had died at age 41 of angiosarcoma—17 years after his exposure. This confirms the belief that the cancer process is irreversible and continues for many years, even after exposure to the carcinogen has ceased.

There is an ironic footnote to the tragedy at Goodrich. Years earlier, scientists had found liver cancer, as well as tumors of the brain, kidney, lung, and lymphatic system, among laboratory animals exposed to vinyl chloride. This underscores the need for prompt recognition by industry of scientific evidence of hazardous substances and for rapid implementation of protective measures for workers.

Foot-dragging in acknowledging that a danger exists—and consequently not doing anything about it—is often the result of studies that appear to be contradictory. Some studies of job hazards, including vinyl chloride, have shown fewer deaths among workers than would be expected in the general population, at least for the first 5 to 10 years covered by the study. This is often the result of what has been called the "healthy worker effect." In other words, the healthiest members of the population are the ones most likely to be hired and the least likely to show early ill effects.

People in poor health tend to shun, and properly so, jobs in which they might be exposed to substances and working conditions that would aggravate their conditions. This is especially true of jobs that generate dust and fumes. Furthermore, employers often refuse to hire these people on the basis of preemployment health examinations.

The NIOSH study avoided clouding its results with the healthy worker effect by restricting its study to workers whose first exposure to vinyl chloride had been at least 10 years earlier. This tends to equalize the advantage of good health enjoyed by some workers at the start of employment over others not so fortunate.

Even before the cancers in the Louisville plant came to light, vinyl chloride had come under suspicion. Widely used in the late 1960s in aerosol sprays and the manufacture of plastics, the chemical became implicated in May 1970 when P.L. Viola of the Cancer Institute in Rome reported that high doses of aerosol sprays caused cancer in animals. Its use in aerosols has since been banned, and plastics manufacturers have altered various processes to avoid worker exposure.

Vinyl chloride is an important ingredient in phonograph records, product packaging, medical tubing, household utensils, bathroom fixtures, and a number of other plastic products. The plastic products themselves pose no danger. But workers in a vinyl chloride factory had a 200 times greater risk than the general public of developing liver cancer.

A close relative of vinyl chloride—*chloroprene*, used in manufacturing polychloroprene rubber—is now also under suspicion.

Benzene is another chemical that signaled its harmful potential to scientists long before it began to be detected as the causative agent for specific diseases. Medical researchers knew more than 100 years ago that benzene was a powerful poisoner of bone marrow, destroying its ability to produce blood cells. Later, repeated exposure was shown to produce a noncancerous but often fatal condition known as aplastic anemia. Over the long term this can lead to leukemia; the first case of "benzene leukemia" was identified in 1928.

Corroborating evidence that benzene is an occupational hazard has come from studies in other countries. Before Italy banned the use of benzene in 1963, scientists had reported that the risk of leukemia among workers in rotogravure and shoe manufacturing plants was 20 times higher than for the general population. However, since the Italian rotogravure (a printing process) industry began using toluene instead of benzene as a solvent, no cases of job-related leukemia or aplastic anemia have come to light.

A Japanese study of the possible link between benzene and leukemia provides another interesting sidelight. Among adult survivors of the atomic bomb blasts at Hiroshima and Nagasaki who had leukemia, the researchers found that the risk of the disease was two and one half times higher for those who had a history of job exposure to benzene or medical x-ray films.

The rubber industry has been a major source of exposure to benzene, once the most commonly used solvent. In a study of various jobs in that industry, researchers at the University of North Carolina School of Public Health found that workers exposed to solvents have three times the normal risk of leukemia. This rate rises to five times normal for those with high levels of exposure.

In addition to benzene, other known or suspected carcinogens now used or used in the past by the rubber tire industry include *beta-naphthylamine, talc dust containing asbestos,* and various *nitrosamines*. Furthermore, the extremely high temperatures required in several rubber manufacturing processes release any number of unidentified chemical substances.

The North Carolina scientists also sought to link other types of cancers besides leukemia with specific jobs and chemicals in the rubber industry. Analyzing cancer deaths over a 10-year period, they found higher than expected numbers of deaths from cancer in general and especially high rates of cancers of the stomach, colon, prostate, and the lymph- and blood-forming systems.

The study also indicated a connection between lung cancer and work in the curing room. Stomach cancer was most common among people who had worked in compounding, mixing, and milling and in jobs that brought the workers in contact with "green rubber." One of the possible causes of stomach cancer, the researchers believed, might be the result of swallowing *carbon black*, a compound containing the carcinogen benzpyrene, as well as asbestos and nitrosamines.

Bladder cancer was most prevalent among rubber workers likely to come in contact with raw-ingredient chemicals. These people are generally working at the beginning of the production line, such as in shipping and receiving, compounding, mixing, milling, and colendering.

The study showed no clear connection between cancer of the prostate and any specific job. However, such cancers did show up among workers in the compounding and mixing areas where metallic oxides are used as accelerators in the vulcanizing process. Among the compounds used is *cadmium oxide*, which has been linked with prostate cancer in the past.

Although the rubber, plastics, and paint industries are users of a wide variety of chemicals, they are by no means the only industrial sources of potential carcinogens. *Benzpyrene*, found in asphalt and hot pitch, has been linked to a high rate of cancer among roofers and waterproofers. *Bis (chloromethyl) ether (BCME),* an alkylating agent used in a number of industrial processes and for killing bacteria and fungi, is known to cause lung cancer. Machine operators exposed to lubricating and cooling fluids while cutting and grinding metals have developed cancers of the hands, arms, and scrotum. Scientists are also concerned that the oil mists released during machine operations may pose an additional hazard to workers who inhale them.

It is not only in dirty, dusty, and oily environments, however, that the risk of cancer lurks. In what should be the cleanest of all places to work—the hospital operating room—there is danger from anesthetic gases that leak from operating room equipment. A nationwide survey showed that physicians, anesthesiologists, and nurse anesthetists are exposed to small amounts of such gases and that they develop cancer, especially leukemia and lymphoma, at rates nearly twice as high as medical personnel who do not work in operating rooms.

Occupational cancer is by no means a worry only for people who work in factories, offices, or an urban environment in general. Agricultural workers are exposed to a wide range of pesticides, herbicides, and fertilizers. Many of these materials are a veritable "witches' brew" of chemical components. Some of these are known to cause human cancer (arsenic, for example) or have proved to be carcinogenic in animal studies or have been shown to be mutagenic in short-term tests. Agricultural pesticides find their way into the food chain and often accumulate in biologic systems, possibly far "downstream" from the original site of application.

How can we prevent, or at least substantially reduce, chemically caused cancer in the workplace? There are several viable ways of controlling carcinogens, short of outright banning:

1. Where there are good animal data or good human data or both, we should encourage industry explicitly, rather than implicitly, to substitute noncarcinogenic chemicals for carcinogenic ones.
2. If there are no substitutes, or if it is alleged that there are none, then industry should use the hazardous substance only with adequate and sensitive monitoring.
3. We should make the fullest use of our monitoring technology, which is capable of going down to the part-per-billion level. It is essential that these steps are coupled with full and honest disclosure of information and adequate and retrievable record retention.

RADIATION

Radiation—the fourth potential cause of environmental and occupational cancer—is the process by which energy is propagated through space or matter in the form of waves. It has been with us since the dawn of time. More than half of the radiation we receive is from natural sources: the sun bombards the earth constantly with radioactive particles, and the earth itself subjects us to radiation from such widely distributed materials as granite, phosphates, and natural gas. Even our bodies contain tiny traces of radioactive elements.

There are two kinds of radiation: ionizing and nonionizing. Nonionizing radiation comes from that part of the electromagnetic spectrum consisting of relatively low-frequency waves. This is the sort of radiation we get from radio waves, microwaves, infrared (heat) radiation, visible light, and ultraviolet light. Nonionizing radiation is less powerful than ionizing radiation, but it can harm cells by breaking chemical bonds.

Ionizing radiation, on the other hand, is powerful enough to knock electrons off atoms or molecules. Ions are formed in this process, which in turn may create harmful compounds in the body that can interfere with the normal working of cells. Ionizing radiation includes such things as x-rays, gamma rays, and particulate radiation.

Natural background radiation includes cosmic rays from outer space and radiation from naturally occurring cosmic rays from radioisotopes in our bodies and in rocks and water. The amount we receive varies according to such factors as the altitudes at which we live; the higher the elevation, the greater the amount of radiation. The average in the United States is about 0.08 rem per year (a rem is a unit of radiation). By the time a person is 70 years old, he or she will have received, on the average, about 14 rem.

Medical radiation exposure is mainly from diagnostic radiology. The amount of radiation given for one x-ray film may be quite large, such as 2 rem for a lateral lumbar spine film, but the average for the entire body and the whole population for routine diagnostic tests is only about 0.1 rem per year. The body has some ability to neutralize the effect of minor x-ray films, and a number of small exposures spread over the years is not as harmful as a single large dose.

When a medical or dental x-ray examination is necessary, you can insist that exposure be limited to what is necessary and useful. Here are some suggestions:

1. Ask how the x-ray film will help with the diagnosis. You have a right to know this.
2. Tell your physician if you are or might be pregnant.
3. Ask if it is possible to use a lead apron to protect the rest of your body, particularly the reproductive organs. This may not always be possible, however, since the shield may cover an area that the doctor needs to see on the x-ray film.
4. Be especially careful whenever a child is involved. Children are at least five times more sensitive to radiation-induced cancer than adults.
5. Keep a record of all x-ray films, showing the date given, name of the physician, type of examination, and place where the film is kept on file. If an x-ray film is suggested for the same part of the body, tell your physician about the previous films. If a new film is still needed, the earlier ones might help to show any changes in your medical problem.
6. Finally, do not insist on an x-ray film. Sometimes physicians may give in to patients who ask for films although they are not medically needed.

Other man-made sources of radiation include such diverse items as color TV sets, airport baggage inspection systems, luminous dial watches, tobacco, and some types of glass and ceramics (the latter usually from various pigments that may contain small amounts of radioactive material). All of these sources may contribute small amounts of radiation, with an average exposure for the whole population of about 0.002 rem.

The probabilities of getting cancer from radiation in everyday life (excluding a nuclear war) are slight. Many studies are now in agreement that if a woman, for example, receives abdominal x-ray films during pregnancy, the child's subsequent risk of developing leukemia is increased from four cases per 100,000 children to about six cases. Although this additional risk is very small, present practice is to avoid x-ray films during pregnancy except for emergencies.

Nuclear power plants release radiation into air and water. Although the effect is believed to be minimal—less than the contamination from a coal-burning power plant—there is still a great deal of uncertainty in this relatively new field. We will have to await the test of time to be certain. The maximum radiation known to be received by anyone living near the Three Mile Island power station, for example, was 0.04 rem—one-half the average person's annual dose. The potential risk from fatal cancer from this dose is 1:100,000, or one additional death from cancer in the Three Mile Island vicinity. This should be compared to the normal risk of fatal cancer of 1:7.

Ultraviolet rays of sunshine penetrate the skin and can cause damage ranging from premature aging of the skin to wrinkles and dryness. The dangers include benign skin conditions, keratoses, and skin cancers, the most virulent being malignant melanoma. The risk and range of susceptibility depend on several factors: where you live, length of exposure and strength of the rays, thickness and color of the skin, and parts of the body exposed. Darker skin pigments contain melanin, a brown skin pigment that is a natural filter against the sun's rays. Blue-eyed blonds and redheads and people with light-colored skin have less melanin and therefore burn more easily. Melanoma is rare in blacks and most prevalent in fair-skinned whites. Superficial skin cancers, primarily basal cell and squamous cell cancers, are curable about 95% of the time.

Here are some suggestions for avoiding skin cancer caused by undue exposure to sunlight:

1. Avoid the sun during midday, when the rays are strongest. About 60% of each day's carcinogenic radiation is received between 10 AM and 2 PM. A suntan may prevent further sunburn, but it does not protect the skin from sun damage, which may not be visible for many years.
2. Remember that burning ultraviolet rays occur even on overcast days. They are invisible and not screened by clouds.
3. Cover exposed areas of the body; when feasible, wear a hat and long-sleeved shirt.
4. Do not depend on beach umbrellas. They offer little protection from sun rays reflected by sand, water, or snow.
5. Use a sunscreen according to PABA (paraminobenzoic acid) rating. Sunscreens are numbered from 2 to 15, with the higher rating giving ing better protection. The more expensive sunscreens offer no advantage over the inexpensive ones; only the rating matters. The ideal sunscreen should penetrate the skin's outer layer and not be lost in perspiration or easily washed or rubbed off. No preparation remains effective during prolonged swimming; therefore, it should be reapplied when you come out of the water.
6. Avoid mineral, olive, or baby oil. Oils magnify the sun's burning effect.

7. Dermatologists agree that sunlamps and taning salons produce skin damage and must be used with great caution.

WORKPLACE PREVENTION AND RECOMMENDATIONS

Cancer's reach is indeed long. Its agents can come at us from many different directions—our jobs, our food and water, the air we breathe, the sun, even our present life-styles and, further back, our genetic inheritance from distant ancestors.

So, what can you as an individual do to prevent becoming a victim of this many tentacled menace?

In a larger context, what can industry and labor unions do to control cancer hazards in the workplace? Since all control methods are variations on the basic principle of avoidance of contact, here are some strategies:

1. Substitute a different, safer substance, or change the dangerous substance to a different and safer form. Dusty powders, for example, are often available in bricks that do not stir up dust when handled.
2. Change the hazardous way of doing a job. Use detergents or steam, for instance, instead of organic solvents for cleaning.
3. Mechanize the process. Can an automatic parts dipper, for example, be used on a vapor degreaser instead of having a worker manually dip parts into a tank?
4. Isolate the process. Hazardous-exposure jobs often can be moved to a different part of the plant where fewer people are working. Can the job be done at a different time—on weekends or the midnight shift?
5. Enclose the operation. This puts a barrier between the worker and the hazard. An example is a splash guard and hoods over machining operations involving cutting fluids. Pumping solvents instead of manually dumping them from one container to another is also sometimes feasible.
6. Provide exhaust ventilation. If none of the pre-

vious techniques can be used, local exhaust ventilation can often be used to control the hazard. This is a common solution to many health hazard problems, such as occur in spray painting and grinding operations.

7. Improve housekeeping. Failure to perform this simple but absolutely essential job can cause toxic materials to be reintroduced into the air, causing additional and needless exposure. Vacuuming is the best way to clean up dusts. Dry sweeping often makes the problem worse. Of course, the best way to avoid poor housekeeping is to have the toxic materials contained *before* they can become a problem.

8. Provide personal protective equipment—but only as an added margin of safety or in an emergency. Good industrial hygiene and OSHA regulations insist that engineering controls must be tried first.

9. Conduct periodic and appropriate medical examinations for high-risk populations at periodic intervals.

While not a cancer preventive measure in the strictest sense, since it would come after the fact, we can prevent the tragedy from deepening by providing adequate and appropriate compensation to assist victims and their families.

SUMMARY

At the highest level of concern, our national organizations, both government and nongovernment, should reverse the present course of responding to the cancer problem on a crisis-to-crisis basis. We have tended to become so agitated over effects (the vinyl chloride story is a good example) that we lose sight of the causes and the urgent need to prevent such crises from arising in the first place.

The federal government has been handicapped in its efforts to come to grips with the problem of occupational cancer by a number of factors, including:

1. The lack of a national consensus on funding research.
2. The large number of individual agencies with separate authority and different approaches to cancer control.
3. Major gaps in data available to the government and in the government's power to obtain data from private industry. (Vigorously used, the Toxic Substances Control Act could go a long way toward closing these gaps.)
4. The long latency period for occupational cancer, which makes causes and effects difficult to identify and prove. Most of our laws are tilted toward dealing with immediate health effects.

The need—and it is being recognized among government agencies and various scientific groups—is for adherence to three basic principles:

1. Any substance that definitely causes tumors in animals should be considered carcinogenic and a potential cancer hazard in humans.
2. It makes no difference whether the substance causes benign or cancerous tumors. A benign tumor often turns cancerous. There is no chemical substance known that produces *only* benign tumors.
3. There is no known way of determining a safe level of exposure to any substance that is shown to cause cancer in animals.

The real issue in occupational/environmental cancer is not so much *if* we can prevent it, but whether we are *willing*. We are dealing with a "social disease" in the truest sense, a disease deeply rooted in the economy, politics, and the technology of our society—the values given highest priority by us. Cancer prevention in the workplace and elsewhere is largely an attainable goal, but reaching that goal will require the coordinated efforts of all parts of society—government, industry, labor, the scientific community, and an informed public.

CHAPTER 9

Stress, Personality, and Cancer

Well, I don't get angry, okay?
I mean, I have a tendency to internalize.
I can't express anger.
That's one of the problems I have.
I . . . I grow a tumor instead.

WOODY ALLEN
MARSHALL BRICKMAN
from *Manhattan*

STEVEN E. LOCKE

In recent years it has become popular to "psychologize" medical illnesses. This has partly been caused by the tendency of physicians for many years to overemphasize the technical aspects of patient care. Currently, the pendulum is swinging the other way—perhaps even too far—so that some people have claimed that all illnesses are "psychosomatic." Clearly, we have underestimated the importance of behavioral factors in disease risk in the past. The role of type A behavior (high-pressured, overly aggressive, overly ambitious) in determining risk of coronary heart disease is a good example.

In the case of cancer, several such ideas have gained widespread popularity despite the scarcity of scientific evidence. These ideas include:

1. There is a cancer-prone personality type.
2. Stress, especially bereavement, can cause cancer.
3. Among patients having cancer, "positive" mental attitudes improve outcome of the disease, whereas "negative" outlooks lead to more rapid progression.
4. Mental strategies and treatments can strengthen the body's resistance and thereby control or even cure cancer.

Since the focus of this book is on the *prevention* of cancer, this discussion will concentrate on the first two ideas.

The popular appeal of these ideas has been remarkable. Although such beliefs may offer hope to many patients, they can also increase the burden of guilt already felt by many cancer patients because of the impact of the illness on their loved ones. The belief that one is responsible for contributing to the cause of one's cancer is a double-edged sword; whereas for some this belief can create a sense of hope for self-control, for others it can produce painful feelings of guilt.

There are several theoretical ways through

This work was supported in part by a Young Investigator Award from the National Cancer Institute (CA-29155).

213

which human behavior could influence the risk or outcome of cancer. These possibilities can be broken down into several categories. First, behavioral factors could cause a new cancer to develop or they could allow a preexisting tumor either to grow or spread more rapidly. Second, behavioral factors can have either a direct or an indirect effect. Through a *direct* effect aspects of behavior such as personality traits, stress, or moods might act directly to encourage tumor development and growth, presumably by affecting the body's endocrine system and suppressing natural cancer immunity. In contrast, *indirect* behavioral effects are those that result from things people do to themselves, such as smoking, drinking, or consuming excessive fat in the diet, thereby secondarily exposing themselves to known carcinogens. Given these possible mechanisms of action, we can explore the ways in which behavioral factors such as personality, stress, and life-style might increase cancer risk. To start, we should consider the nature of these behavioral factors.

Personality traits are enduring qualities of character that reflect our uniqueness and determine the quality of our relationships with others. These traits can be measured quite easily with paper and pencil tests called personality inventories; the Minnesota Multiphasic Personality Inventory (MMPI) is the best known of these. *Moods*, on the other hand, are emotional states that change from moment to moment and reflect how we "feel."

Stress is a popular word currently in vogue. However, its use has been widely criticized by physicians and scientists because the term is too vague and poorly defined. For example, some people use the word "stress" to refer to something external that happens to them and has an impact requiring readjustment. Others use the term to mean a collection of internal symptoms experienced by people when they feel they cannot cope. We favor the latter definition—namely, that *stress is the preception by individuals that their life circumstances have overwhelmed* *their capacity to cope.* Depression, anxiety, and certain minor physical complaints such as headache are often symptoms of stress.

Life-style is a vague term encompassing all the behaviors that collectively reflect how a particular person grapples with modern living from day to day. It includes community and social ties, as well as work, play, diet, and exercise habits. Certain of these factors, acting either alone or together, are known to have an important bearing on risk of cancer. Examples are dietary habits, occupational health hazards, and cigarette smoking.

PERSONALITY AS A RISK FACTOR FOR CANCER

The notion that some people, because of their personality, are more likely to get cancer is an ancient idea. The Greek physician Galen is reported to have said in the 2nd century that "melancholic" women were more prone to develop breast cancer. In the modern era research on personality and cancer was pioneered by psychologist L. LeShan, who concluded after interviewing hundreds of patients with cancer that cancer patients lead lonely, emotionally isolated lives and tend to be self-condemning. Another early researcher was C. Bahnson, who also asked cancer patients about their lives before the development of their disease. According to Bahnson, cancer patients were more likely to describe their parents as having been neglecting and cold than were patients with other diseases. D. Kissen concluded from his studies of cancer patients that they suppressed their expression of feelings more than other patients.

These types of studies—called *retrospective* studies—are limited in what they can tell us about the personality characteristics of people who develop cancer because the "backward view" through the patient's life is colored by the present experience of living with the disease. Chronic diseases often slant our view of the past so that a cancer patient's memories of childhood may be distorted.

The best solution to this problem is to evaluate the personality characteristics of large numbers of healthy people and then wait 20 or 30 years until a portion of them go on to develop cancer. The researcher can then check the records obtained many years earlier to see which personality characteristics predicted the later development of the disease. This may sound easy, but there is a big problem with this type of research: it is extremely expensive. Only a small portion of the group may actually develop cancer during the period of the study. Thus the lives and health status of a large number of healthy people must be followed for many years. To determine just how unwieldy and expensive such *prospective* studies can be, B. Fox, a behavioral epidemiologist at the National Cancer Institute, used statistical methods to determine just how many people would be needed. He calculated that more than 10,000 people would have to be followed for 20 years or more!

One way of reducing the cost of these types of studies is to use research data from groups of people studied for other reasons. Two such studies have been conducted and have yielded results that are surprisingly similar.

For the past 35 years C. Thomas of the Johns Hopkins Medical School has been following the health status of over 1300 medical school graduates who had completed a battery of psychologic tests administered during medical school. As of 1978, 200 out of 913 male graduates had developed certain medical illnesses: cancer, coronary heart disease, high blood pressure, benign tumors, and mental illness.

Among these men, the group who later developed cancer reported different family attitudes in youth from those of their healthy classmates. The items checked on a questionnaire about family attitudes by the future cancer group indicated a lack of closeness to parents when compared with the items checked by the healthy group. The family attitudes of the cancer group resembled those of the group who later developed mental illness or committed suicide. In contrast, the family attitudes of the coronary heart disease and the high blood pressure groups were similar to those of the healthy group. These findings, initially based on a small number of cancer cases, have held up as new cancer cases have been added over the years. Although they support some of the ideas suggested by the older retrospective studies, these findings are not free of controversy. Critics have pointed out that the researchers had evaluated the contributions of so many psychologic factors that it was probable that some accidental connections would turn up just by chance alone.

In another study of a large group of individuals by R. Shekelle and his colleagues at the University of Chicago, the health of more than 2000 male industrial employees was followed for 20 years. When they compared the personality profiles of those who had died from cancer with those who died from other causes, the cancer victims were twice as likely to have had depressive character traits measured 20 years earlier — long before they developed cancer. Furthermore, this increased cancer risk could not be explained away by increased rates of smoking or drinking among those men who were more depressed.

These two studies are the largest prospective attempts to find psychologic predictors for the later development of cancer. Taken together, they suggest that depression may be a risk factor for human cancer. B. Fox, however, after reviewing almost a dozen studies of personality traits and cancer, believes that the evidence supporting depression as a risk factor for cancer is very weak.

To avoid the problems hindering these prospective studies, some researchers have used a shortcut approach. They have studied the personality characteristics of patients who already have a problem — a lump, for example — that has not yet been diagnosed. Using the information gathered from interviews, the researcher tries to predict at a rate better than chance who will turn out to have cancer, basing his guesses on psychologic traits. In one such study women who had responded to a recent major life trauma with feelings of helplessness and hopelessness— the so-called given up–giving up complex—were more likely to have biopsy-confirmed cancer following a suspicious Pap smear. Since a detectable cancer takes months or even years to develop, these tumors must have already been present before the life trauma occurred. Therefore, if the helpless/hopeless response was a factor, it must have been the result of an influence on resistance to the growth of an already established tumor rather than a cancer-causing effect.

A logical extension of this approach is to study the behavioral characteristics of people just diagnosed as having cancer to see if behavior traits bear any relation to the course of the disease. In other words, why do two people with the same disease and the same treatment have different outcomes? Could psychologic factors play a role? S. Greer and his colleagues in England have been asking such questions in following a group of women with breast cancer for several years. They have observed that those women who reacted with feelings of helplessness and hopelessness or stoic acceptance at the time their breast cancer was just diagnosed were more likely to have recurrence and shorter survival rates than those who responded with a fighting spirit or denial. If similar findings turn up in other studies presently underway, the results will be evidence for the importance of a patient's attitude in shaping the course of the disease. If true, such factors will have to be given greater importance in planning treatment for cancer patients.

STRESS AS A RISK FACTOR FOR CANCER

Today the concept that stress is a promoter of disease has become very popular. A variety of medical illnesses occur more often during periods in peoples' lives when they feel stressed.

Examples of such stress-related conditions are tension headache, migraine headache, and irritable bowel syndrome (or spastic colon).

Research has shown that when individuals undergo many life changes in a brief time, especially when the changes are deemed undesirable (such as death of a spouse or being fired), they are more prone to a wide range of illnesses. However, the evidence that cancer can be *caused* by stress is extremely weak and is probably a popular myth.

Stress and cancer in animals

Some research studies have tried to determine the extent of the influence of stress in either the development or growth of cancer. Most of the research has been done with animals because animals can be experimentally stressed.

A pioneer in the field of stress and cancer research was the late V. Riley. He realized that most laboratory animal facilities are already stressful for animals, so he went to considerable trouble and expense to design and build a low-stress sheltered animal facility. He found that when he injected mice raised in the sheltered facility with tumor-causing viruses, they developed tumors more slowly than their counterparts raised in the standard animal facility. In other studies spanning a decade, Riley was able to demonstrate that a variety of stressors inhibited the growth of experimental tumors in animals.

Other researchers have studied how coping ability can modify the impact of stress on experimental tumor growth. L. Sklar and H. Anisman of Carleton University in Ontario, Canada, set up an intriguing experiment in which one group of rats was given a painful electric shock that they could turn off, while another group received the same shock but had no control over it. A third group of rats—the control group—got no shock. All the rats were first injected with tumor cells just before being placed in the apparatus. Tumors grew more rapidly and death occurred more quickly in the rats who had no control over the shock than in those who could turn it off, even though both groups received the same amount of shock. The only difference between them was that one had ability to control the shock, whereas the other rat was a helpless victim. The tumors in the group of rats with control over the shock grew at roughly the same rate as those in the control animals receiving no shock at all. Thus it seems that *being able to cope actively with a stress reduces the impact of the stress on tumor growth.*

The accumulated evidence from many similar experiments confirms that a variety of stressors can actually change the rate of growth of experimental tumors in animals. Furthermore, experimental stress has been shown to alter function of the immune system, the main line of defense against cancer development. However, *there is absolutely no evidence that stress can cause the spontaneous development of new cancerous growths in otherwise normal and healthy animals.* *

Stress and cancer in humans

Research with humans on the role of stress has centered on either the ability of stress to cause cancer or the role of stress during the disease to encourage a preexisting cancer to spread more rapidly.

Several types of naturally occurring stressful life experiences have been considered as possible contributing factors in the development of cancer. These have included:

1. The loss of an important relationship preceding the development of the tumor
2. Disturbance in the cancer patient's relationship to his parents
3. The lack of satisfactory outlets for emotional expression

4. Stressful life changes and impaired coping abilities
5. A history of depression that precedes the development of cancer

As mentioned earlier, the weakest evidence for the role of behavior in cancer development comes from retrospective research on patients who already have the disease. The studies of far greater significance are prospective ones. Let us examine these five ideas for such evidence.

Loss of an important relationship. Although there are many stories about bereaved people who developed cancer following the death of their spouse, there is no scientific evidence to support this popular idea. It is true that widowers (but probably not widows) have a higher death rate from all causes following bereavement, but there is insufficient evidence to implicate cancer specifically. Recently two different groups of researchers have shown that certain laboratory measures of immune function are suppressed in recently bereaved persons, although the relevance of these findings to cancer is questionable. Other research has investigated the effects of the experience of early childhood losses on adult cancer development.

Whereas memories about the *quality* of a childhood relationship may be distorted by the cancer experience, it is less likely that specific facts about deaths or births will be changed during recollection. In this regard there is some evidence that traumatic early childhood experiences can predispose to cancer. Women with breast cancer report with greater frequency the death of a brother or sister occurring in infancy than their healthy counterparts. In a separate study a shorter interval before the birth of the next younger sibling was found. These events are both traumatic experiences in the life of a developing child. Not all of the research on childhood stress and adult cancer development found these relationships. In some studies no connection was found between childhood loss or separation and adult cancer. It must be concluded that the relationship between stress in-

---

*Some researchers have reported increased rates of spontaneous tumor development in experimentally stressed animals that were already at high risk for the development of spontaneous tumors for genetic reasons.

duced by childhood loss and adult cancer is at best uncertain.

A frequently overlooked fact is that tumors develop slowly. The time lag from the moment the first cancerous cell escapes detection, begins to multiply, and grows to a detectable size is generally many months or even years. Therefore, if loss of a loved one could have an effect on cancer development, it would most likely affect the *rate of growth* of a preexisting tumor, not directly cause the development of a new cancer.

Disturbance in parental relationship. Psychologist L. LeShan interviewed hundreds of cancer patients about their lives before they developed cancer. He compared the lives of the cancer patients to a group of similar patients who suffered from other medical illnesses. The cancer patients were far more likely to report a pattern of emotional trauma in early childhood that had affected their ability to relate to others. Traumas such as the loss of a parent through death or divorce typically left the child with guilt feelings and a sense of failure or unworthiness. Later on in adult life, when another loss such as divorce or losing a job occurred, feelings of failure, helplessness, and even doom emerged and preceded the development of cancer by 6 to 18 months. Other researchers have also suggested on the basis of interviews with cancer patients that the patients suffered from disturbed relationships with their parents in early childhood. However, only one such study has tackled this question using the most powerful tool of all—the prospective study.

The ongoing study of C. Thomas of the Johns Hopkins medical graduates described earlier is of particular interest because the cancer victims were queried about their childhood relationships while they were healthy medical students. Thomas and her collaborators found no evidence that a history of childhood trauma was more common in those physicians who developed cancer than in those who remained healthy. However, they did find that the cancer victims had reported poorer family relationships during childhood, particularly between fathers and sons.

Lack of satisfactory outlet for emotional expression. A number of retrospective studies have suggested that people with a diminished ability to express their feelings are more prone to develop cancer. D. Kissen repeatedly found in his studies that lung cancer patients suppressed emotional conflicts and had "poor outlets for emotional expression" in comparison to cancer-free patients with other lung diseases. C. Bahnson and M. Bahnson observed that cancer patients repressed and denied unpleasant feelings such as anger, anxiety, and guilt more than other patients. L. LeShan found cancer patients described themselves as unable to express hostile feelings toward others. However, this is a classic "chicken and egg" problem. Perhaps cancer patients suppress their emotions more *because* of the disease. To get around this problem, we must study the patterns of emotional expression of patients before they know they have cancer.

S. Greer and T. Morris of Kings College Hospital in London interviewed a group of women with undiagnosed breast lumps about to undergo biopsy. They found that those women whose biopsies turned out to be malignant suppressed anger and other emotions more than the women whose lumps proved to be benign. However, it is possible that although the women and their physicians were *consciously* unaware of the diagnosis, on some level the existence of the cancer was influencing their emotional responses. Since some tumors are known to produce mood-altering hormones, this latter possibility is not so far-fetched.

The suppression of emotions may also alter the course of cancer. Patients with metastatic breast cancer who were angrier and who complained more of being anxious or depressed lived longer than patients who were less angry and reported more positive moods. In another study among patients with malignant melanoma (a virulent skin cancer), those who seemed to minimize the psychologic distress accompanying their disease were more likely to suffer a relapse during the year after the surgical removal of the cancer. Other research has shown that patients with malignant melanoma deny and repress their emotions more than patients with coronary heart disease or healthy individuals of similar sex and age.

If the expression of disturbing feelings is related to cancer susceptibility or to the course of the disease, then perhaps complaints about such symptoms as depression, anxiety, or hostility might be related to how well a person's immune system functions. S. Levy, Chief of the Behavioral Medicine Branch at the National Cancer Institute, has found that among patients with metastatic breast cancer, those who complain of more psychiatric symptoms have cancer-fighting white blood cells with a greater ability to kill tumor cells in laboratory tests. On the other hand, my colleagues and I have found exactly the opposite relationship in a group of healthy college students we have studied. We observed that the more our students complained of depression or anxiety, the lower was the tumor-killing activity of their blood cells measured in the laboratory. A possible explanation for these seemingly conflicting results was recently proposed by L. Bieliauskas. He pointed out that it is normal for well-adjusted cancer patients to complain about psychiatric symptoms such as depression and anxiety, because of the stress of living with the disease. It is the suppression or denial of emotional symptoms that is pathologic. The reverse is true for healthy young adults; their self-reporting of psychiatric symptoms is evidence of poor coping.

In conclusion, despite the popularity of the idea that suppression of emotions causes cancer, at present there is insufficient evidence to conclude that it is true.

Stressful life changes and coping ability. The research of Schmale and Iker mentioned earlier revealed that a skilled psychiatric interviewer can predict the outcome of a biopsy for cancer of the cervix more than half the time. Patients who reported that they felt like giving up after a major loss or stress during the 6 months before the biopsy had fewer positive biopsies than their counterparts who coped better. However, the malignancy probably had already started growing before the stressful event occurred. This "giving-up complex" is similar in some ways to depression.

Depression. Depression can be a personality trait (present for most of someone's life) and/or a temporary state. We discussed the role of depressive traits as a risk factor for cancer earlier; there is no evidence that acute depression can cause cancer. Recently, a number of researchers have found that people suffering from depression have impaired immunity. As just mentioned, my research found that healthy college students who reported many symptoms of depression (along with other minor psychiatric symptoms) had a diminished tumor-killing ability of their white blood cells in the laboratory. However, there is no evidence that this means they are more susceptible to cancer.

A number of studies have shown that people are more likely to become ill following a large number of life changes, especially when these life events were judged to be stressful, undesirable, and unexpected. Several studies have shown that a variety of experimental or naturally occurring stressors may impair immunity, as measured by laboratory tests. However, it has not been shown that cancer is a stress-related disorder.

LIFE-STYLE AS A RISK FACTOR FOR CANCER

Of all the ways in which psychologic or behavioral factors could influence cancer risk, life-style factors are by far the most important. Life-style encompasses a variety of complex interactions between an individual and the social environment and includes aspects of personality and stress already covered. For example, it is well known that the risk for lung cancer among smokers is 20 times higher than for nonsmokers, and yet personality and stress factors may partially determine someone's choice to smoke or not to smoke.

The important point is that despite the popular appeal of the notion that "stress causes cancer" or that there is a cancer-prone personality pattern, the evidence is overwhelming that it is the choices we make and the abusive things we do to our bodies that are really the behavioral causes of cancer. The fascination with stress and cancer-prone personalities is a diversion, distracting us from the far more important need for aggressive public health measures essential to preventing cancer.

SUMMARY AND RECOMMENDATIONS

It is widely believed that "stress" increases the risk of physical illness. The major problem with research on the health effects of stress is the lack of agreement among clinicians and researchers as to what "stress" is and how to measure it. A considerable body of medical research implicates life changes, especially those experiences rated as undesirable and stressful, in increasing the risk of physical and mental diseases. Even so, many physicians are not convinced of the scientific validity of this purported connection because much of the research on human stress and disease is flawed.

In any case there is no scientific evidence that stress can *cause* human cancer. Several lines of evidence suggest that certain behavioral factors may influence the regulation of human immunity and that this could in theory alter susceptibility to cancer or the growth of an established tumor. However, this argument remains

conjecture for lack of evidence at present.

What is clear is that certain models of human stress such as bereavement are associated with (and probably cause, although this is unproved) depression of human immune function. Furthermore, experimental stress can alter immunity and cancer growth in animals, with stress generally favoring increased tumor growth in most experimental studies. Supportive evidence in both animals and humans suggests that access to effective coping strategies may blunt the deleterious effects of stress on the immune system. In the final analysis, however, whether or not these observed changes in laboratory measures of immunity have clinical relevance to resistance to human cancer growth remains to be proved.

The role of personality factors in cancer risk is another matter. Suggestive evidence links disturbed family relationships and depression with altered immunity and increased later risk of adult cancer. However, once more the evidence supporting these links is weak and deserves further study. The scientific underpinnings of these beliefs are far too uncertain to justify the widespread public acceptance of these ideas. In a world often seemingly out of our control, a belief system that emphasizes our native capacity to consciously self-regulate our body's defenses has considerable appeal. Consequently, it is important to keep a clear perspective as to what constitutes "scientific fact" and what represents "belief." In clinical practice faith and science are partners in the art of healing. However, it is important to maintain a distinction between the two.

The two sets of boxed material give recommendations concerning stress and personality and possible indicators of stress.

**Recommendations related to stress and personality
and possible cancer prevention**

1. Make active health maintenance an important priority in your life. Regular meditation and exercise, coupled with adherence to healthful dietary recommendations described elsewhere in this book, must become important priorities.
2. Increase your self-awareness of symptoms and signs of excessive stress. (These are listed in the other boxed material.)
3. During periods with many stressful life changes, alter your life-style to reduce known risk factors and introduce stress-reducing activities such as meditation and exercise.
4. When self-help approaches to stress management are not enough and signs of excessive stress persist, seek professional help from someone specializing in behavioral or psychosomatic medicine.
5. Cigarette smoking and alcohol abuse can often be helped with behavioral modification treatments. Consult a behavioral medicine specialist or a psychologist or psychiatrist who has experience with behavior therapy.
6. Do not permit severely troubled and conflict-laden relationships to go on indefinitely without resolution. Seek professional help from a competent mental health professional, if necessary.
7. If you habitually respond to life stresses with feelings of helplessness and hopelessness or are prone to depression or anxiety when under stress, you may be at increased risk for illness, including cancer. Seek professional help from a mental health professional. More effective means of coping can be learned. Psychiatric consultation may lead to effective drug treatment for severe depression or anxiety, in addition to the possible benefits from psychotherapy.
8. If you are someone who has difficulty expressing negative emotions and tends to keep angry feelings bottled up, do not focus your concerns on the fear of getting cancer. The added risk of this behavior pattern to the expected risk for cancer is very small, if real at all. Far more important is the destructive effect this behavior pattern has on many other aspects of your life, especially personal relationships. Concentrate your self-improvement efforts on improving your relationships, not on trying to avoid cancer.

Stress warning signals*

Feeling unable to slow down and relax

Explosive anger in response to minor
  irritation

Anxiety or tension lasting more than
  a few days

Feeling that things frequently go wrong

Inability to focus attention

Frequent or prolonged feelings of
  boredom

Fatigue

Sexual problems

Sleep disturbances

Tension headaches

Migraine headaches

Cold hands or feet

Aching neck and shoulder muscles

Indigestion

Menstrual distress

Nausea or vomiting

Loss of appetite

Diarrhea

Ulcers

Heart palpitations

Constipation

Lower back pain

Allergy or asthma attacks

Shortness of breath

Frequent colds

Frequent low-grade infections

Frequent minor accidents

Overeating

Increased consumption of alcohol

Increased dependence on drugs

*Some of these signs and/or symptoms may indicate the presence of an underlying physical or mental disorder. Be sure
to consult a physician if such symptoms persist.
From Miller, L.H., Ross, R., and Cohen, S.I.: Stress: what can be done? Bostonia Magazine **56** (4 & 5): 13, 1982.
Reprinted with permission of Boston University Alumni House Publications.

CHAPTER 10

Life-style and Cancer

Cancer is a disease of civilization.

DAVID LIVINGSTONE

ERNEST H. ROSENBAUM

It has become painfully obvious that our life-style plays a major role in many diseases, including cardiovascular disease, hypertension, ulcers, asthma, and cancer. Our culture and religious beliefs, the substances we ingest such as tobacco, alcohol, and drugs, and even our sexual activities and childbearing patterns all play various roles in our health.

We know that there are many associations between our life-style choices and cancer. Unfortunately, however, we have not solved all the cancer riddles clearly enough to always be able to point to specific substances. Because of this and because our knowledge is growing and changing as research becomes more detailed and accurate, the public gets confused. Reports come out in the media that are not truly authoritative or mature, and the end result is that people wonder why more cannot be done, when in fact much is being done.

We do know that cancer is caused by many forces that either act alone or in concert with other forces to result in the disease. We also know the factors that influence or determine cancer incidence. It is important (1) *how you live* and (2) *where you live*. If you lived in a poor country, you might actually benefit because you avoid the affluent diet of the richer countries, which has been linked to cancer. Some countries also have a high incidence of a particular virus or cancer. For example, in Asia or Africa hepatitis B infections are prevalent, and they start occurring even among young children. The liver is further affected by aflatoxin. Aflatoxin can stimulate cancer. (In the United States special precautions have successfully prevented fungal aflatoxin contamination of food.) These combined factors have a strong association with liver cancer in certain areas of the world.

Another factor is (3) *exposure*, either on the job, in a geographic area (near a factory or chemical plant), or in your home. You may be exposed to various synthetics, chemicals, radiation, as well as other substances that can induce cancer in humans. You may also, through choice, occupation, and geography, be exposed to more of the sun's ultraviolet rays.

A more general factor is (4) *your social and cultural habits*, such as smoking, drinking, or—in Asia and India—chewing betel nuts. The age at which one gets married and has children

223

and the kind of sexual activity experienced are other examples of social habits.

A personal factor is one's (5) *genetic resistance or susceptibility*, the tendency an individual has to either contract or resist cancer because of the genes inherited from ancestors. This may explain why two people exposed to the same carcinogenic stimulus do not both get the disease. Another, clearer example is the higher incidence of skin cancers among fair-skinned people, who in general are more susceptible to damage from the sun's rays.

A further factor may be (6) *religious beliefs and practices*. Jewish women, for example, have a low incidence of cervical cancer. The reason for this is unknown, with speculations including male circumcision and a fairly strict observance of monogamy among Jewish females and males. Mormons and Seventh Day Adventists who follow a healthy diet with restricted tobacco and alcohol, as well as other healthy observances in their lives, have a lower incidence of cancer, especially the cancers specifically related to alcohol and tobacco use.

Finally, (7) *ethnic characteristics* may play some part in cancer susceptibility and resistance. This is genetics on a larger scale than individually inherited characteristics. For example, prostate cancer in black males is twice as common as it is in white males. The reason for this is not known, although it may have more to do with occupational exposure than genetic inheritance, since many blacks work in dangerous industrial jobs.

Just as there are certain known factors about cancer, there are also myths about dangers. For example, air pollution is often believed to be a considerable cancer risk to the population; yet Geneva, Switzerland, which has fairly clean air, has a higher incidence of cancer than urbanized Birmingham, England, which has a high level of industrial toxins and other airborne pollutants. This is not to say that pollution is not a factor, but rather that there is rarely a simple cause-and-effect relationship (except for smoking and lung cancer).

Many elements affect cancer rates. The behavior of people varies with their culture, religious attitudes, where they live, and where they migrate. Sexual habits, such as age at first intercourse, number of partners, number of children, and age at first pregnancy, can also influence cancer. Diet is known to be a contributing factor.

In addition, two more elements need to be included in the cancer equation—the unknown risks and the potential for known risks to interact with one another. Many of the substances we are exposed to might cause cancer, but because of the time lag between exposure and development of the disease, it is hard to pinpoint the original risk factor. We know that the combination of alcohol and cigarettes or of obesity and smoking increases the risk factor of either alone. In other words, in the realm of cancer susceptibility, one and one can total more than two.

Our life-styles include our total cultural behavior, life patterns, eating, smoking, and sexuality, and these vary considerably with age, education, background, religion, sex, and income level. Regardless of the patterns that emerge, the main point about life-style risks is that they involve choice. In this respect cancer risks resulting from our life-styles are the opposite of a genetic or inherited risk, which is simply a matter of what family you were born into and what genes you inherited. As discussed in Chapter 3, we now know that most cancers are caused by the interaction of a person's genes and the environment—external factors such as smoking, diet, sexuality, occupational exposures, and so on. Of these, the first two, smoking and diet, may be largely responsible for as much as 50% to 60% of our cancers.

The essence of life-style risks is that most of the factors involved can be avoided or altered to reduce the risk. This is not to say that choices toward a healthier life-style are easy or simple to make: tobacco is addictive and so are other drugs, alcohol dependence is a real malady, and eating habits become deeply ingrained in us from a very early age. Most of our daily habits are difficult to change.

What people in the past did not realize, however, was the price they would have to pay for these habits. A lot of our daily patterns are acquired rather subtly over time for reasons or motivations that do not take future health into consideration. A young man wanting to seem worldly and mature gives no thought to his body 40 years later when he starts smoking at age 17. A child who naturally enjoys sweets may more easily grow obese, thus starting a lifetime habit with a higher risk of cancer, unless the parent lays down some limits. A young woman may feel happy to be sexually liberated and enjoy many partners, only to find that she has contracted herpes simplex II, genital herpes, which up to now has no cure and which may increase her risk of cervical cancer.

Many things are beyond our control, but our personal choices are not. Unfortunately, we often do things, not realizing that we are starting a pattern or habit that may have negative effects later on in time. That first cigarette, that habit of three colas a day, and that pattern of eating meat several times a day—these do not seem like such momentous things, but they may be if they are repeated enough. The way we live will certainly influence and possibly determine how and when we die: before our time from a serious illness or comfortably after we have lived out our full measure with vigor and health.

In learning about the health risks of certain habits and the benefits of others, you are beginning to take control of your health and your life. That is why good health education and information are so important. In choosing to educate yourself and then make life-style choices accordingly, you are also making it easier for the world around you—your family, friends, and associates—to make the right choices as well. If you are lucky, you may even be a good example for a younger person, so that he or she will establish a positive habit first and not need to struggle with overcoming a bad choice later in life.

Although life-style choices involve things such as smoking, drinking, diet, and the environment we live in, we are not referring to these subjects in the present chapter, because they have been discussed individually in separate chapters. This chapter deals specifically with other aspects of our mode of life, both cultural and social. Included are obesity and sexuality, including pregnancies, multiple partners, and exposure to sexually transmitted viral diseases. Viruses that have been associated with cancer are also discussed.

OBESITY*

Obesity is a chronic problem for many Americans. In our society, with its abundance of food and many food treats that tempt us to overindulgence, it is understandably difficult to control weight. Over the past 100 years in the United States, obesity has been constantly increasing. Obesity is defined as being 20% to 25% over ideal weight standards as established by the Metropolitan Life Insurance Company. (These standards are currently being revised slightly upward for men.) An example would be a woman weighing in at 144 pounds, when she should, according to her height, age, and frame size, weigh around 115.

Many people do, however, control their weight. Interestingly enough, more women than men are in the underweight-to-normal category. Men predominate in the 10% to 20% overweight category, but two thirds of those in the 30% to 40% category are women. The worst potentially dangerous ages for obesity seem to be between 45 and 64.

*See also Chapter 5.

Obesity is implicated in many diseases because of the body's extra load, which strains the functioning of many organs and systems, including, of course, the heart. Obesity is specifically a risk factor for cardiovascular disease, diabetes, and hyperlipidemia. The specific risk factor between overweight—that is, how much extra weight—and cancer is not known; yet obesity is associated with uterine, ovarian, and breast cancer in women, and it may be a contributing factor to colorectal cancer in men. The American Cancer Society has found that when people are more than 40% above their ideal weight, cancer rises dramatically: 55% higher than normal for women and 33% for men.

The exact causative process (if there is one) between obesity and cancer is not known. Only this simple fact is known: "Obesity is related to cancer," according to J. Higginson, worldwide cancer expert. One of the possible reasons may be that people who are grossly overweight eat a lot more and so may consume more food products or additives that could have a carcinogenic effect. Most obese people would also tend to consume a high-fat, high-red-meat diet, which has been associated with cancer.

Many people apparently realize the multiple dangers of being so much over their ideal weight, and they try to do something about it. Currently, more than 1 million people participate in weight reduction clinics that promise inexpensive and painless methods of weight reduction; $2 billion per year are spent on diet aids (books, over-the-counter medications, diet clinics, non-nutritional food supplements, and so on). Unfortunately, the claims made by some of these clinics are unrealistic, such as losing 30 pounds in 30 days. The statistics from one weight-reduction clinic show that by 6 weeks 50% of the original clients had dropped out, and by 12 weeks 70% had quit. Many clinics offer no refunds, but rather free supplementary treatment, which actually encourages dropouts. Only 20% of the individuals at the clinic mentioned who started the program remained long enough to reduce their weight significantly.

There have not been enough physician-directed weight-reduction clinics that have developed and provided successful weight reduction programs with long-lasting results. People who need to lose weight often think in terms of a quick and easy diet that will do the trick so they can get down to a normal weight and then forget about the diet. Losing large quantities of weight and keeping it off involves major behavioral changes—in what people eat, how they eat, and, of course, how much they eat. (See boxed material.)

Individuals attempting substantial weight loss need guidance from their physicians that includes:

1. Improved education
2. Improved regimes (diets and eating habits)
3. Improved psychologic support
4. Improved maintenance techniques once weight is lost

A workable weight-loss program would include (1) a diet analysis and history of prior attempts at weight loss, (2) a baseline calorie intake and planned program, (3) an assessment and recommendations for exercise behavior and a metabolic assessment, (4) dietary restrictions and an intense behavior-modification program and advice to help reduce failures, and (5) state-of-the-art weight-loss programs with close medical supervision to maintain essential nutrients and good health.

These recommendations come from *The Dietary Goals of the United States* prepared by the Select Committee on Nutrition and Human Needs of the United States Senate—Senator McGovern; *Diet, Nutrition and Cancer* by the Committee on Diet, Nutrition, and Cancer from the Assembly of Life Sciences, National Research Council, National Academy Press, 1982, Chairman Clifford Grobstein, M.D.; *The*

> **Recommendations for successful weight loss**
>
> 1. Increase physical activity.
> 2. Eat less fat and fatty foods. Try to reduce fat consumption from 40% to 30% of total calories.
> 3. Eat less sugars and sweets and try to eat a balanced diet that includes the recommended daily allowances of vitamins such as A and C. This should include fruits, vegetables, and dietary fiber.
> 4. Avoid alcohol.

> **Recommendations for reducing obesity**
>
> 1. Use diets that reduce the efficiency with which the body utilizes the calories consumed (for example, carbohydrates and fat contribute just as much as protein to the amount of energy dissipated in heat loss.
> 2. Losing a lot of weight and keeping it off is very difficult. *Your physician should be involved in any weight reduction program you use.*
> 3. High-fiber diets have *minimal* effect on weight loss.
> 4. Exercise helps, but it should be pursued consistently and actively, not only to maintain body tone but also to burn up additional calories. No diet program works without an exercise program. But more important than an exercise program alone is a good low-calorie regimen, calorie counting, and a specific weight-reduction program. (See Chapter 5 on nutrition.)
> 5. Unbalanced low-calorie diets may be used *with caution* and care under medical supervision. Many are popular but dangerous to humans, since they have an imbalance of protein, carbohydrates, or fat, which may create an imbalance of micronutrients, vitamins and minerals. An example of a low-calorie diet is the Pritikin diet, which is reasonable. Most of the others, known as "fad of the month" diets, are rarely successful after a few weeks and many are frankly dangerous.

Prudent Diet, published by the American Heart Association; and *Toward Healthful Diets,* published by the Food and Nutrition Board of the National Academy of Sciences.

The situation with obesity differs from that of a person trying to lose 5 to 10 pounds. For this reason, our recommendations differ.

Try out a fully nutritious, well-balanced, lower-calorie diet. Some hints are to:

1. Plan the total number of calories per day and keep a calorie and protein count for 1 month (get a calorie counter). A lower calorie diet that is also a balanced diet makes sense.
2. Avoid nighttime snacks.
3. Plan your meals and use smaller portions. Reduce total calories and proteins. Use exchange lists. Try 1000 to 1200 calories as a good guide for a starter.
4. Set goals for weight loss and provide yourself with low-calorie "bonus" or a nonfood present when successful.
5. Compete with a friend with a prize for the winner.

Not all health and cancer problems are associated with being obese and overweight. Underweight and malnutrition also have implications for cancer, but not all of them are negative. For example, women who are undernourished tend to have less breast cancer. These women often have a later onset of menstruation (and an earlier menopause), which is thought to result in reduced cancer risk. However, malnutrition can lead to a general weakening of the immune system or an overall physical deterioration. This may in turn make a person more susceptible to the effects of cancer-causing agents or less able to fight off a precancerous or cancerous condition once it has begun. For additional information, refer to the material on obesity in Chapter 5.

In the balance, probably being slightly underweight is better than being substantially overweight, *if the overall nutrition is good.* Some of the poor people in the world who live on a sparse diet that is rich in complex carbohydrates such as whole grains, rice, and corn, with only occasional small amounts of meat, are by virtue of their "poor" diets richer in health. They do not suffer the diseases of the rich.

SEXUALITY

Several years ago, when giving a lecture on breast cancer to the sophomore class at the University of California, I mentioned that most of the pleasurable things we enjoy during our lifetime may lead to cancer — an affluent diet, cigarettes, and alcohol. I concluded the introduction on a note of optimism, saying, "Sex is okay," only to have second thoughts after that spontaneous statement was made. Later in the talk I added some supporting evidence, pointing out that women who have babies, obviously the result of sexual experience, have less breast cancer and that nuns, who are celibate, have a higher incidence. This fact was first reported by Bernardino Ramazzini in 1713.

Over the last 15 years, the relationship between sexuality and cancer risk has undergone extensive research. It has been shown that certain sexual patterns are associated with a higher incidence of some cancers. For example, not having children is a known risk factor for breast cancer, but it is unlikely that anyone would decide to have a child primarily to avoid the risk of breast cancer, since the additional

risk is small. Yet a person might take definite steps to avoid contracting herpes simplex II virus, which has been associated with cervical cancer in women, by at least inquiring if your sexual partner has had herpes.

Childbearing and cancer

Pregnancy and childbirth may play a role in decreasing a person's risk of ovarian, breast, and endometrial cancer. These occur less commonly in women who have children than in those who have had no children. Another factor is that women who are younger at the time of their first pregnancy are even less likely to develop breast cancer than women who were older at first pregnancy. Just becoming pregnant is not enough, however; women who have had an abortion and never carried a child to term do not gain the protective effects of pregnancy. This may be because the protection is a side effect of the lactation process milk production that begins at the end of pregnancy.

Women who start menstruating at later ages (after 12 or 13) have a slightly decreased risk of breast cancer compared to women who began menstruating before age 12.

Heterosexuality

The relationship between cervical cancer in women and infectious agents has been known for many years. Population studies relate cervical cancer to several sexual risk factors: (1) beginning sexual activity at an early age, (2) having multiple partners, and (3) being pregnant at least once. Recent evidence has led to the speculation that male semen may be the carrier for infectious agents, as well as other agents (viral and bacterial strains have been identified), and that repeated exposure to a partner with a symptomless urogenital infection or else exposure to many different partners may lead to cervical cancer for women.

There is evidence supporting this theory. Among men whose first wives had cervical cancer and who later remarried, the second wives had a three- to fourfold higher risk of developing cervical cancer than the general population. This could be explained if there were some agent or virus in the ejaculate semen of these men that affected their wives. There are several other theories about the causes of cervical cancer, but at present nothing has been proved conclusively. Interestingly, cervical cancer is extremely rare in virgins and Jewish women. In Jewish women this is most likely due to monogamous marriages rather than to male circumcision.

Sexual viruses and cancer

The most dramatic recent findings that relate to sexuality have been those of an association between cancer and viruses. The viruses in question are the *herpes simplex II,* papilloma wart virus, and other sexually transmitted viruses. Several theories exist about the relationship. It is possible that viral disease causes a prolonged inflammation that may develop into a carcinoma on the same site, or that the virus itself may be a cocarcinogen that induces precancerous changes.

Laboratory studies have shown herpes II virus to be related to cervical cancer in mice. One study at Emory University done by Thomas and Rawls in 1978 showed that 60% of those women sampled who had cancer also had herpes II antibodies, and it was thought that the percentage would be higher if better testing methods were available. This means that these women had been exposed to herpes II, and their blood had developed antibodies to the virus.

Herpes II causes genital sores, whereas herpes I usually causes sores in and around the mouth, commonly called "cold sores." However, type I can cause genital sores, and type II can cause oral sores. When type I virus causes sores in the genital region, however, they *do not* tend to recur. This is not so with type II genital sores, which *do* recur. The genital lesions are painful, and as yet there is no known cure for this viral infection, which presently affects more than 20 million Americans.

Recent research suggests that cervicitis, cervical dysplasia, and possibly cervical carcinoma may be linked to the papilloma wart virus, rather than to the herpes virus. Thus the evidence that a sexually transmitted virus is linked with cervical

TABLE 10-1   Sexually transmitted viruses with cancer-causing potential

Virus	Tumor or location	Carcinogenic potential— 1 to 4 + range
EBV (Epstein-Barr virus)	Burkitt's*	4 +
	Nasopharynx	4 +
HBV (hepatitis B virus)	Hepatoma	3 +
CMV (cytomegalovirus)	Kaposi's†	2 +
HSV-II (herpes simplex II)	Cervix	1(?)
HSV-I (herpes simplex I)	Head and neck	?
Papilloma	Genital warts	4 +
	Condyloma	4 +
	Rectal	2 +
	Penile	?
	Cervix	?

Adapted from John L. Ziegler, personal communication
*A lymph node tumor usually present in equatorial Africa, associated with Epstein-Barr virus.
†A reddish, pigmented skin and soft tissue tumor.

cancer is increasing. However, it will probably require years of further research to pinpoint the exact agent and to determine whether one or more viruses are required to transform healthy cells into cancer.

Table 10-1 lists other sexually transmitted viruses that potentially may cause cancer.

AIDS, homosexuality, and cancer

One of the most striking occurrences in the cancer field in the last few years has been among the male homosexual population, particularly in New York, San Francisco, and Los Angeles. Homosexual men in these cities are experiencing a high-mortality epidemic of acquired immune-deficiency syndrome, called AIDS by medical practitioners. Hardly a day goes by without the mention of AIDS in a newspaper or magazine. There have been many recent radio and television programs concerning some new medical fact or story. AIDS is now the leading cause of death among gay men in their thirties and forties.

Currently unknown is whether the cause of this problem is a sexually transmitted infectious agent encountered in the homosexual life-style, an environmental agent (drugs, semen, and so on), or a combination of several factors working together. AIDS is, however, now being considered a new disease that was not seen in the United States before 1979.

The current working medical definition of AIDS is that it is a disease associated with a defect in cell-mediated immunity, occurring in a person with no known reason for diminished resistance to that disease. *Pneumocystis carinii* pneumonia, *Kaposi's sarcoma*, a skin cancer, and other serious opportunistic infections are common manifestations. Table 10-2 shows a breakdown of AIDS cases and deaths according to these malignancies as of July 1983. By July 1983, the Centers for Disease Control in Atlanta have counted more than 1750 cases and over 700 deaths from AIDS; the current mortality rate of AIDS victims is between 50% and 70% of cases. New cases continue to be reported at the rate of 3 to 5 per day. The total number of cases reported has been doubling every 5 to 6 months. With 1750 cases and a 5 to 6 month doubling rate, there may be 10,000 to 20,000 cases in the next 5 years. The number may not seem significant, but AIDS is not widely distributed at present: 70% to 75% of its victims are homosexual men. The other 25% of the cases occur in hemophiliacs who received blood products, intravenous drug abusers, Haitian immigrants, female sexual partners of patients with AIDS, and male prisoners (many of whom have used intravenous drugs or have had homosexual contact in prison). More cases of AIDS have been reported than the total number of cases of toxic shock syndrome and Legionnaires' disease. It is not a disease that is casually transmitted; rather, it is spread predominantly by intimate sexual contact.

What is AIDS?

Perhaps the easiest way to understand AIDs is to analyze the term word-by-word.

Acquired   Indicates that it is not an inherited or genetic condition and not the result of an accident or birth defect

Immune   Refers to the body's natural mechanism to protect itself from disease or to fight infection

Deficiency   Indicates that the immune mechanism is malfunctioning and therefore "deficient" in its ability to protect the body

Syndrome   The state in which the body is vulnerable to a number of diseases *only* because it has literally acquired an immune deficiency

From San Francisco Department of Public Health, Bureau of Communicable Disease Control, May, 83.

Symptoms of AIDS are:

- Unexplained weight loss–over 10 pounds.
- Swollen glands (lymph nodes) in neck, underarms, and groin.
- Prolonged fevers, unexplained by acute illness.
- Prolonged flulike symptoms—generalized aches.
- Night sweats
- Skin changes—persistent red or purple skin rashes, often painless, flat or raised
- Prolonged diarrhea

Among homosexual males, those at risk generally seem to be men between the ages of 25 and 40 who have had many sexual partners, possibly up to a thousand or more in a lifetime. The significance of multiple sexual partners among male homosexuals can be the same as for promiscuous women or female prostitutes. Imagine, for example, that one person is firing a rifle at you from a distance of 100 yards; your chances of getting hit are small. However, if 100 people are shooting at you, at least one has a good chance of hitting you. Specifically, a person who chooses a life-style involving many sexual contacts increases the odds of being exposed to a virus that may possibly initiate or encourage cancer.

The life-style choices of the homosexual men who develop AIDS often involve repeated insults to their immune systems:

1. About 90% have had venereal disease.
2. Two-thirds have had hepatitis.
3. Most have had a variety of intestinal infections and feces exposures.
4. Most have used drugs recreationally, sometimes mixing them—marijuana, alcohol, cocaine, and nitrites ("poppers").
5. Most have had a large number of sexual partners, both strangers and friends, which may number from hundreds to a 1000 or more in a lifetime.
6. Most engage in sexual practices that lead to recurring rectal damage or anal-oral contact.

Of the other AIDS victims, some 35 have been Haitian immigrants who moved to Miami and New York. Thus far, 50 cases have been diagnosed in Haiti as of May 1983. These Haitian cases initially denied intravenous drug use or abuse, hemophilia, or homosexuality, but recent evidence suggests that a substantial number were homosexuals or drug users. Of note is that Haiti is often visited by vacationing homosexual men. It is possible that AIDS originated in Haiti and was introduced into the United States by returning visitors. The reverse is also possible: that American visitors may have introduced AIDS into Haiti.

Hemophiliacs are another risk group for AIDS. There are approximately 20,000 hemophiliacs in the United States who require periodic commercial blood product transfusions. In the past, a blood protein product known as cryoprecipitate was used. Multiple donors were needed since the hemophilia patient may require 5 or 10 units of cryoprecipitate at a time to prevent hemorrhage. A new way of producing this factor is in the form of a freeze-dried factor VIII concentrate, which is made from a pool of up to 20,000 donors. It has the advantage of being very concentrated; thus, a small quantity will work and can be given by rapid injection after reconstitution. It may also carry various viral-type products, and problems such as hepatitis have been implicated. As of July 1983, 16 hemophiliacs who have used factor VIII concentrate have acquired AIDS.

Roughly another 3 million Americans receive blood products every year for anemia, infections, or other medical reasons. Thus far, two patients have developed AIDS following transfusion. One was an infant in San Francisco who had an Rh incompatibility. The donor, who was healthy at the time of blood donation, subsequently died of AIDS.

According to Dr. Herbert Perkins of the Irwin Memorial Blood Bank, San Francisco, most people can be exposed to the agent and not contract AIDS; thus AIDS may affect some blood recipients and skip others who have received blood from the same donor.

Because of the connection between AIDS and users of blood products, there has been conflict over who is the safest or best donor for blood. In Los Angeles, 400 homosexual donors were rejected in 1 month. In New York, one of the blood donation centers gave a written description of the symptoms of AIDS to the potential donors, who then had the option of choosing to donate blood for transfusion or only be used for studies. What is needed is a simple medical test that can detect AIDS in the blood, but thus far no such test has been devised.

The U.S. Public Health Service has suggested that a person might:

1. Donate his own blood ahead of time for elective surgery, so that the blood could be administered as needed during surgery
2. Screen out donors at high risk for developing AIDS.

The highest risk group, however, remains homosexual males, so that AIDS is commonly termed the "gay cancer." Many medical practitioners are currently trying to understand what the disease is, how it works in the system, and how it is transmitted.

The development of "gay cancer," as it has been called, seems to involve two steps. Fir the immune system of the individual is impaired in some way, possibly by a sexually transmitted agent such as a virus. Then, either the same virus or another virus may subsequently induce a cancer.

Recent speculation has centered around the possible relationship of *cytomegalovirus (CMV)* infection to AIDS. A high percentage of healthy male homosexuals in the United States have CMV in their systems. CMV is found in almost all people suffering from AIDS syndrome, but we do not know if the virus is a cause or just a fellow traveller. While this is still unknown, CMV does have the intriguing property of being potentially *oncogenic*, that is, tumor causing. In addition, acute CMV infection has been shown to transiently suppress cell-mediated immunity. In other words, this is a virus that is almost universally present in homosexual men, may simultaneously suppress immunity, and then foster some change in the cell's DNA leading to a tumor, such as Kaposi's sarcoma. This, however, is speculation, and much more research is required. In the next few years, advanced techniques in research will be able to reveal which cancers are caused by viruses and possibly how a virus acts to produce cancer. Meanwhile, the evidence linking viruses to cancer is circumstantial, but several viruses seem implicated (see Table 10-2).

It will be necessary to try to isolate the agent

TABLE 10-2   AIDS cases and deaths in United States and San Francisco Bay Area according to malignancy—July 1983

Malignancy	Cases*		Deaths*	
	U.S. (%)	S.F. (%)	U.S. (%)	S.F. (%)
Kaposi sarcoma (KS) only	438 (26)	124 (43.5)	93 (21)	17 (20)
Pneumocystis carinii pneumonia (PCP) only	857 (51)	107 (37.5)	373 (43.5)	41 (47)
Both KS and PCP	125 (7.5)	36 (73)	73 (58)	21 (24)
Other opportunistic infections	256 (15)	18 (6)	111 (43)	8 (9)
Total	1676	285	650	87

Modified from an update by Lawrence Mintz, M.D., Laurence Drew, M.D., and Selma Dritz, M.D.
*Approximate percentages in parentheses.

and develop a vaccine or a way of approaching this disease. So far, no vaccines have evolved, although if the AIDS agent is proved to be a virus, a vaccine could possibly be produced. Even in this case, it would probably take at least 3 years to develop a satisfactory vaccine. The incubation period for AIDS is approximately 18 months, thus most likely some 5 years would have to elapse before one could even begin to determine whether the vaccine was effective in preventing AIDS.

Interferon is now being tried at many centers, both in New York and in San Francisco. A recent report by Dr. Susan Krown and her associates from Sloan-Kettering Cancer Center *(New England Journal of Medicine)* stated: "Although Interferon treatment does appear to restore some aspects of immunity in some patients with Kaposi's sarcoma, we do not have evidence in this study that Interferon consistently or permanently reverses the underlying immunologic defects that characterize AIDS." Interferon, which was produced through genetic engineering, was given to 12 homosexual men who had Kaposi's sarcoma. The disease completely disappeared in three and partially disappeared in two; three had a minor but temporary response. However, the interferon seemed to have little effect on the destruction that AIDS caused on the defective immune system.

In the meantime, one has to consider maximum precautions as a way of dealing with this problem. Homosexual men interested in protecting themselves may need to alter their sexual life-style to reduce the incidence of this disease. This has already begun to happen among gay men in San Francisco, where daily conversations about AIDS are common. Almost all these men know something about the disease and the evidence of its probable sexual transmissability. Each man knows at least one person, possibly a friend or lover, who has AIDS.

One survey showed that 30% of the gay men in the San Francisco area had already changed their sexual life-styles to limit the number of their sexual partners. Some were asking specific questions before sexual contact, in effect screening their potential partners for AIDS. Many of the gay bars and bath houses, once the meeting places for making casual sexual connections, have closed down, primarily because of a decrease in business and in part for moral reasons. Louis Gaspar, who closed his gay bathhouse, stated: "I just couldn't stay open when I might be responsible for people getting AIDS" *(San Francisco Chronicle,* July 11, 1983). A recent newspaper article stated that some of the men are substituting cultural outlets such as music, raising exotic plants, or other interests for their former promiscuous life-style. An upsurge in monogamy and traditional "courting" was also reported. More homosexual men are seeing their medical practitioners more often for check-ups and choosing to reduce their use of recreational drugs. All this is to the good as life-style changes are currently the only known preventative steps one can take to limit the possibility of contracting AIDS.

The fear of contracting AIDS has at times reached hysterical proportions both within and outside the homosexual community. The evidence to date suggests that AIDS is transmitted by *intimate* contact, such as sexual intercourse, or by transfusions or exposure to contaminated needles.

There is no evidence out at this time to suggest that AIDS is transmitted by:

1. Toilet seats
2. Swimming pools
3. Shaking hands
4. Sitting next to an AIDS patient in a movie theater, bus, or at work
5. Eating food prepared or served by a person with AIDS

So far, in the past 3½ years healthy doctors, nurses, and hospital medical personnel have worked with AIDS cases; thus far no one has acquired AIDS.

The situation is different for individuals who have intimate contact with an AIDS victim. At

---

Recommendations for avoidance of AIDS (homosexual males)

1. Reduce the number of partners and sexual contacts, thus reducing potential exposure to sexually transmitted diseases.
2. Reduce the contact of one's sexual partner with semen by use of condoms.
3. Eliminate anonymous sexual contacts, and even ask one's potential partner whether he has had herpes, AIDS, and so on.
4. Avoid sexual activity that may cause bleeding. Refrain from sex that may tear, pierce or abrade delicate tissues. Anorectal tissues, even hemorrhoids, can easily be stretched or torn by fisting and other vigorous sexual acts, causing bleeding that may not be apparent to either party and introducing AIDS infection through the torn tissues. Even cuts, sores, or abrasions on the hands and arms can be an entry port for infection. Basically, sex of any kind involving the possibility of bleeding—even in the smallest amounts—should be avoided.
5. Eliminate (or at least minimize) recreational drug use. Many drugs popular with gays (and nongays of course) can damage the immune system. Shooting heroin, speed, and cocaine *with a shared needle* is especially damaging. Alcohol, marijuana, and other street drugs can blur your ability to make good decisions about your sexual conduct; when taken in excess they damage your overall good health.
6. Avoid prolonged kissing.
7. Maximize one's health with rest, good diet, and physical exercise.
8. Have more careful physical evaluations and checkups.
9. Consider avoidance of steroid therapy (with cortisone) because this may lead to dissemination of infections in cases such as idiopathic thrombocytopenic purpura (low blood platelets of unknown cause).
10. (For victims, potential victims, and physicians alike.) Regulate blood transfusions. There is a great controversy concerning the safety of blood transfusions from homosexual donors because they may be potential carriers of AIDS. Blood recipients have developed symptoms of AIDS, and potential AIDS victims are urged *not* to donate blood.

Points 4 and 5 from San Francisco Department of Public Health, Bureau of Communicable Disease Control.

---

this point, there are no proven ways of protecting yourself *if your partner has AIDS*. There are, however, several common sense precautions you can take:

1. Reduce hygienic contact such as prolonged kissing and body secretion contact, such as with saliva, stool, and semen.
2. Use condoms.
3. Reduce sexual practices or have no sexual relations.
4. Avoid new partners, as there is a potential chance that as the partner of an AIDS patient you may already be infected and would therefore help to disseminate the infection.

Counseling, discussion groups, blood screening, and diagnostic clinics are now all available in high-risk areas and should be used without hesitation.

Recommendations

In spite of what remains unknown, some general guidelines concerning sexuality and cancer prevention are valid, based on the incidence of certain patterns. Both heterosexuals and homosexuals can minimize their exposure to herpes simplex II. Reducing exposure to viruses can be done by restricting the number of sexual partners and/or making sure that they do not have genital herpes in an active stage. One of the first questions now asked before heterosexual relations is "do you have herpes?" Some people even wear "I do not have herpes" T shirts. Romantic, no—practical, yes. An interesting sidenote to this serious issue involves the case of Susan Liptrot, who was trying to sue a man she slept with once after she developed herpes. After moral reflection she thought the law should compel the man to give her more than $100,000.

It may also be possible to restrict the transmission of herpesvirus and other sexually transmitted viruses by the use of a condom. Among homosexuals, practices such as rectal intercourse may be more apt to facilitate transmission of viruses such as CMV and hepatitis B than other forms of sexual behavior.

Conclusion

In the past two decades there have been many changes in our moral values and our sexual practices. It is now evident that multiple sexual exposures increase the risks of getting AIDS and/or sexually transmitted viruses. Because of this medical evidence, people are becoming more cautious in choosing their sexual partners and are limiting the number of people with whom they are sexually intimate. Monogamous relationships are again increasing in popularity.

LIFE-STYLE RECOMMENDATIONS

Although it is easy to make specific recommendations with regard to certain dietary practices, such as high-fiber, low-fat diet, or smoking cessation, the term "life-style" is more vague, and it is somewhat difficult to make specific suggestions. However, there is no question that our life-style choices do play a role in cancer causation or prevention, as well as in many other diseases, such as cardiovascular disease, ulcers, or asthma. The following paragraphs may be considered guidelines for life-style changes that may prevent cancer.

Environment

In certain geographic areas or on certain job sites there is a high toxic exposure, with asbestos, radiation, or synthetic compounds. One might consider the importance and extent of this exposure and its potential cancer risk and review the risk with one's physician. If the risk is high, if there are other complicating factors, or if one has small children, one might wish to move or change employment.

Culture

Each society has certain practices that are observed, almost without thinking, by its members. Some of these may be detrimental to health, and specifically in this discussion, may be said to promote cancer. If one lives in such a culture, one may wish to consider the benefits or possible hazards of such practices as chewing betel nuts in India or the American tradition of a cocktail and a cigarette before the evening meal. If we are aware of the risks inherent in these practices, we can take steps to eliminate them from our lives. It is an irony of 20th century Western life that our very affluence can lead us into habits of overconsumption of rich food and drink, which can ultimately lead to diseases such as cancer. However, a person does not *have* to consume high-fat meals or consume alcohol in excessive quantities simply because he can afford to do so. The members of certain religious groups, such as the Mormons or the Seventh Day Adventists, follow rules concerning diet and alcohol and tobacco consumption and statistically have very low rates of cancer per population. One might do well to consider adopting some of these measures oneself.

Obesity

In the United States, as has been stated, this condition is related to our affluence and our life-style choices. It is a chronic problem and not only causes cardiovascular disease, diabetes, and hyperlipidemia, but may also be associated with cancer of the uterus, ovary, and breast and may possibly be a cofactor in colon cancer. Therefore, in addition to certain specific recommended food choices, such as the high-fiber, low-fat diet, it is generally considered advisable to maintain a normal body weight and to avoid the accumulation of fat in the tissues.

Suntanning

In the United States and Western Europe, having an intense suntan is considered attractive. Likewise, certain populations work out of doors in all weather. These persons, especially those who are very light-skinned, are at high risk for skin cancers. It would be advisable for these persons to use sunscreens and avoid the most intense sunlight during the day to reduce cancer incidence, as well as to prevent premature aging of the skin.

Ethnic groups

Certain ethnic groups have a higher incidence of certain types of cancers, but the cause is not primarily genetic. Ethnic groups in certain areas may have high-risk jobs or follow practices detrimental to their health. A good example of this is the breast cancer incidence of Japanese women. It is extremely low in Japan, but when these women move to the United States and adapt to the American life-style and diet, the incidence becomes similar to that of whites. If a person is a member of a racial or ethnic group at risk for a specific cancer, then he or she would be well advised to get routine, yearly screening examinations for this cancer.

Sexuality

It is becoming apparent that our sexual habits play a role in the development of certain cancers. For example, a woman who delays starting a family until after age 30 may be increasing her risk for breast cancer. No one should have children simply to avoid cancer, but knowing about the protective effect of a fairly early pregnancy may influence a woman's decision about *when* to start her family. Likewise, the risks of multiple partners, whether heterosexual or homosexual, and the risk of early intercourse should be known. A person who has multiple sexual partners should be aware of the increased incidence of cancer — cervical cancer in women and Kaposi's sarcoma, Burkitt's lymphoma, and rectal cancer in male homosexuals. The occurrence of a new disease, AIDS, has been discussed in this chapter, as well as a possible connection between the herpesvirus and cancer, especially cervical cancer. The major recommendations are to avoid herpes or other viral exposures by asking sexual partners if they have herpes or by using condoms and to consider hepatitis vaccination when indicated (see recommendations provided earlier in the chapter). See also p. 296.

Smoking

Smoking, especially while drinking alcohol, is so interwoven into our life-style in the United States that it sometimes seems inescapable. However, the evidence is overwhelming and conclusive that smoking, particularly at the same time as one is consuming alcoholic beverages, is extremely dangerous and should be eliminated from our lives. Taking an occasional drink without a cigarette may do no harm, but the effects of doing the two together considerably increase the cancer risks. Smoking should be avoided entirely.

SUMMARY

Thus it can be seen that one has to pay a price for a long, healthy, and hopefully cancer-free life. But is it really too high a price? Is that cigarette, that constant overindulgence in rich foods, or that avoidance of adequate preventive screening really worth more to you than the benefits of improved health, a sense of security about your body, and an overall lessening of the risks of cancer? Of course, it is each person's decision to make, but it is our hope that we have clarified these issues in such a way that the decisions you make regarding your health will be educated decisions and decisions in favor of health.

CHAPTER 11

Drugs, Immunity, Vaccination, and Cancer

Ten enemies can't harm a man as much as he harms himself.

JEWISH PROVERB

ERNEST H. ROSENBAUM

Many of us take drugs to improve our health status. Sometimes these drugs have an adverse side effect that can affect our body with allergic reactions, toxicity, or depression of the immune system. In addition, certain drugs damage normal cells and keep these cells from functioning properly. They may cause temporary or permanent genetic defects in the DNA mechanism, which may lead to cancer. Sometimes such effects result from *prolonged* use of drugs, and other times a spontaneous allergic reaction or idiosyncrasy can cause cell damage within a short period of time.

The immune system, which is discussed extensively in Chapter 10, plays an important role in protection and in maintenance of our body to keep it in a homeostatic or normal status. Viruses may alter cells by damaging DNA and may cause cancer. Since this is a possibility, vaccines made to protect our bodies against such viral or bacterial infections may play a role in cancer prevention. This chapter deals with the relationships that have been found between cancer and drugs, immunity, and vaccination.

DRUGS

It has been known for years that certain drugs are carcinogens. It is ironic that a person might need to take a therapeutic drug to control or limit a disease that may in turn cause another disease. The most difficult of these situations is when a drug is used to treat one cancer and then may cause another cancer years later. One has to balance the physical and emotional damages — health versus risk of cancer — when choosing a drug. There is little doubt that the healing potential of a drug when one's life is threatened is worth the small risk of facing cancer again later.

During the years 1971 to 1977 the International Agency for Research on Cancer (IARC) evaluated 368 chemicals and drugs. Of these, 26 were found to be carcinogenic in humans, and 221 showed some evidence of causing cancer in animals. The drugs in Table 11-1 have a proven carcinogenic activity.

"The pill"

One of the drugs people are most concerned about is "the pill," or oral contraceptive, which

TABLE 11-1 Drugs with proven carcinogenic activity

Drug	Organ or site of cancer
DES (diethylstilbestrol), sex hormones	Vagina Uterus Breast
Androgens (17-methyl substituted) Oxymetholone	Liver
Conjugated estrogens	Uterus
Aniline dyes—chlornaphazine, 2-naphthylamine	Bladder
Arsenic, arsenicals	Skin
Alkylating anticancer agents (mustards)	Leukemia, lymphoma
Immunosuppressive drugs—Cytoxan (cyclophosphamide), Imuran (azathioprine), Leukeran (chlorambucil), corticosteroids	Histiocytic lymphoma Blood disease
Butazolidin (phenylbutazone)	Possible leukemia
Chloramphenicol	Possible leukemia
Amphetamines (suspicious—not rated by the IARC)	Possible Hodgkin's disease; increased risk

has been widely used for years now. Many studies have investigated birth-control pills in terms of their potential for causing cancer. Several papers of the World Health Organization in 1978 suggested a possible increased risk of uterine cancer, as well as benign adenomas or malignant liver cancer. Reviewing the question of birth-control pills and breast cancer, recent studies reported from the Centers for Disease Control in Atlanta have stated that cancer and steroid hormone research showed no evidence that oral contraceptives, when used as medically recommended for more than 10 years, increased the risk of breast cancer.

Other research indicated no increased risk of breast cancer from oral contraceptives even in high-risk women with a family history of breast cancer or in those who had previous biopsies for benign breast disease. Also, a negative finding was reported for women who used oral contraceptives before their first pregnancy. If one already has breast cancer, however, it would be unwise to use hormones of any type, unless prescribed by one's physician.

Estrogen

A number of years after physicians started to treat women with estrogen supplements for premenopausal symptoms, an increase in endometrial cancer was noted. This cancer of the inner lining of the uterus was increasing mostly among affluent white women, in contrast to poorer white and black women. These women were the ones most likely to seek out a physician's care for menopausal symptoms and to be treated for their symptoms with estrogen. It soon became clear that the estrogen supplements were a factor in fostering endometrial cancer, and the dosage used was reduced or the estrogen was cycled with progesterone to counteract its negative and potentially cancerous effects.

This is an excellent example of causing one problem while curing another. Since the initial discovery, estrogen supplements have been studied and found to increase the risk of uterine carcinoma between four to eight times above normal. However, some of these studies have been criticized by other researchers, who thought there was no excess risk of endometrial cancer after estrogen supplements. Yet the National Institute of Health found, after 2 to 4 years of daily use of conjugated estrogens (0.625 or 1.25 milligrams of, for example, Premarin), an increased risk of up to seven times above normal. The risk also related to the duration of use.

DES

From the 1940s to the middle 1960s, the drug stilbestrol, or diethylstilbesterol (DES), was used during pregnancy for women who had a history of previous miscarriages. It is difficult to know with certainty how many women were given the drug, possibly 100,000 or even 150,000. The daughters of women given DES during pregnancy can develop an unusual form of adenocarcinoma of the vagina. This cancer of the vagina may require hysterectomy or vaginectomy in young women who have not yet had children. There is also some preliminary evidence that the sons born of women who took high-dose DES during pregnancy have smaller testes, possible cysts in the reproductive tract, undescended testes, and a higher incidence of infertility. The first DES-linked testicular cancer was reported in 1983 by Conley and associates. Research studies continue, and a nationwide search is still going on to find the children of women who took high-dose DES during pregnancy before it was contraindicated for pregnancy by the U.S. Food and Drug Administration.

Anticancer agents

Antineoplastic agents, or anticancer agents, are not only used to treat cancer; they are also used to treat benign diseases such as psoriasis and to prevent kidney or heart transplant rejection. There are many types of antineoplastic agents; those in the widely used *alkylating* or *mustard* group have been related to acute leukemias occurring years later in some myeloma and lymphoma patients treated with *melphalan*. However, the initial treatment was essentially to prevent the original cancer from progressing and causing death. There is little doubt that the curative effect far outweighed the risks. Fortunately, new drugs have been developed that may have less carcinogenic effects, and they are now undergoing clinical trials.

In one study anticancer drugs were found to act as a cocarcinogen. Anticancer drugs such as *methotrexate, Imuran (azathioprine), Cytoxan (cyclophosphamide)*, and the *cortisone* group are also used in transplant surgery.

One estimate is that cancers have been found to occur approximately 100 times more frequently in patients who received immunosuppressive drugs for kidney transplants than in the normal population. This means that a small percentage of transplant patients who receive daily immunosuppressive drugs may have approximately a 3% chance of developing cancer later in life. New and safer drug treatments are being developed.

Miscellaneous drugs

Therapeutic *radioactive phosphorus*, P-32, often used to treat a disease called polycythemia vera (rich blood), has been related to increased incidence of acute myelogenous leukemia. *Thoratrast*, a 25% colloidal suspension of *thorium dioxide*, was used as a radiographic contrast medium years ago to help visualize the blood/bone marrow system. Thoratrast can be retained for long periods in bone marrow, liver, spleen, and lymph nodes and can deliver constant local irradiation, which has led to several forms of cancer: liver tumors, angiosarcomas, leukemias, and Thoratrast-associated sarcomas of the bone. *Thoratrast has not been used for many years.*

Metronidazole (Flagyl), an effective antibiotic against amebiasis and *Trichomonas* infection, has had an association with lung tumors and lymphomas in experimental animals when used in very high doses. Under clinical studies this drug was not considered a carcinogen for humans.

Chloramphenicol, one of the most widely used antibiotics many years ago, has had a relationship to aplastic anemia (marrow damage). A relationship to possible human leukemia has been found since about 1955, when 17 cases were reported.

Arsenic compounds

Patients who live in areas where the local water is very high in *arsenicoles* seem to be at higher risk for skin cancer, especially noted on the trunk, palms, feet, and extremities. Also, a specific remedy known as *Fowler's solution* showed an association to a definite increase in skin cancers; this solution is no longer used.

Hydantoin derivatives such as *Dilantin*, which has been used for epilepsy since about 1948, showed a relationship to malignant lymphomas and psuedolymphomas in one major study. The study had poor controls, however, and the results cannot be considered conclusive. More recent studies found excessive lymphomas in children with epileptic mothers, and four reported cases of children exposed to hydantoin in utero developed a neuroblastoma or ganglioneuroblastoma, but the incidence is *extremely* rare.

Amphetamine (Dexedrine), a common antidepressant and appetite suppressant, has been associated with an increased incidence of Hodgkin's disease. Further studies are in progress to confirm or deny this finding, as these drugs are very widely used.

Recommendations

An effort is underway worldwide to identify those drugs that might have a potential for causing cancer. Certainly researchers are trying to establish more concrete information on the subject of drugs and cancer. At this point, although much is known, a lot more remains unknown. Nonetheless, an individual can follow some sensible guidelines (see boxed material) for the use of medications.

Remember that studies are continuously being made to help detect the true risks of drugs. These are being done using laboratory animals as well as using epidemiologic studies to see if there are any associations between the use of a specific drug and later cancer cases. In the meantime a healthy caution is advised when using medications.

IMMUNITY AND CANCER

Immunity is the body's ability to prevent certain disease organisms from invading the body or to counteract the effects of a disease once it is established. Some people seem naturally to have a more powerful immunity system and rarely get ill; others are just the opposite. The

---

Recommendations regarding drug use

1. Never use over-the-counter drugs casually for minor symptoms. Reduce the use of all over-the-counter drugs, as well as prescription drugs, whenever possible. (Under carefully assessed conditions, a drug with some risk may be worth taking when its beneficial effects are considered. This is a decision for you to make with your physician after you have discussed all the facts, including potential side effects.)
2. Women who are pregnant should not take drugs or hormones unless they are specifically prescribed by the physician caring for them during pregnancy.
3. Women with breast or uterine cancer should avoid all use of hormone supplements.
4. If you did take stilbesterol (DES) during pregnancy for previous miscarriages, your children, both male and female, should know this, and they should be closely followed by a physician who knows of their history of exposure to DES.
5. Never hesitate to question your physician thoroughly when a drug is prescribed about its known side effects, its risk potential, and the necessity for its use for the illness in question. Physicians will appreciate your intelligent concern.

interesting question is whether this health system, the body's immunity, can work against cancer, either preventively or as a means of recovery when used along with medical therapies after a cancer has become established.

This is still an area open to conjecture. We do know from various studies that people who are immune deficient (for one reason or another) have greater cancer risks. The clearest example is patients receiving drug therapy to suppress the immune system so they can undergo a successful organ transplant and not have their immune system reject the organ from another person's body. Other examples include those who already have one cancer that impairs their immunity and children and adults with immune-deficiency diseases who also have a higher rate of cancer.

To say that there is an association between a weakened immune system and cancer is not the same, however, as saying that cancers are caused by a deficiency in the body's immune system. The only fact that we are sure of is that immune-suppressed individuals have a higher risk of cancer than the general population. (See Chapter 10.)

The relationship between immunity and lifestyle can be looked at in two ways — biomedically and with commonsense. Biomedically, we know some things about the immune system. It can be injured by disease and malnutrition, and it can be affected by stress. On a commonsense level these biologic changes are experienced as feeling weak, rundown, or on-the-verge of catching something. Most people intuitively know when their health is below par, when they are more susceptible to any disease "going around." If we take corrective steps at this stage, when we get those "early warning signals," we are often able to maintain the overall working strength of our body's immune system, and not "get the bug." This may not have any direct impact on our cancer risk, but it can certainly keep us free from more transitory illnesses such as colds, flu, and the like. It can also maintain our body's strength and health, enabling it to better fight off threats from more serious diseases.

With advancing age, the immune system loses some of its functional capacity to protect and maintain a normal body status, as well as to detect, control, and destroy cells that are not normal — many of which could develop into cancer. The body's control of cancer is obviously far more complex than immune regulation alone; it seems to require many factors to initiate a cancer, such as repeated injuries from a carcinogen. It may take many years to initiate DNA changes and cell damage, as discussed in Chapters 1 and 3. Nevertheless, as one ages the immune system is less protective and under the constant bombardment of a toxic environment that may include tobacco smoke, alcohol, drugs, environmental and occupational exposures to chemicals, and infections.

A general approach to cancer prevention involves mainly common sense and following healthy life-style practices to try to maintain your body. As stated before, prevention through good health techniques is far better than therapy after a medical disaster.

To summarize the ways to maintain a properly functioning immune system:

1. Maintain good nutrition. Balance protein, carbohydrate, and fats with appropriate calorie and adequate vitamin and mineral intake. Experimental work has shown that zinc — 15 mg per day — might be helpful in maintaining a more normal immune status if cancer or deficiency states exist.
2. Exercise daily and get adequate sleep.
3. Maintain a normal vaccination program through your physician. This would include a DPT, measles, mumps, rubella, and polio immunization programs. Flu and hepatitis control should be used when indicated and specific vaccines taken when one is traveling to an area where the risk

of infections is increased. *There are no known anticancer vaccines, foods, or drugs that have been proved to prevent cancer.* The current hepatitis vaccine (discussed next) may potentially become the first specific anticancer vaccine.

4. Review recommendations on AIDS—see Chapter 10.

VIRUS VACCINATION

In view of the evidence that several viruses have been associated with cancer, the development of a vaccine against a virus is a major medical step. The virus in question is for hepatitis B virus (HBV). This virus could not be grown in a test tube, and thus required special techniques for a final pure antigen preparation to be obtained. The vaccine was then developed from this, and safety tests were conducted, initially on chimpanzees and then later on human populations. The vaccines were uniformly successful with no subsequent negative results several years later.

Among men vaccinated, 77% have detectable anti–hepatitis B antibodies within 2 months of their initial innoculation. This increased to 96% after a 6-month booster. The few cases of HBV found in the vaccine group were believed to be caused by infection that had occurred before they received the vaccine.

This vaccine may also be the first anticancer vaccine because of the relationship between HBV infection and primary hepatocellular (liver) carcinoma. In South African blacks, a population with the world's highest incidence of hepatocellular carcinoma, a full 95% showed positive serologic evidence of a prior HBV infection. A study of 2000 men in Taiwan showed that the relative risk for hepatocellular carcinoma was 223 times greater among those who had the HBV antigen and were carriers than among noncarriers.

Although not conclusive, the evidence is mounting that there is a relationship between HBV and hepatocellular carcinoma, which is an endemic disease in Asia and parts of Africa. Thus it will be possible to achieve, if the vaccine continues to prove successful, a potential control for this form of cancer. The implications for conquering HBV are similar to the conquest of smallpox. Approximately 200,000 new cases of HBV are diagnosed each year, and there are an estimated 800,000 HBV carriers in the United States alone, with another 10,000 to 20,000 becoming chronic carriers each year. A further implication is that the success of this one antiviral vaccine may lead to the development of other types of antiviral vaccines that would work to control cancers that are viral related.

Certain populations are more at risk for hepatitis and should be considered for the vaccine, according to H. J. Alter of the National Institute of Health. These include the following:

1. Health workers exposed to hepatitis patients or to hepatitis-infected blood or blood products, including dentists, oral surgeons, laboratory technicians, physicians, and nurses.
2. Renal dialysis patients and all negative dialysis patients.
3. Institutional patients, especially the mentally retarded.
4. Patients with hereditary or acquired disorders such as hemoglobinopathies, who require repeated transfusions; for example, those with sickle cell, thalassemia, hemolytic anemias.
5. Patients with leukemia or malignant disorders, who may have chemotherapeutically induced marrow aplasia and require multiple transfusions. (NOTE: Specialized vaccine dose regimens have been recommended for those with malignant diseases as well as patients on dialysis.)
6. Male homosexuals, who have a 12% to 19% annual attack rate of HBV infection, which is 100 to 200 times higher than the national average in the United States.

7. The sexual partners and household contacts of HBV antigen carriers, who require protection because they are more heavily exposed.

8. Infants born to HBV-antigen-positive mothers. Globally, it has been estimated that at least 50% of the world's chronic carriers evolve from virus *transfer at the time of delivery*. Infants older than 3 months of age respond well to the vaccine, and 95% of neonates developed HBV antibody response to three innoculations of the hepatitis vaccine.

9. Children and susceptible adults in regions with epidemic HBV.

10. Military and foreign service personnel who are assigned to epidemic-HBV areas in the Third World nations.

CHAPTER 12

Can You Prevent Cancer?

Approximately 60 to 80 percent of cancers are man-made.

JUSTIN STEIN
Emeritus Professor of Radiotherapy
University of California at Los Angeles

ERNEST H. ROSENBAUM

The objective of this book has been to address the question of whether or not cancer can be prevented. By now you realize that our answer is a qualified "Yes." We have described or outlined the potential causes of cancer, and we know these factors can be avoided or reduced. We can also make educated guesses about another 30% of the causes of cancer. These risk factors have been discussed throughout the book; you should now be fairly well acquainted with them.

Simply knowing about and understanding the problem of cancer will not, however, solve it. It will take the sustained efforts of many individuals, the general public, the media, and all levels of government to help reduce the risk and incidence of cancer.

To begin with, there are certain qualifications to cancer prevention. By our personal choices we can radically reduce our chances of getting cancer, but there are some things that are outside our control, such as heredity, a defective immune system, and numerous environmental factors. In addition, many things remain unknown, including many of the causes of cancer. Scientific knowledge is limited, although present research is turning up important new data at a fast pace. We will probably never be able to cure all diseases, but we can try through the most effective means — prevention — to conquer cancer.

Reducing cancer risk is primarily a personal decision. It cannot be made for you; it cannot be done for you by anyone else because it involves a choice of life-styles, and only you can make those choices. Had your parents guided you and had you adopted specific health practices such as not smoking or drinking, while eating a high-fiber, low-fat diet with appropriate vitamins in fresh fruit and vegetables, your risk for cancer would be reduced. For you, your children, and your family, this can still be done, by following the good health practices suggested. Although pollution of the air and water, industrial exposure and contamination, and radiation or pesticides receive the greatest media coverage as cancer threats, the most effective approach to avoiding cancer comes from personal life-style choices. Probably no more than 10% of cancers relate to occupational/environmental hazards, and another 2% may be caused by heredity. Prudent daily living patterns with appropriate changes in personal behavior toward a more healthy life-style seem

245

The Seven Personal Health Practices

1. Never smoke cigarettes.
2. Perform regular physical activity.
3. Moderate or no use of alcohol.
4. Sleep 7 or 8 hours per day regularly.
5. Maintain a proper weight.
6. Eat breakfast daily.
7. Do not eat between meals.

---

to be the most important preventative steps you can take. Yet noncompliance, a poor cooperation, in a cancer prevention program remains a problem. The best example is that most smokers don't quit.

An example of the positive effects of good life-style choices appears in a study done by L. Breslow and J. Enstrom reported in *Preventative Medicine* in 1980. A group of people in Alameda County, California, who practiced a set of rules known as the Seven Personal Health Practices (see boxed material) were followed for 9½ years. The goal of the study was to find out if a person would live longer by taking an active and responsible role in his or her health and body care. The group who followed most or all these personal health practices were compared to the group who followed three or less.

Males who practices six or seven of these practiced for 5½ years had a mortality rate only 28% of the rate of those who followed three or less of these practices. Females who followed six or seven of the health practices had a mortality rate that was 43% of those who followed three or less of the health practices.

In the population followed 5½ years, those who adhered to six or seven personal health practices had a longer life expectancy at age 45 than those who practiced zero to three health practices — 33.1 years versus 21.6 years, respectively. This is a means of an average of 11½ ad-

ditional years of LIFE. Women who followed the guidelines showed a 7-year life prolongation when compared to those who followed zero to three health practices.

The conclusion of the study was that poor health habits led to earlier death, and good health habits prolonged life. Good health practices were even more important to longevity than one's initial health status. This was a simple study with a few elementary guidelines that relate to health — nothing exotic or esoteric. Anyone can follow these straightforward guidelines; they require no additional expense and little investment of time.

Only three of the recommendations involved in this study relate directly to cancer prevention: not smoking, minimal alcohol consumption, and maintaining proper weight. These are possibly the three most important general guidelines for cancer prevention (unless you fall into a special risk category such as having a family history of a certain cancer or having a specific industrial or occupational exposure). The remaining cancer guidelines that could be added are general: (1) avoid a high-fat, high-red meat diet and add fiber and vitamins A, C, and E as well as minerals selenium and zinc to your diet; (2) avoid or reduce exposure to viruses, especially sexually transmitted ones; (3) reduce exposure to sunlight and radiation; and (4) maintain the strength of your immune system by reducing insults to it.

The reason that these guidelines must remain general is that we know enough to make some recommendations, but much of the information we have is not yet specific enough for us to pinpoint causative factors except in certain areas such as tobacco consumption. The best examples of what we know about cancer incidence come from the field of cancer epidemiology, which studies cancer worldwide, comparing the cancer rates among certain populations and life-styles. Epidemiologists such as Daniels, Higginson, Muir, Petrakis, Wynder, and others have already given us a tremendous amount of information, but some of what they turn up leads to further puzzles.

A good example comes from J. Higginson, who compared the colon cancer rate of the Danes with that of the neighboring Finns. The Danes show four times the colon cancer rate of the Finns, yet both populations are considered equally affluent, living quite well compared to the rest of the world. In addition, the Finns (compared to the Danes and the rest of Europe) have the highest rate of cardiovascular disease. One of the differences noted between the two groups was dietary: the Finns, with the lower colon cancer rate, eat more fiber, but they also eat more fat, which may account for their higher rate of cardiovascular disease and their lower rate of colon cancer, although colon cancer is thought to be associated with a high-fat diet. Obviously, we cannot yet say that a high-fat diet automatically causes colon cancer because in the case of the Finns this does not hold up.

Another set of facts turned up by Higginson was that the incidence of breast cancer was higher in urban Denmark compared to rural Denmark. Increased fat intake is thought to have a relationship with breast as well as colon cancer. Given this thesis, one would assume that the urban Danes ate more fat, since they had a higher incidence of breast cancer. In fact, however, it is the other way around—the rural Danes eat approximately 50% more fat than the urban Danes. Therefore, the cause does not seem to be diet alone, and just cutting down on fat alone may not solve the problem.

These examples illustrate a major point of the entire book—cancer is probably in most cases not caused by a single factor or exposure. Cancer risk most likely results from multiple factors that are sometimes related or interrelated. These exposures somehow add up over a period of time to produce changes in the body chemistry–DNA that lead to cancer.

The risk factors we have studied and know about can be broken down into two general categories: internal and external. Internal fac-tors are more limited than external ones, and they include such things as genetic susceptibility, an inherited disease pattern or immunity weakness, and possibly an inherited cellular pattern so that the cells that are damaged over years or a lifetime cannot repair their DNA damage and thus survive intact. The internal metabolic balance of an individual is complex and difficult to characterize simply, but there may be both biologic inhibitors to internal damages as well as promotors that allow damage to be more extensive. All of these factors relate to a person's physical equipment rather than external events.

The external influences or risk factors are more varied and complex, as shown by the following paragraphs.

1. The *geographic area* of the world in which a person lives is a determining factor due to physical and cultural practices. In some parts of the world, the soil may be high or low in selenium. If the selenium level in the soil and diet is low, an increase in cancer has been noted. Thus the increased or decreased amount of selenium in food may affect the occurrence of cancer.

The diet of a country may include little or no meat and lots of vegetables and grain, and this might reduce colon cancer. In some countries a specific cultural pattern, such as betel nut chewing in India, can increase the cancer rate. In another country certain viruses that are associated with cancer can flourish, such as the hepatitis B virus in parts of Africa and Asia.

2. Specific *cultural and religious practices* relate to cancer prevention and incidence. Early or late marriages, age at first pregnancy, monogamy, the number of sexual partners, patterns of sexual hygiene, and the dietary patterns and prohibitions for some religious groups can all play a part in cancer and cancer prevention.

3. *Environmental exposures* that are cancer producing, including pollutants and pesticides, are a concern of many people, but this factor is often overrated compared to others. Air pollution, for example, is a minor problem, but it be-

comes a major problem if you smoke.

4. *Occupational risks* relate to specific groups of people who are exposed to agents such as asbestos, nickel, cadmium, and uranium. It is thought that there is a relationship to the length of time exposed, with longer exposure posing a greater risk. Although specific exposures do seem to promote cancers, industrialization as a whole is not correlated to the patterns of cancer incidence. An example is Japan, which has become a highly industrialized nation, but the rate of cancer in Japan did not change as it industrialized.

5. *Time* is a factor, since usually a long time elapses between the exposure to a carcinogen or carcinogens and the development of the disease. The exception to this may be the current explosion of specific cancers among male homosexuals, but even in these cases, where the cancer appears to develop very quickly (approximately 18 months), the individual may have had a multiyear exposure or multiple assaults to his DNA or immune system involving multiple partners and frequent sex (as seen in women with cervical cancer or homosexual men with AIDS), including practices that damage rectal tissue and the use of common recreational drugs. Because of the lag time, it is often difficult to establish which exposure to what agent actually caused a cancer to develop.

6. *Viruses* play a part in the risk of cancer. We now know of six that are associated with tumor production, both benign and malignant (see Chapter 10).

7. *Diet* is a general risk factor; we know it is related to cancer risk, but highly specific correlations have not yet been made (see Chapter 5). Diet is influenced by one's culture; the location of one's country; the local surroundings, whether they are rural or urban; and the relative lifestyle of the surroundings—rich or poor. A definite relationship has been established between cancer and a high-fat diet. A diet high in total fat (especially beef and pork) has been associated with an increased risk of breast, colorectal, ovarian, endometrial, prostate, pancreatic and renal cancer. A diet high in fiber, conversely, seems to have a preventive influence on colon cancer. Vitamins may play a protective role, including vitamin A or beta-carotene, which may reduce or partially control cell growth; vitamin C, which can neutralize nitrosamines; and vitamin E and selenium, which act as antioxidant agents. All of these may help protect cells from becoming malignant. An example of the geographic influence is exposure to toxic foodstuffs, such as those containing the fungus aflatoxin that is common in Africa and Asia and increases the incidence of cancer in those exposed.

Obesity is a specific risk factor for cancer that is related to diet. Obesity has been associated with tumors of the breast and uterus. It is thought that the cancer risk of obesity may be caused by estrogen, which is produced in the fatty tissues of an obese person from a hormone of the adrenal gland called epiandrosterone. Estrogen does not seem carcinogenic when it occurs in a normal estrous cycle and alternates with progesterone production, as in a normal menstrual cycle. However, an obese person experiences a constant barrage of estrogens, and this relates to that other risk factor of time—the chronic long-term exposure to a potential carcinogen. (See also Chapters 5 and 10.)

8. *Hormones* such as estrogen, as well as other *chemicals,* and *medications* have been associated with cancer. These are reviewed in Chapter 11. This association was first noted when menopausal women on estrogen therapy started showing an increased incidence of endometrial cancer.

9. *Smoking* tobacco is clearly identified as one of the most important factors causing cancer (lung, bladder, oral, pharyngeal, esophageal, laryngeal, pancreatic, and possibly renal). The evidence is clear: at least 30% of all cancers are smoking and tobacco related, including chewing and sniffing the stuff (see Chapter 7).

10. *Alcohol* is a factor in approximately 2%

to 4% of cancers, usually those of the head and neck area and of the liver. The risk factor of alcohol is markedly increased by smoking. (See Chapter 6.)

11. *Psychologic states* can have a biochemical effect on our body, releasing certain hormones, increasing heart and respiratory rate, and tightening muscles. (See Chapter 9.)

It has not been shown that cancer is a stress-related disorder, but stress can result in an impaired immune response, as measured by laboratory tests which could affect a cancer growth rate. Behavioral factors or life-style can influence cancer risk directly by affecting immune competence and also, in part, by determining whether one smokes or not, which will alter a person's cancer risk. The evidence is *weak* that stress can cause cancer or that there is a cancer-prone personality. It is our choice on how we live and/or abuse our body that results in the life-style/behavioral cause of cancer.

12. *Sunlight* and other ultraviolet exposure influences the incidence of skin cancers, both squamous cell and the more dangerous melanomas. Those with fair skin are at higher risk. Patients with pigmented skin that changes color, grows or itches should be evaluated by their physician. The risk can be reduced by appropriate use of a sunscreen. (See Chapter 4.)

13. *Sexuality* relates to cancer in specific areas, including the age of a woman at first pregnancy, the age at the beginning of intercourse (for a woman), large numbers of sexual partners and consequent increased risk of exposure to sexually transmitted viral diseases (cervical cancer), and nulliparity (breast cancer). For male homosexuals the cancer risk includes many partners, exposure to viruses and feces, and rectal damage through sexual practices (Kaposi's sarcoma, Burkitt's lymphoma, AIDS, rectal cancer.) (See Chapter 10.)

14. *Radiation exposure* can also be a factor; cancer is a health risk from low-dose ionizing radiation. Radiation is both from the earth (natural) as well as cosmic exposure (air travel).

Over a lifetime the total dose from background (0.1 rem per year) is added to medical radiation (0.08 rem per year) to add up to about 14 rem average life dose. The increased risk is when the lifetime cumulative dose exceeds 40 to 50 rem, thus we need not fear normal low-level radiation exposure. The exceptions are fetal injury during x-ray filming and occupational hazards (radiologists, x-ray technicians). When possible, try to limit the amount of dental and medical x-ray films, and when x-ray films are done, use a lead apron shield in areas exposed but not being evaluated. (See Chapter 8.)

15. *Affluence* is a catch-all risk factor because it describes the fact that cancer rates are related to growing affluence, which seems to involve the temptations or opportunities to overindulge in eating, drinking, smoking, and so on. This overindulgence and increased cancer rate is not, however, necessary. One can live a very comfortable life and still not put oneself at risk for cancer through exposures that may be entirely avoidable.

These are the major external risk factors for cancer, but as you can see, they constantly interrelate and augment each other. For example, we are all exposed to some sunlight, although darker people have more built-in protection. We all have varied dietary and smoking patterns as well as occupational exposures.

Some of our exposures to carcinogenic agents are very brief; others are long-term or chronic. Cancer is above all a multifactorial event. One example might be:

Alcohol—cirrhosis of the liver, plus

Geography—Africa or Asia, with exposure to a virus such as hepatitis;

Virus—hepatitis is present in almost 100% of babies during first year of life, plus

Aflatoxin—a fungoid carcinogenic by-product of contaminated food in parts of Africa and Asia, plus

Genes—increased hereditary susceptibility in some individuals.

These all lead to a highly increased risk for a primary liver cancer.

Another example would be a male homosexual who has exposure to a cytomegalovirus (widespread in the homosexual population) and also has multiple partners and frequent sexual relations that may lead to exposure to other viruses and rectal damage. It is suspected that the interrelationship of these factors can lead to an increase in AIDS and rectal cancer risk. (See Chapter 10.)

Further examples are exposure to asbestos (a known carcinogen) and being a heavy smoker and possibly a moderate to heavy drinker—again, multiple risk factors.

Risk factor analysis is, therefore, very difficult because many variables are involved. To begin with, one would have to do a risk factor analysis for each culture. As an example, Higginson has suggested a scale for worldwide incidence of prostate cancer. In his scale, the Japanese would be 1, white Americans 30, and black Americans 60. The rate of prostate cancer varies between the United States and Japan, yet both countries show about a 10% incidence of latent prostatic cancer in men over age 75. Why is it then that prostate cancer occurs in a more virulent and aggressive state in American males, particularly blacks, compared to the Japanese?

When Japanese men migrate to the United States, where they adopt the American lifestyle, their incidence of prostate cancer increases toward the American incidence. The same is true for the incidence of breast cancer in Japanese women who migrate to the United States. It is believed that the factor explaining the difference is dietary; this is speculation about this one factor with respect to two particular cancers. There are many risk factors and a few hundred cancers, which makes pinpointing specific risks difficult to impossible unless large groups show significant patterns, such as smokers and lung cancer.

It seems safe to conclude that *most* of the risk factors relate to life-style rather than air and water pollution and industrial exposure. It is in the area of life-style risks that we have the greatest chance to make changes. We do, after all, control our own lives in terms of what we eat, drink, or whether we smoke, how much time we sunbathe, and who we have sex with; these all involve choices that we can make—perhaps not easily, but they are within reach. We do not have to petition our politicians or pay exorbitant fees to specialists in medicine to make life-style changes. The choices for prevention of cancer are simple and readily available to all of us.

In addition to the general guidelines offered throughout this book, individuals interested in determining if they are at high cancer risk for some reason might want to fill out the self-history questionnaire in Appendix C.* If the results indicate that you have multiple risk factors, you may want to consider a program of experimental chemoprevention *under medical supervision.* These programs involve dietary intake of vitamin A/beta-carotene, vitamin C, vitamin E, selenium, and zinc.

Private life-style changes are not the only approach we have available to reduce cancer risks, although they are the most immediate and effective actions we can take. Social changes will also be necessary to prevent cancer and reduce the effects of cancer.

The U.S. government can fulfill its protective functions more fully by pursuing research into dangerous exposures and controlling toxic wastes that are known to cause cancer. *It can free itself of the domination by the tobacco industry and eliminate all tobacco advertising,* as has been done with great effectiveness in several other countries.

Educational programs should be started in grade school to influence young people not to become smokers when they grow older. The

---

*If you are interested in information on cancer risk analysis, write to The Claire Zellerbach Saroni Tumor Institute of Mount Zion Hospital and Medical Center, P.O. Box 7921, San Francisco, CA 94120.

video *Death in the West* (Chapter 6) should be shown and discussed annually in elementary, high, and prep schools all over the country as well as monthly on prime time television. Additional efforts should be directed toward reducing alcoholic drinking, improving nutritional awareness, and eliminating the casual use of drugs from our culture. These educational programs can be effectively directed toward specific populations and altered or translated for Americans who speak a language other than English.

Health services can be improved with nationwide miniscreening and preventative education programs for cancer. This would involve a health history and a current health practices questionnaire, including an analysis of patterns such as smoking, drinking, diet, and toxic habits, with education on the risks involved. The physical examination would include weight, blood pressure, mouth, lymph node, liver, spleen, breast, and genital examination and Pap smear as indicated.

General health information on smoking, diet modification, reducing alcohol consumption, and guidelines for positive health can be offered in multilingual brochures, videos, movies, and TV spots. Local governments can help coordinate community services, and local media can be used to promote periodic health evaluations such as community health fairs; mass screening evaluation, however, should not replace the routine medical evaluation by your physician.

It is unrealistic to expect industry to pursue research on the toxic effects of the substances used because of the costs involved, which would reduce the margin of profit; nor can a farmer be expected to understand everything about the pesticides and fertilizers used, so he must have some guidelines. The government should take a more responsible role in doing research, making consistent recommendations, and giving constant guidance to improve the quality of our lives. Money spent to pursue health is money well spent by government—it can save billions of dollars lost to illness and incapacity. Cancer could be reduced in this way by reducing the risk factors we are exposed to over our lifetimes. It is the duty of each elected official to insist on higher standards, better education, and honest objective programs for improved health practices, screening, and prevention as well as provide protective legislation and funds for research and health programs. It is our duty to insist on cancer prevention legislation and strong government protective policies from our elected officials. Political pressures should be exerted to reduce smoking and alcohol intake and to encourage dietary modifications for better health.

Imagine a people who are dedicated to maintaining their health and vigor, whose tax monies are wisely spent for this purpose, whose government works through education, guidelines, and regulation to promote the health and well-being of its people; imagine individuals who choose what is best for themselves and so become examples of strength and good sense to their young. Most measures used to prevent cancer will also reduce the risk of heart disease and stroke, the number one and number three killers.

This is not an unattainable dream by any means. Because we are now beginning to understand the mechanisms and causes of cancer and other diseases, we are gaining information that enables us to remove what once seemed an inevitable threat. We have many options as individuals and as citizens to prevent cancer and improve the quality of our lives.

The guidelines for cancer prevention are not meant to restrict one's enjoyment of life. On the contrary, we can still relish the fruits of our civilization—we need not do away with industrialization or modern conveniences. We do need, however, to choose which fruits are good for us and which are not. Medical science can provide the information, but only informed human intelligence and determination can make the choices that count. A commonsense and practical approach to reduce toxic and carcinogenic exposure is important. Implementation of such common sense is even more important.

Cancer prevention begins with you at home and at work. *You* are responsible for your health. *You* have the capacity to act and implement a safer life-style and thus reduce your cancer risk.

> Life is meant to be lived, and curiosity must be kept alive; one must never, for whatever reason, turn his back on life.
> ELEANOR ROOSEVELT

Glossary

acute infection An infection of viral or bacterial origin that develops and progresses rapidly, as opposed to a *chronic infection,* which may have a prolonged course.

acute lymphocytic leukemia A disorder of blood cell production in which abnormal white blood cells accumulate in the blood and bone marrow. Called also *acute lymphatic leukemia* or *acute lymphoblastic leukemia.*

adenocarcinoma A cancer whose cells resemble those of glands.

adjuvant programs The administration of radiotherapy or chemotherapy to patients from whom all known cancer has been surgically removed, in an effort to destroy undetected cancer.

adrenaline An excitatory chemical produced by the adrenal glands that plays a major role in the arousal of the human system.

aflatoxin A toxic factor and carcinogen produced by the pathogenic mold *Aspergillusflavus.*

alcoholism A chronic relapsing disease ending in death, characterized by tolerance for alcohol, the presence of an alcohol withdrawal syndrome on the cessation or diminution of alcohol intake, and/or physical diseases consequent to alcohol ingestion.

alkalating agents A family of chemotherapeutic drugs that combine with the genetic substance DNA to prevent normal cell division.

Ames test A laboratory bacterial growth test to detect cancer-causing agents. This is done by using mutant strains of *Salmonella typhimurium* on culture mediums containing the chemicals in question along with a rat-liver enzyme that is capable of converting carcinogen and mutagen precursors into active metabolites.

amphetamines Drugs that stimulate the human nervous system.

analgesic A drug used for reducing pain.

androgens Male sex hormones.

anemia The condition of having less than the normal amount of hemoglobin or red cells in the blood.

angiogram The process of visualizing an x-ray image of the blood vessel through the introduction of a substance that renders the blood vessels radiopaque (capable of blocking x-rays).

antibody A substance, probably made by lymphocytes and certain other specialized cells, that helps defend the body against infections from viruses, bacteria, and other foreign organisms.

antigens Chemical structures in a cell that can be recognized by the body as foreign and thus stimulate immune reactions.

antioxidant Any substance that delays the process of oxidation.

arterial system A branching pattern of vessels by which blood is distributed from the heart to all tissues of the body.

asbestosis Scarring of the lungs from prolonged inhalation of asbestos dust.

bacille Calmette-Guerin (BCG) A form of the tuberculosis bacterium, used primarily for TB vaccination, which can act as an excellent stimulant to the immune system.

253

bacteria   One-celled primitive plant organisms widely encountered in nature, sometimes capable of causing disease in humans.

barbiturates   A specific class of drugs capable of inducing relaxation, narcosis, sleep, or unconsciousness.

barium   A substance through which x-rays cannot pass.

basal cell carcinoma   The most common form of skin cancer; it rarely spreads beneath the skin and is easily treated and cured. Basal cells are found in small numbers in the lowest layer of the epidermis, the surface of the skin.

benign   Not malignant.

benign prostatic hyperplasia (BPH)   A benign condition in which the prostate swells, crowding against the urethra and the bladder and blocking the flow of urine.

biopsy   The surgical removal of a small portion of tissue for diagnosis.

bladder   The body's container for urine (waste water). It is found in front of the rectum in the pelvis.

blast cells   An immature stage in cellular development before the appearance of mature cells.

blood chemistry panels   Multiple chemical determinations prepared by an automated method from a single sample of blood serum.

blood count   A laboratory study to evaluate the amount of white cells, red cells, and platelets in the blood.

bone marrow   A soft substance found within bone cavities, ordinarily composed of fat and developing red cells, white cells, and platelets.

Bowen's disease   A precancerous scaly skin disease.

breast self-examination (BSE)   Self-examination of the breast by a woman to find early signs of breast cancer.

bronchi   The large air tubes of the lung.

bronchioles   The tiny branches of air tubes of the lung.

bronchogram   A procedure for outlining the inside of lung passages to make it visible.

Burkitt's lymphoma   A lymph node tumor originally found in equatorial Africa; many can now be cured by chemotherapy.

cancer   The proliferation of malignant cells that have the capability for invasion of normal tissues.

carcinogen   any cancer-producing substance or agent.

carcinogenicity   The potential to produce cancer.

carcinoid   A potentially malignant tumor arising in the wall of the gastrointestinal tract or bronchial tree, capable of secreting substances causing diarrhea, flushing, or rapid heartbeat.

carcinoma   A cancer that begins in tissue that lines an organ or duct.

carcinoma in situ   Cancer that involves only the top layer of tissue without invasion to deeper tissue.

case-control study   Study of a suspected cancer-causing factor that occurs commonly among people who have a specific type of cancer (cases); compared to persons who do not have cancer (controls).

cervical canal   The passage in the cervix that connects the main part of the uterus with the upper vagina.

cervix   The lower portion of the uterus, which protrudes into the vagina and forms a portion of the birth canal during delivery.

chemotherapy   The treatment of disease by chemicals (drugs) introduced into the bloodstream by injection or taken by mouth as tablets.

chromosomes   Material in a cell made of DNA that carries the genes.

chronic   Defining a disease process that develops over a long period and progresses slowly.

cirrhosis of the liver   The laying down of scar tissue causing decreased liver function; symptoms include jaundice, fluid retention, and enlarged liver.

cobalt-60   A radioactive isotope of the element cobalt used in radiation treatment.

cobalt treatment   Radiotherapy using gamma rays generated from the breakdown of radioactive cobalt-60.

cocarcinogen   An agent that increases the effect of a carcinogen to cause cancer.

colitis   Inflammation of the large intestine.

colon   The lower 5 to 6 feet of the intestine. Called also the *large bowel*.

colonoscope   A highly flexible fiberoptic telescopic instrument used for examination of the colon.

colonoscopy   An examination with a colonoscope.

colostomy   Formation of an artificial anus in the abdominal wall, allowing the colon to drain feces (stool) into a bag.

conization   The surgical removal of a cone-shaped section of tissue from the cervix and cervical canal. Conization may be performed to diagnose or to treat a cervical condition.

consultation   The formal process of soliciting the opinion of a specialist.

crossover   An exchange of genes between two close chromosomes.

cyst   A fluid-filled sac of tissue; a cyst may be malignant or benign.

cystoscope   An instrument that enables the physician to see the interior of the bladder, to remove a tissue sample or a small tumor, and to cauterize tissue.

D and C   An abbreviation for *dilation and curettage.* A D and C is a minor operation in which the cervix is expanded (dilated) enough to permit the cervical canal and uterine lining to be scraped with a spoon-shaped instrument called a curette (curettage).

diagnosis   The process by which a disease is identified.

diagnostic procedures   Studies designed to yield information about the nature and extent of disease in a patient.

digestive tract   The esophagus, stomach, and intestines and colon, and other organs involved in digestion such as the liver and pancreas.

DNA   Abbreviation for *deoxyribonucleic acid,* the building block of the genes, responsible for the passing of hereditary characteristics from cell to cell.

double-blind   A clinical study comparing two agents—a placebo (inert substance) and a specific substance—by using a code number, but neither physician, patient, nor medical team know which drug is the active and which is the placebo.

dysplasia   The presence of abnormal cells. Cervical dysplasia may be classified as mild, moderate, or severe.

edema   The accumulation of fluid within the tissues.

electrons   Negatively charged particles making up the outer shell of atoms; electron beam is a form of radiotherapy used for treating the skin.

endometrium   The inner lining of the body of the uterus.

endoscopic retrograde cholangiopancreatography (E.R.C.P.)   An endoscopic examination of the bile duct system from the small intestine.

enzymes   Proteins that assist the occurrence of specific chemical reactions; the increase of certain enzymes in the blood may be a measure of certain diseases.

epidemiology   The study of a disease and its relationship to other diseases through such factors as cause, rate of occurrence, and distribution in a human community.

epidermoid carcinoma   A cancer that begins on the epidermis, or surface, or organ lining of, for example, skin, lung, and bladder.

Epstein-Barr virus   A virus that is known to cause infectious mononucleosis and has been associated with Burkitt's lymphoma and certain cancers of the head and neck.

esophagoscope   A long, slender, hollow instrument that is passed through the mouth into the esophagus, enabling the physician to see the interior of the esophagus, to biopsy a suspected area, and to collect cell specimens by means of a washing solution introduced and removed through the instrument.

estrogens   Female sex hormones.

estrogen therapy   Treatment with estrogens.

excision   Surgical removal of tissue.

exploratory   Surgery undertaken to investigate a situation that diagnostic tests have failed to clarify.

extrinsic   Situated or coming from outside an organ or body.

fallopian tube   The tube on each ovary that conducts the egg from the ovary to the uterus.

familial polyposis   An inherited tendency to develop polyps in the intestine and rectum.

fiberoptic bronchoscope   A medical instrument used to view many air passages of the lung. It is a thin, flexible tube that can be maneuvered into branching air passages of the lungs.

fibroid   Called also *Leiomyoma.* Benign tumor of the uterus composed of muscle tissue.

fluoroscope   An instrument used for observing the internal structure of the body by means of x-rays.

food additives   Substances or agents added to food.

gamma rays   A unit of radium or radiation dosage.

Gardner's syndrome   A familial disease characterized by colon polyps.

gastrointestinal tract   The digestive tract, including the esophagus, stomach, small and large intestines, and the rectum.

gene   A portion of DNA capable of transmitting a single characteristic from parent to progeny.

genetics   A branch of biology that deals with heredity and the study of the differences and disease risk between parents and children.

gynecomastia   Enlargement of breasts in the male.

hematology   The study of theblood and blood-forming tissues.

herpes   An acute viral inflammation of the skin or mucous membranes characterized by the development of groups of vesicles or blisters.

high-density lipoprotein   A high-molecular-weight fat-protein complex.

history and physical examination   The routine by which information is obtained from patients and their physical characteristics are assessed.

Hodgkin's disease   A form of lymphoma that arises in a single lymph node and may spread to local, then distant, lymph nodes and finally to other tissues, commonly including the spleen, liver, and bone marrow.

hormonal anticancer therapy   A form of therapy based on certain cancers stabilizing or shrinking if a specific hormone is added or removed.

hormones   Naturally occurring substances that are released by the endocrine organs and circulate in the blood, stimulating or turning off the growth or activity of specific target cells or organs.

hyperplasia   An increase or growth in normal cells.

hysterectomy   Surgical removal of the uterus.

immune   Identifies the state of adequate defense against a particular infection or possibly against a certain cancer.

immunogenetic   Pertaining to interrelationships of immune reactions and a person's genetic constitution.

immunology   The study of the body's natural defense mechanisms and of the diseases that result from deficient or inappropriate defense responses.

immunotherapy   A method of cancer therapy that stimulates the body defenses (the immune system) to attack cancer cells or modify a specific disease status.

immunotoxicity   A toxic reaction of the immune defense system.

in vitro   Occurring within laboratory apparatus; observable in a test tube.

in vivo   Occurring within a living organism.

incidence   An expression of the rate at which a certain event occurs.

infectious mononucleosis   A viral infection involving the blood and organs.

inflammation   The triggering of local body defenses resulting in the outpouring of defensive cells (leukocytes) from the circulation into the tissues, frequently with associated pain and swelling.

intestinal tract   Esophagus, stomach, small bowel, and colon.

intravenous pyelogram   The intravenous administration of a radiopaque dye that is concentrated and excreted by the kidneys, making the kidneys and drainage system visible with x-rays.

intrinsic   Situated inside or within.

isotopic scan   A class of diagnostic procedures for assessing organs (liver, bone, brain) in which particular radioactive substances are introduced intravenously; the relative concentrations of these substances are detected by their radioactivity, yielding information about cancerous involvement of specific structures.

jaundice   The accumulation of bilirubin, a breakdown product of hemoglobin, resulting in yellowish discoloration of the skin and of the white portion of the eyes; this is indicative of liver disease or blockage of the major bile ducts.

keratosis   A skin disease characterized by an overgrowth of the top layer of the skin.

large cell carcinoma   A lung cancer characterized by large cancer cells that do not resemble the cells of other types of lung cancer.

laryngectomy   The surgical removal of the larynx or voice box.

leiomyoma   See *fibroid*.

leukemia   A malignant proliferation of white blood-forming cells in the bone marrow; cancer of the blood cells. There are two types of acute leukemia: *lymphocytic* and *myelogenous*.

localized   With reference to cancer, confined to the site of origin, without evidence of spread or metastasis.

low-density lipoproteins   A low-molecular-weight protein-fat complex.

lung   The part of the respiratory system that enables a person to breathe.

lymph   The clear fluid that bathes body cells.

lymph nodes   Organized clusters of lymphocytes through which the tissue fluids drain on returning to the blood circulation; they act as the first line of defense, filtering out and destroying infective organisms or cancer cells and initiating the generalized immune response.

lymphangiogram   A diagnostic method by which radiopaque dye is introduced into the lymph channels that drain tissue fluids to the blood circulation; this dye is filtered by the lymph nodes, making them visible on x-ray film, and cancerous involvement of lymph nodes is evaluated by this test.

lymphatic system   Circulatory network of vessels that carry lymph and of the lymphoid organs such as the lymph nodes, spleen, and thymus that produce and store infection-fighting cells.

lymphocytes   A family of white blood cells responsible for the production of antibodies and for the direct destruction of invading organisms or cancer cells.

lymphoma   A group of malignant diseases of the lymph nodes or lymphatic tissues, which are divided into Hodgkin's disease and nonHodgkin's lymphoma (histiocytic, nodular, and diffuse lymphomas and Burkitt's lymphoma).

macrodose   A very large dose that exceeds many times the normal dose.

macronutrient   Dietary nutrients: carbohydrates, fats, and proteins.

mainstream smoke   That portion of the smoke drawn from the mouthpiece of a tobacco product during puffing.

malignant   Having the potential of being lethal if not successfully treated. All cancers are malignant by definition.

mammography   An x-ray technique for checking the breast.

melanocytes   Skin cells that produce melanin, a dark brown or black substance that gives the skin its color.

melanoma   A cancer of the pigment cells of the skin, usually arising in a preexisting pigmented area (mole).

menopause   The time of a woman's life when menstrual periods permanently stop, usually between the ages of 45 and 50. Called also the "change of life."

menstrual cycle   The 4-week intervals from female puberty to menopause during which the lining of the uterus expands and the ovary releases the egg. During the final phase of the cycle, if the egg is not fertilized, menstrual bleeding occurs.

mesothelioma   A primary tumor of the covering of the lungs or heart, associated with asbestos.

metabolism   The process of transformation of foods or compounds into substances needed for body function or energy resources.

metaplasia   The stage at which cells have attained complete growth.

metastases   The spread of cancer from one part of the body to another; cells in the new cancer are like those in the original tumor.

micronutrients   Dietary nutrients: vitamins, minerals, and water.

modality   A general class or method of treatment. The basic modalities of cancer therapy include surgery, radiation, medical (chemotherapy or hormonal) therapy, and experimental immunotherapy.

mutagen   A chemical or physical agent that induces genetic mutations; a factor that can transform a normal cell into a malignant cell.

mutation   A change in the DNA of a cell that alters the genetic potential of chromosomes in animals and their offspring; it may be a response to a chemical substance, and the daughter cells may be cancerous.

mycotoxins   Toxic substances produced by certain fungi.

myelogram   The introduction of radiopaque dye into the sac surrounding the spinal cord, a process that makes it possible to see tumor involvement of the spinal canal or nerve roots on x-ray film.

narcotics   A legal term defining euphoric and analgesic substances whose use is closely regulated by the U.S. Government; natural and synthetic relatives of morphine make up the major class of narcotics.

nausea   Stomach distress and an urge to vomit.

neoplasia   The formation of a new growth or tumor.

neurologic   Pertaining to the nervous system.

nicotine   A colorless alkaloid present in tobacco; it exerts a stimulating effect if tobacco is inhaled, chewed or snuffed. The nicotine effect is thought to be the major addicting incentive for habitual tobacco users.

nitrates, nitrites   Compounds of the salt of nitric acid that are used to preserve food.

nodes   See *lymph nodes.*

nude mice   A genetically bred species of mice that lack the thymic immune system and are thus born without the normal defenses against disease. Nude mice are hairless and will accept a transplant or tumor without rejection.

oncologist   An internist who has subspecialized in cancer therapy and has expertise in both chemotherapy and the handling of problems arising during the course of the disease.

oophorectomy   The surgical removal of an ovary.

osteosarcoma   Tumor of the bone.

ovarian carcinoma   Cancer of the ovary.

ovary   The female gonad, responsible for the production of ova (eggs) and of female sex hormones.

palpation   Examination with the hand of internal body structures or growths.

pancreas   A large gland lying behind the stomach that secretes digestive enzymes and the hormone insulin.

Pap smear   Papanicoulaou smear; a screening diagnostic procedure for the rapid detection of precancerous and cancerous conditions of the cervix.

papillary tumor   The most common type of bladder tumor; it is shaped like a small mushroom, with a stem attached to the inner lining of the bladder.

passive inhalation   Involuntary exposure to tobacco smoke by a nonsmoker in the presence of smokers.

pathologist   A physician skilled in the examination of tissues and in the performance and interpretation of laboratory slides.

pelvic area   The area of the body lying within the pelvic bone; organs of the female in this area include the uterus, vagina, ovaries, fallopian tubes, bladder, and rectum.

pentosan   A member of a group of five carbon sugars.

peritoneoscope   A slender, flexible instrument used to examine the internal organs and to take samples of suspicious tissue.

peritoneoscopy   A small incision of the abdomen to examine the internal organs with a peritoneoscope.

perivascular   About or surrounding blood vessels.

pi mesons   Subatomic particles of an element.

polyps   Nodular growths of tissue from the lining of nasal, gastrointestinal, urinary tract, or uterine tissues that can be benign or malignant.

prevalence   The number of cases of a disease in existence at a certain time in a designated area.

primipara   A woman who has had one successful pregnancy.

procarcinogen   Precancerous reducing agent.

proctosigmoidoscope   A tube through which the physician examines the lower 10 to 12 inches of intestine.

prognosis   An estimate of the outcome of a disease process based on the status of the patient and accumulated information about the disease and its treatment.

progression   The advancement or worsening of a cancer with respect to size.

promotors, promoters   Factors that act in combination with carcinogens to initiate cancer.

prostate   An organ located at the bladder neck in males; it produces some components of the semen.

radiation   Energy propagated through space or matter in the form of waves or particles.

radiation therapy   The use of radiation for control or cure of cancer.

radioactive isotope   An element that has undergone spontaneous or artificial decomposition and may emit radiation.

radioactivity   The emission of radiation resulting from the spontaneous rearrangement of the nucleus of an atom.

radiotherapist   A physician who specializes in the treatment of disease by means of radiation therapy.

receptor   A protein inside a cell that determines if the cell or cancer will respond to hormonal treatment.

rectum   The terminal section of the large intestine.

regression   The diminution of cancerous involvement, usually as a result of therapy; it is manifested by decreased size of the tumor(s) or its clinical evidence in fewer locations.

relapse   The reappearance of cancer following a period of remission or absence of evident active disease.

remission The temporary disappearance of evident active cancer occurring either spontaneously or as a result of therapy.

resection The surgical removal of tissue.

residual disease, residual tumor Cancer left behind following the palliative removal of cancerous tissue.

sarcoma A cancer of the connective tissue; for example, osteogenic sarcoma (bone), rhabdomyosarcoma (muscle), and Ewing's sarcoma (long bones).

scan See *isotopic scan.*

scrotum The external bag or pouch containing the testes.

selenium An element resembling sulfur.

sepsis Bacterial growth within the bloodstream.

sidestream smoke That smoke emitted from the smoldering tobacco product in a steady stream. Smoke particles and selected smoke constituents are found in sidestream smoke and in even greater concentrations than in mainstream smoke.

small cell carcinoma A lung cancer whose cells are small and round. Called also *oat cell carcinoma.*

spleen An organ adjacent to the stomach, composed mainly of lymphocytes.

sputum Mucus and pus from the bronchial tubes.

squamous cell carcinoma A form of surface cell cancer. In the skin it is easily cured when treated promptly. Most of the surface of the skin is composed of squamous cells. If it involves lung, bladder, or other organs, it may be highly malignant.

staging An organized process of ascertaining the extent of spread of a cancer.

stress The nonspecific response of the body to any demand made on it; the generalized arousal of the psychologic and physical systems aimed at adapting to or coping with internal and external change.

stressor The triggering event making demands on the human system for psychologic and physical adaptation.

stress-related disorders Also known as the diseases of adaptation or of "coping," these are the functional disorders that result directly or indirectly from the chronic excitation of the stress response.

symptom A manifestation or complaint of disease as described by the patient, as opposed to one found by the doctor's examination, referred to as a *sign.*

synergy A joining of two or more agents that work together for a cooperative result, often greater than the effects of either alone.

systemic disease Disease that involves virtually all parts of the body.

tar More properly called "particulate matter" or "smoke condensate"; it consists of aerosol particles that are the dark brown residue present in tobacco smoke. This condensate, not nicotine, causes the yellowish brown stain on the fingers and teeth of some cigarette smokers. The cancer-inducing potential of tobacco smoke lies mainly in its "tar."

teleologic Pertaining to an ultimate purpose in development.

teratogenicity Production of physical defects in embryo.

testicular mass A firm swelling involving a testis, or testicle, the male gonad.

testes, or **testicles** The paired glands in which male germ cells (sperm) are formed.

therapeutic procedure A procedure intended to offer palliation or cure of a condition or a disease.

thermography A technique in which heat from the breast or organ is measured and recorded; increased temperature in one breast may indicate an abnormal condition.

thoracic Of or pertaining to the thorax, or chest —the rib cage and all organs within it.

thoracotomy A major surgical procedure in which an incision is made into the chest and the lung to examine the lung for cancer or other disease.

tobacco The origin of the word probably comes from the name of the hollow tube, *toboca* or *tobago*, through which the Carib Indians of the West Indies inhaled or snuffed a mixture of dried leaves.

tomogram A series of special x-ray films which are slices through a part of the body that give a three-dimensional view of body structures.

toxicity The property of producing unpleasant or dangerous side effects.

trachea The windpipe, the air passageway between the larynx and the lungs.

tumor   A mass or swelling. In itself, the word "tumor" carries no connotation of either benignity or malignancy.

tumor initiator   An agent that stimulates the growth or activity of a tumor.

tumor promoter   An agent that increases the rate of activity or growth of a tumor.

ulcer   An erosion of normal tissue resulting from corrosive chemicals (acids), infection, impaired circulation, or cancerous involvement.

ulcerative colitis   Chronic, recurrent ulceration in the colon.

ureter   The tube that carries urine from the kidney to the bladder.

urethra   The male urethra is about 8 inches long, extending from the neck of the bladder through the full length of the penis; it is part of both the urinary and reproductive systems.

urinary tract infection (UTI)   An infectious disease in the kidneys, ureters, bladder, or urethra, caused by bacteria or viruses; such infections are common and usually not serious.

uterine cervix   The neck or lower part of the uterus.

uterus   The womb; the organ that holds a baby before birth.

vagina   The hollow, muscular organ below the uterus that receives the male penis during sexual intercourse.

virus   One of a group of minute (microscopic) infectious agents, which consist of either RNA (ribonucleic acid) or DNA.

vocal cords   Two small shelves of muscular tissue within the larynx; they vibrate against each other and generate sound.

white blood cells   Nearly colorless blood cells that fight infection and can be stimulated to fight some cancers.

x-ray   Radiation with high enough energy to destroy cancer, or, in low doses, to diagnose disease.

xeromammogram   X-ray examination of the breasts by a new method that improves the detail representation of soft tissues and facilitates the diagnosis of minute areas of cancer.

1983 Cancer Data and Figures

ADAPTED FROM CANCER FACTS AND FIGURES: 1983, NEW YORK, 1982, AMERICAN CANCER SOCIETY.

General cancer data
Who gets cancer?

Cancer strikes at any age. It kills more children aged 3 to 14 than any other disease, and cancer strikes more frequently with advancing age. In the 1970s there were an estimated 3.5 million cancer deaths, over 6.5 million new cancer cases, and more than 10 million people under medical care for cancer.

How many people alive today will get cancer?

About 66 million Americans now living will eventually have cancer — about 30%, according to present rates. Over the years, cancer will strike in approximately three out of four families.

How many people alive today have ever had cancer?

There are more than 5 million Americans alive today who have a history of cancer, 3 million of them with diagnosis 5 or more years ago. Most of these 3 million can be considered cured, whereas others still have evidence of cancer. By "cured" it is meant that a patient has no evidence of disease and has the same life expectancy as a person who never had cancer.

The decision as to when a patient may be considered cured is one that must be made by the physician after examining the individual patient. For most forms of cancer, 5 years without symptoms following treatment is the accepted time. However, some patients can be considered cured after 1 year, others after 3 years, whereas some have to be followed much longer than 5 years.

How many new cases will there be this year?

In 1983 about 855,000 people will be diagnosed as having cancer.*

How many people are surviving cancer?

In the early 1900s few cancer patients had any hope of long-term survival. In the 1930s less than 1:5 was alive at least 5 years after treatment. In the 1940s it was 1:4, and in the 1960s, until recently, it was 1:3.

Today about 320,000 Americans, or 3:8 patients who get cancer this year, will be alive 5 years after diagnosis. The gain from 1:3 to 3:8 represents about 40,000 persons this year. This 3:8, or about 38%, is called the "observed" survival rate. The observed survival rate is the proportion of people alive 5 years after diagnosis of cancer. When normal life expectancy is taken into consideration (factors such as dying of heart disease, accidents, and diseases of old age) 46% will be alive 5 years after diagnosis. This is the "relative" survival rate, and is a more commonly used yardstick to measure progress against cancer.

Could more people be saved?

Yes. About 145,000 people with cancer will probably die in 1983 who might have been saved by earlier diagnosis and prompt treatment.

*These estimates of the incidence of cancer are based on data from the National Cancer Institute's SEER Program (1973-1979). Nonmelanoma skin cancer and carcinoma in situ have not been included in the statistics. The incidence of nonmelanoma skin cancer is estimated to be about 400,000.

How many people will die?

This year about 440,000 will die of the disease—1,205 people a day, about one every 72 seconds. Of every five deaths from all causes in the United States, one is from cancer. In 1982 an estimated 431,000 Americans died of cancer. In 1981 it was 423,000; in 1980, 414,000.

What is the national death rate?

There has been a steady rise in the age-adjusted* national death rate. In 1930 the number of cancer deaths per 100,000 population was 143. In 1940 it was 152. By 1950 it had risen to 158, and in 1978 the number was 176. The major cause of these increases has been cancer of the lung. Except for that form of cancer, age-adjusted cancer death rates for major sites are leveling off, and in some cases declining.

Can cancer be prevented?

Many cancers, but not all, can be prevented. Most lung cancers are caused by cigarette smoking, and most skin cancers by frequent overexposure to direct sunlight. These cancers can be prevented by avoiding their causes. Certain cancers caused by occupational/environmental factors can be prevented by eliminating or reducing contact with carcinogenic agents. Examples include bladder cancer among workers in the dye industry, and lung cancer in asbestos workers—especially those who are also smokers.

Cancer rates in blacks and whites†

A study of cancer rates over several decades shows that the cancer incidence rate for blacks is higher than for whites, and that blacks also have a higher death rate than whites.

Male incidence and mortality rates in each race increased, whereas female rates decreased.

The overall cancer incidence rate for blacks went

*A method used to make valid statistical comparisons by assuming the same age distribution among different groups being compared.
†Figures for cancer incidence are from the National Cancer Institute National Surveys, 1947-50 and SEER program 1975-76; those for cancer mortality from the National Center for Health Statistics, 1953-1978.

up 27%; for whites it increased 12%. Cancer mortality has increased in both races, but the rate for blacks is greater than for whites. In the last 25 years cancer death rates in whites have increased 9% and black rates have increased 34%. The rates were virtually the same 25 years ago.

Cancer sites where blacks had significantly higher increases in incidence and mortality rates included the lung, colon/rectum, prostate, and esophagus. Esophageal cancer, long considered mainly a disease of males, declined in whites and rose rapidly in blacks of both sexes.

The incidence of invasive cancer of the uterine cervix dropped in both black and white women, although the incidence in blacks is still more than double that in whites. However, the rate for endometrial cancer—or cancer of the body of the uterus—for white women is double that of black women.

Survival for patients diagnosed between 1967 and 1973 was compared. More whites than blacks had cancer diagnosed in an early, localized stage when the chances of cure are best: 37% versus 28% for men, and 42% versus 31% for women.

A recent ACS-sponsored survey by the black-owned New York firm of Evaxx, Inc., showed that urban black Americans tend to be much less knowledgeable than whites about cancer's warning signals, and less apt to see a physician if they experience those symptoms. Specifically, the blacks interviewed knew little about three of the cancers that have seen a sharp increase in mortality: colorectal, prostate, and esophageal. The survey also showed that blacks tend to underestimate both the prevalence of cancer and the chances of cure.

In both studies most of the differences between whites and blacks were attributed to economic, environmental, and social factors rather than to inherent biologic characteristics. Because a higher percentage of blacks than whites are in the lower socioeconomic group, risk of exposure to industrial carcinogens is increased. Also, limited educational opportunities may prevent early detection because the less educated are less likely to know the importance of symptoms that could lead to an early diagnosis.

TABLE A-1 Estimated new cases and deaths for major sites of cancer — 1983*

Site	Cases	Deaths
Lung	135,000	117,000
Colon/rectum	126,000	58,000
Breast	115,000	38,000
Prostate	75,000	24,000
Uterus	55,000†	10,000
Urinary	57,000	19,000
Oral	27,000	9,200
Pancreas	25,000	23,000
Leukemia	24,000	16,000
Ovary	18,000	12,000
Skin	17,000‡	7000

Incidence estimates are based on rates from N.C.I. SEER program 1973-1979. From Cancer facts and figures: 1983, New York, 1982, American Cancer Society.
*Figures rounded to nearest 1000.
†If carcinoma in situ is included, cases total more than 99,000.
‡Estimated new cases of nonmelanoma about 400,000.

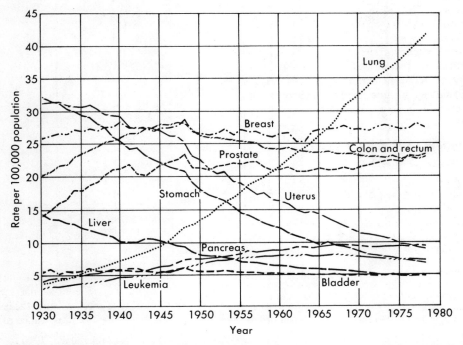

FIG. A-1 Cancer death rates by site — United States, 1930 to 1978. Rate for population standardized for age on 1970 U.S. population. Rates are for both sexes combined except breast and uterus (female population only) and prostate (male population only). (From Cancer facts and figures: 1983, American Cancer Society; data sources: National Center for Health Statistics and Bureau of the Census, United States.)

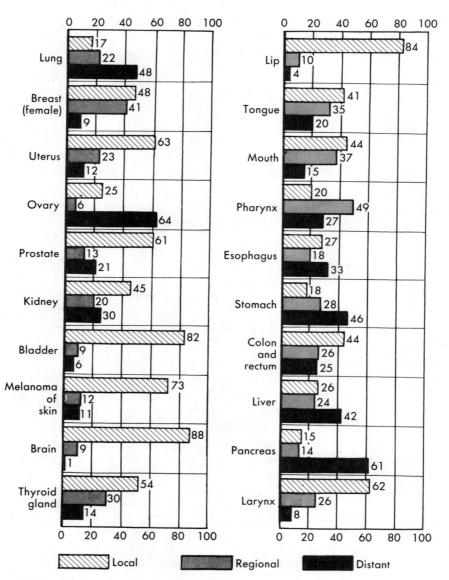

FIG. A-2 Percentage of cancer cases by site and by stage in cases diagnosed, 1970 to 1973. (From Cancer patient survival, Report No. 5, DHEW Pub. No. [NIH] 77-992.)

Cancer incidence by site and sex

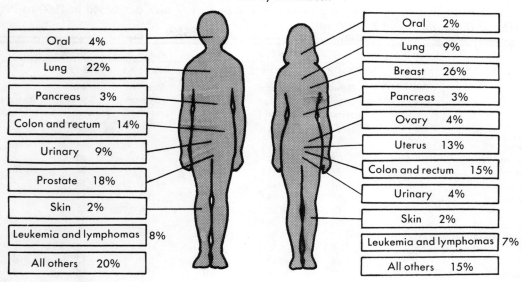

Oral	4%
Lung	22%
Pancreas	3%
Colon and rectum	14%
Urinary	9%
Prostate	18%
Skin	2%
Leukemia and lymphomas	8%
All others	20%

Oral	2%
Lung	9%
Breast	26%
Pancreas	3%
Ovary	4%
Uterus	13%
Colon and rectum	15%
Urinary	4%
Skin	2%
Leukemia and lymphomas	7%
All others	15%

Cancer death by site and sex

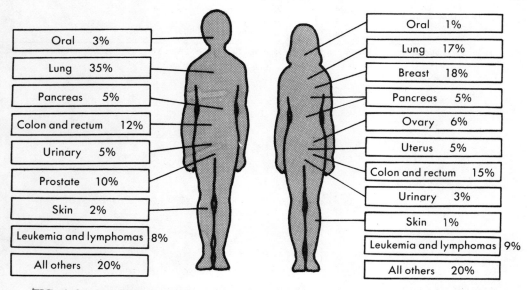

Oral	3%
Lung	35%
Pancreas	5%
Colon and rectum	12%
Urinary	5%
Prostate	10%
Skin	2%
Leukemia and lymphomas	8%
All others	20%

Oral	1%
Lung	17%
Breast	18%
Pancreas	5%
Ovary	6%
Uterus	5%
Colon and rectum	15%
Urinary	3%
Skin	1%
Leukemia and lymphomas	9%
All others	20%

FIG. A-3 American Cancer Society's 1983 United States estimates. **A,** Cancer incidence by site and sex (excluding nonmelanoma skin cancer and carcinoma in situ). **B,** Cancer deaths by site and sex. (Redrawn from Cancer facts and figures: 1983, American Cancer Society.)

TABLE A-2   Trends in survival by site of cancer and by race—cases diagnosed in 1960 to 1963 compared to those diagnosed in 1970 to 1973

Site	White			Black		
	1960-1963	1970-1973		1960-1963	1970-1973	
	Relative 5-year survival (%)	Relative 5-year survival (%)	Increase (%)	Relative 5-year survival (%)	Relative 5-year survival (%)	Increase (%)
Prostate	50	63	13	35	55	20
Kidney	37	46	9	38	44	6
Uterine corpus	73	81	8	31	44	13
Bladder	53	61	8	24	34	10
Colon/rectum	41	48	7	31	35	4
Uterine cervix	58	64	6	47	61	14
Breast	63	68	5	46	51	5
Ovary	32	36	4	32	32	0
Brain and central nervous system	18	20	2	19	19	0
Lung and bronchus	8	10	2	5	7	2
Stomach	11	13	2	8	13	5
Esophagus	4	4	0	1	4	3
Hodgkin's disease	40	67	27			
Lymphocytic leukemia—acute	4	28	24			
Lymphocytic leukemia—chronic	35	51	16			
NonHodgkin's lymphoma	31	41	10			
Larynx	53	62	9			
Tongue	28	37	9			
Melanoma of skin	60	68	8			
Pharynx	24	28	4			
Thyroid	83	86	3			
Mouth	44	44	0			

Source: Biometry Branch, National Cancer Institute. From Cancer facts and figures: 1983, New York, 1982, American Cancer Society.

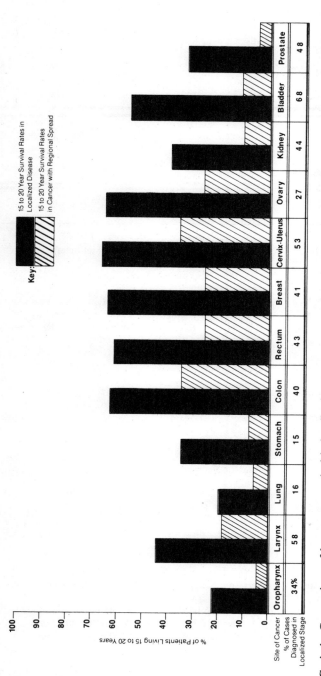

FIG. A-4 Comparison of long-term survival in localized cancer versus regional spread. (From Miller, D.:Your Patient and Cancer, July 1981.)

Quitting Resources and Information Sources for Smokers

TABLE B-1 Quitting resources

Resources	Duration	Cost (approximate)
Group therapy		
American Lung Association (ALA)	ALA groups meet twice a month, for an indefinite period.	No fee or minimal fee
American Cancer Society (ACS)	ACS groups meet approximately 2 hours, twice a week, for 4 weeks.	
American Heart Association (AHA)	AHA groups meet for 1½ hours. (Helping Smokers Quit)	
SmokEnders 37 N. 3rd St. Easton, PA 18042 800-423-5900	SmokEnder participants attend nine weekly meetings of 2 hours each. Reunions and other reinforcement contact is provided after the last meeting.	Average cost: $395 per program
5-day plans		
General Conference of Seventh Day Adventists Health and Temperance Department 6840 Eastern Ave. NW Washington, DC 20012 202-723-0800	1½ to 2 hours for 5 consecutive days.	$0 to $25
Schick Laboratories	1 hour for 5 consecutive days.	$625, with a money back guarantee
5-day live-in program—Seventh Day Adventist	1 week at St. Helena Hospital, Deer Park, Calif.	$795, which covers room and board, tests, and so on
Commercial aids		
Cigarette filters Waterpik One Step At A Time	Filters are used for 2 weeks. Four reusable filters.	$10.50
Nu-Life Stop Smoking Kit	One filter is to be used each day; 44 disposable filters.	$10.00
Aqua-Filter	Each filter is to be used for 20 cigarettes; 10 filters.	$1.99
Venturi Tar Guard	Each cartridge is good for 15 to 20 cigarettes; 10 cartridges.	$3.95

Modified from Calling it quits, U.S. Department of Health, Education, and Welfare, Public Health Service, National Institutes of Health.

Information sources

Books (see also References)

Holbrook, J.: The changing cigarette: a state-of-the-art paper. In National Conference on Smoking or Health: Developing a blueprint for action, Nov. 18-20, 1981.

National Conference on Smoking or Health: Developing a blueprint for action. Nov. 18-20, 1981.

Agencies

The Office on Smoking and Health
Public Health Service
Park Building, Room 1-58
5600 Fischer's Lane
Rockville, MD 28057
301-443-1575
Selected materials/publications available from the Office include:
Teenage Self-test
Smoking, Tobacco & Health: A Fact Book
Two Things Women Should Know
Slim and Smokeless
Tar and Nicotine Card
We Americans Have Seen the Light
Teenage Self-test Discussion Guide
Smokers Self-test
Unless You Quit
If You Must Smoke
Smokers' Health Book

National Cancer Institute
Office of Cancer Communication
Building 31, Room 10A-18
Bethesda, MD 20205
301-496-5583
Publications include:
Smoking Programs for Youth
A School Bibliography
Clearing the Air (available in Spanish)
Calling it Quits (NIH Pub. No. 82-1824)
Cancer of the Lung—Research Report Series (NIH Pub. No. 82-526)
For physicians:
Helping Smokers Quit—enough material for 50 patients and instructions for using the simple 4-step procedure.
For dentists:
Let's Help Smokers Quit

The American Cancer Institute, American Lung Association, and the American Academy of Family Physicians Committee on Cancer
Stop smoking program called:
Everyone Can Do Something About Smoking
(The kit, designed to be presented to local communities and schools, includes an audiocassette narrated by Dick Cavett, slides, and numerous pamphlets. Kits may be purchased for $33 from the *National Audiovisual Center,* ATT: Order Section, Washington, DC 20409. Checks should be made payable to the *National Archives Trust Fund.* The order *must* include the title of the kit and the title number-[A01800].)

American Cancer Society
(Contact local chapter or affiliate; national number: 212-267-3700.)
Resources include:
How to Quit Cigarettes
Seven Day Plan to Help You Stop Smoking Cigarettes (1978)
I Quit Kit
Helping Smokers Quit

American Heart Association
(Contact local chapter or affiliate; national number: 214-750-5300.)
Major publication:
How to Stop Smoking

American Lung Association
(Contact local chapter or affiliate; national number: 212-245-8000.)
Publications include:
Me Quit Smoking? How?
A Lifetime of Freedom from Smoking
Freedom from Smoking in 20 Days

Coalition on Smoking or Health
National Interagency Council on Smoking and Health
419 Seventh St. NW
Suite 401
Washington, DC 20004
202-393-4446

Group Against Smokers' Pollution (GASP)
P.O. Box 632
College Park, MD 20740
301-577-6427
(Supports the rights of nonsmokers with newsletter and literature.)

The American Health Foundation
Ernst L. Wynder, M.D.
320 E. 43rd St.
New York, NY 10017
212-953-1900

California Nonsmokers' Rights Foundation
2054 University Ave., Suite 500
Berkeley, CA 94704
415-841-3032
Publications include:
Tobacco Smoke and the Nonsmoker
Clearing the Air at Work: Some Essential Background for Employees

Action on Smoking and Health
2013 H. St. NW
Washington, DC 20006
(Citizens' legal action group with newsletter and Congressional Record reprints.)

Other sources

The Smoking Cessation Newsletter
P.O. Box 68511
Indianapolis, IN 46268

Directory of Stop Smoking Clinics
(Periodically updated list of clinics and resources to help the smoker quit: Greater San Francisco Bay Area. Describes approach or method, contact process, and fees.)

Regional Cancer Foundation of San
Francisco and Marin
San Francisco
15th Ave. & Lake Street
Building 1805
San Francisco, CA 94129
Marin
80 Lomita Drive
Suite #9
Mill Valley, CA 94947

A Personal Cancer History and Risk Analysis

Since each person is responsible for his or her health, using the guidance of the medical profession, one would be wise to keep a *Personal Health Record.* * This should be updated every 3 to 5 years. If there are serious illnesses, a card should be in one's wallet or a "Medic Alert" chain should be worn.

*If you are interested in information on personal risk analysis, write to The Claire Zellerbach Saroni Tumor Institute of Mount Zion Hospital and Medical Center, P.O. Box 7921, San Francisco, CA 94120.

NAME _____

ADDRESS _____ TEL NO. _____

RELATIVE TO NOTIFY _____

ADDRESS _____ TEL. NO. _____

DISEASES _____

DRUGS _____

I. PATIENT HISTORY

Name_____

Age _____

Sex   M ____   F ____

Race _____

Occupation _____

Married (year) _____

Last diagnostic
   evaluation_____

Chest x-ray film _____

Pap smear _____

Rectal examination _____

Childhood diseases

   Measles_____

   Mumps _____

   Chickenpox _____

Adult diseases

   Diabetes _____

   Tuberculosis_____

Continued.

I. PATIENT HISTORY — cont'd

Vaccination
			#1	#2			
DPT	☐				Measles	☐	☐
Polio	☐	Booster	_____	_____	Mumps	☐	☐
Hepatitis	☐	Booster	_____	_____	Rubella	☐	☐
Pneumovax	☐	Booster	_____	_____	Other	_____	
Flu shots	☐						

Hypertension _____

Cancer history_____

Family cancer history_____

Major illnesses

Age   Physician   Complications

_____

_____

_____

Surgery

Age   Physician   Complications

_____

_____

_____

Allergies

_____

_____

_____

Transfusions

Age   Reason

_____

_____

_____

X-ray exposure

Diagnostic   Therapeutic

_____

_____

II. HEALTH FORM

Health testing

Breast examination
Frequency of self-examination (BSE)*

Started _____
Age started _____
Frequency _____
Last BSE_____

Frequency by physician (semiannually or annually)

_____
_____
_____

Every _____ year(s)

Mammogram
Frequency   _____
Results   _____
Normal   _____

Pap smear
Frequency   _____
                _____
                _____

Rectal examination

Sigmoidoscopy
(most recent)

_____   _____
_____
_____

Chest x-ray film
Last   _____

Every _____ year(s)

Last physical examination
Frequency of checkups

_____
_____

_____
*Should be done monthly 7 to 10 days after period.

Continued.

II. HEALTH FORM — cont'd

Personal history — life-style

	Age started	Pack-years*	Filter/nonfilter	Approximate years	Quit
Smoking					
Cigarette					
Cigar/pipe					
Chewing tobacco					

Alcohol

Wine	4 oz.	Daily _____	Weekly _____
Liquor	1 oz.	Daily _____	Weekly _____
Beer	1 oz.	Daily _____	Weekly _____

Infections/venereal disease
  Viral infections _____
  _____

Weight   High _____   Current weight _____
        Low _____

Sunshine   Years exposure _____   Hours/week _____

Drugs
  Current medications _____
  Sedatives/sleep   Types _____   Frequency used _____
  For illness _____
  Pain
    Narcotics (Demerol, codeine, morphine, and so on) _____
    Tylenol _____
    Aspirin _____
  Tranquilizers (Miltown, Librium, phenobarbital, Seconal, Nembutal, and so on) _____
  Contraceptives ("pill") _____
  Amphetamines ("pep pills") _____
  Miscellaneous _____

*Pack-years = Number of packs × years smoked.

Mental status

Do you worry or feel blue much of the time?	☐ No	☐ Yes
Do you often feel alone and lonely even when there are others around you?	☐ No	☐ Yes
Have you lost your appetite or have you had decreased desire to eat?	☐ No	☐ Yes
Do you have trouble with waking up too early, or being unable to stay asleep?	☐ No	☐ Yes
Have you ever seriously considered killing yourself?	☐ No	☐ Yes
Has anyone in your immediate family (parents, brothers, sisters) taken his or her own life?	☐ No	☐ Yes

Environmental/industrial exposure — toxic exposure

Pollution _____

_____

_____

Family history
Family history chart

Continued.

II. HEALTH FORM — cont'd

Family names

Father _____

Mother _____

	Type of cancer	Age diag-nosed	Cause and date of death (age)
Paternal (Father's) grandmother	_____	___	_____
Paternal (Father's) grandfather	_____	___	_____
Maternal (Mother's) grandmother	_____	___	_____
Maternal (Mother's) grandfather	_____	___	_____
Mother-in-law	_____	___	_____
Father-in-law	_____	___	_____

Brothers
1. _____   _____   ___   _____
2. _____   _____   ___   _____
3. _____   _____   ___   _____
4. _____   _____   ___   _____

Sisters
1. _____   _____   ___   _____
2. _____   _____   ___   _____
3. _____   _____   ___   _____
4. _____   _____   ___   _____

Screening and prevention

	Performed in last year	
	Yes	No
History	☐	☐
Physical examination	☐	☐
Flexible endoscopes	☐	☐
X-ray tests	☐	☐
Biopsy of suspicious lesions	☐	☐

Exercise _____ Number of times a week _____

Stress
High_____
Medium _____
Low _____

Aggravation and frustration list

_____
_____
_____

Chart for attempts to stop smoking (see Chapter 7)

Date quit or decreased intake	Resources used	Date resumed/reason
_____	_____	_____
_____	_____	_____
_____	_____	_____
_____	_____	_____
_____	_____	_____

American Cancer Society's seven warning signs of cancer

	Yes	No
Change in bowel or bladder habits	☐	☐
Sore that does not heal	☐	☐
Unusual bleeding or discharge	☐	☐
Thickening or lump in breast or elsewhere	☐	☐
Indigestion or difficulty in swallowing	☐	☐
Obvious change in wart or mole	☐	☐
Nagging cough or hoarseness	☐	☐

Continued.

III. CANSCREEN*: HEALTH HISTORY QUESTIONNAIRE FOR CANCER RISK AND PREVENTION ANALYSIS

These questions are a general format to cover most of the pertinent questions that may give clues for an evaluation that could lead to an earlier diagnosis of cancer. They are compiled from:

1. Personal experience (A Personal Cancer History and Risk Analysis)

2. Canscreen—Health History Questionnaire For the 12 most common forms of cancer—causing 85 percent of cancer deaths—the 15- to 20-year long-term survival rates are markedly better when the disease is localized as compared to regional spread. Currently, the localized cancer detection rate is 16%. This can be increased to 37% when an organized detection program is used, as with that employed at the Preventive Medical Institute, Strang Clinic. The early detection for breast cancer is 41%; the Breast Cancer Demonstration Project (BCDP) can increase this to 70%. Colon cancer early detection is 43%; this can be increased to 80% with the methods of Special Program at the Preventive Medicine Institute-Strang Clinic.

NOTE: **The questionnaire and physician evaluation should be done annually.**

---

*Canscreen Program, Preventive Medicine Institute, Strang Clinic, 57 East 34th St., New York, NY 10016. Daniel G. Miller, M.D., Director, Preventive Medicine.

HEALTH HISTORY QUESTIONNAIRE

Cancer Prevention and Detection Screening Program (CANSCREEN)*

		Yes	*No*

SKIN

In the past six months have you noticed bleeding or a change in the size or color of a mole? . . . .   **1.** ☐ ☐

Do you now have a sore that has not healed for one month or more? . . . .   **2.** ☐ ☐

Do you have any skin changes in an area where you had x-ray treatments? . . . .   **3.** ☐ ☐

Do you have a severe burn scar from a burn which happened over a year ago? . . . .   **4.** ☐ ☐

Do you have a mole on the sole of either foot, palm of either hand or in a place where it may be irritated by underwear, a belt, shirt collar, shaving, jewelry, etc.? .   **5.** ☐ ☐

Do you have very fair skin and/or sunburn easily? . . . .   **6.** ☐ ☐

Has a doctor ever told you that you had skin cancer? . . . .   **7.** ☐ ☐

MOUTH & THROAT

Do you now have pain or difficulty swallowing which has lasted more than a month? . . . .   **8.** ☐ ☐

Do you have irritation of your tongue, cheek or gums caused by dentures or a tooth? . . . .   **9.** ☐ ☐

Do you now have pain or tenderness in the mouth which has lasted more than a month? . . . .   **10.** ☐ ☐

Do you now have a sore or a white spot on your lips, tongue, cheek or gums that has lasted more than a month? . . . .   **11.** ☐ ☐

Do you drink beer, wine or hard liquor daily? . . . .   **12.** ☐ ☐

If yes, is it more than 5 beers or 5 glasses of wine or 3 hard liquor drinks a day? . . . .   **13.** ☐ ☐

Has a doctor ever told you that you had cancer of the mouth or throat? . . . .   **14.** ☐ ☐

LARYNX

Have you had any change in the voice, such as hoarseness, which has lasted one month or more? . . . .   **15.** ☐ ☐

Has a doctor ever told you that you had cancer of the larynx (voice box)? . . . .   **16.** ☐ ☐

---

*From Miller, D.G: Your Patient and Cancer, July 1981.

Continued.

HEALTH HISTORY QUESTIONNAIRE — cont'd

THYROID

Do you have a steady pressure or tightness in the lower front of the neck that has lasted more than a month? . . . .   17.   ☐   ☐

Do you have a lump in the lower front of your neck that you can see or feel with your fingers? . . . .   18.   ☐   ☐

As a child or teenager, did you have x-ray *treatment* to your face or front of your neck for acne, a neck tumor, tonsils, enlarged thymus, or for other reasons? . . . . .   19.   ☐   ☐

Has a doctor ever told you that you had thyroid cancer? . . . .   20.   ☐   ☐

LUNGS

In the past month have you coughed blood? . . . .   21.   ☐   ☐

    If yes, are you seeing a doctor for this? . . . .   22.   ☐   ☐

Have you had a daily cough for the past month or more? . . . .   23.   ☐   ☐

Has a doctor ever told you that you had emphysema? . . . .   24.   ☐   ☐

Have you had two or more bouts of pneumonia in the past year? . . . .   25.   ☐   ☐

Have you ever smoked? (If no, go to question 34.) . . . .   26.   ☐   ☐

    If yes:
Have you stopped smoking only within the past year? . . . .   27.   ☐   ☐

Do you smoke now? . . . .   27a.   ☐   ☐

    If yes:
Do you smoke cigarettes? . . . .   28.   ☐   ☐

    Do you smoke 1 or more packs a day? . . . .   29.   ☐   ☐

Do you smoke cigars? . . . .   30.   ☐   ☐

    Do you smoke 5 or more cigars a day? . . . .   31.   ☐   ☐

Do you smoke a pipe? . . . .   32.   ☐   ☐

    Do you smoke 5 or more bowls of tobacco a day? . . . .   33.   ☐   ☐

Has a doctor ever told you that you had lung cancer? . . . .   34.   ☐   ☐

KIDNEY & URINARY BLADDER

In the past six months, have you had blood in your urine? .... 35. ☐ ☐

    If yes, are you seeing a doctor for this? .... 36. ☐ ☐

For the past month have you had pain or burning on urination three or four times a week? .... 37. ☐ ☐

Has a doctor ever told you that you had kidney cancer? .... 38. ☐ ☐

Has a doctor ever told you that you had cancer of the bladder (not gall bladder)? . 39. ☐ ☐

STOMACH

Have you lost more than 10 lbs. in the past six months, *and don't know why*? ..... 40. ☐ ☐

Have you vomited blood in the past month? .... 41. ☐ ☐

    If yes, are you seeing a doctor for this? .... 42. ☐ ☐

In the past six months, have you had black, tarry stools (black, not just dark)? ... 43. ☐ ☐

    If yes, does this happen only when you are taking iron pills, or vitamins with iron? .... 44. ☐ ☐

During the past month, have you had a stomach pain (in the upper abdomen) two or more times a week? .... 45. ☐ ☐

Has a doctor ever told you that you had polyps (growths) in the stomach? .... 46. ☐ ☐

Has a doctor ever told you that you have a gastric ulcer (stomach ulcer)? .... 47. ☐ ☐

Has a doctor ever told you that you had a type of anemia called *pernicious anemia*? .... 48. ☐ ☐

To your knowledge, have any of your blood relatives* ever had cancer of the stomach? .... 49. ☐ ☐

Has a doctor ever told you that you had cancer of the stomach? .... 50. ☐ ☐

---

*By blood relatives we mean: daughters, sisters, sister's children, mother, mother's sisters, mother's brothers, mother's mother, mother's father, sons, brothers, brother's children, father, father's sisters, father's brothers, father's mother, father's father.

Continued.

HEALTH HISTORY QUESTIONNAIRE — cont'd

LARGE INTESTINE & RECTUM

Have you had a change from your usual bowel habits which has now lasted more than one month? .... 51. ☐ ☐

If yes:

Has this change caused you to become constipated, or more constipated than usual? .... 52. ☐ ☐

Has this change caused you to have diarrhea? .... 53. ☐ ☐

In the past six months, has your stool (bowel movement) been becoming progressively narrower in size (like a pencil or ribbon)? .... 54. ☐ ☐

If yes, does this happen with every bowel movement? .... 55. ☐ ☐

In the past month have you had bleeding from the rectum, either with bowel movements or at other times? .... 56. ☐ ☐

In the last month, have you had mucus in your stool every time you had a bowel movement? .... 57. ☐ ☐

Has a doctor ever told you that you had a polyp (growth) in the large intestine (colon, rectum or bowel)? .... 58. ☐ ☐

To your knowledge, have any of your blood relatives* ever had polyps in the large intestine? .... 59. ☐ ☐

To your knowledge, have any of your blood relatives* ever had cancer of the large intestine? .... 60. ☐ ☐

Has a doctor ever told you that you had a type of colitis called *ulcerative colitis*? .. 61. ☐ ☐

Has a doctor ever told you that you had cancer of the large intestine? .... 62. ☐ ☐

*By blood relatives we mean: daughters, sisters, sister's children, mother, mother's sisters, mother's brothers, mother's mother, mother's father, sons, brothers, brother's children, father, father's sisters, father's brothers, father's mother, father's father.

CERVIX, UTERUS & VAGINA

Do you have vaginal bleeding or spotting and don't know why?	63.	☐	☐
If yes:			
Is it between monthly periods?	64.	☐	☐
Is it after menopause (change of life) or hysterectomy?	65.	☐	☐
Is it after sexual intercourse?	66.	☐	☐
Have you stopped having your monthly periods?	67.	☐	☐
If yes, at what age was this? _____	68.		
Since then, have you ever had hormone therapy for treatment of menopause symptoms, for example, Premarin or DES (diethyl-stilbestrol)?	69.	☐	☐
Have you had a hysterectomy (removal of womb)?	70.	☐	☐
Have you ever had sexual relations (intercourse)?	71.	☐	☐
If yes, did you first have intercourse before age 16?	72.	☐	☐
When your mother was pregnant with you, did she use the female hormone DES (diethyl-stilbestrol) to prevent miscarriage?	73.	☐	☐
To your knowledge, have any of your female blood relatives* had cancer of the uterus (womb)?	74.	☐	☐
Has a doctor ever told you that you had cancer of the cervix?	75.	☐	☐
Has a doctor ever told you that you had cancer of the uterus?	76.	☐	☐
Has a doctor ever told you that you had cancer of the vagina?	77.	☐	☐

*By female blood relative we mean: daughters, sisters, sister's daughters, mother, mother's sisters, mother's mother, brother's daughters, father's sisters, father's mother.

Continued.

HEALTH HISTORY QUESTIONNAIRE — cont'd

BREASTS

Do you have a lump in either breast? . . . . 78. ☐ ☐

If yes:
Did you see a doctor for this? . . . . 79. ☐ ☐

Have you had a mammogram (breast x-ray) in the last year? . . . . 80. ☐ ☐

If yes, when? _____
                month   year

Do you now have breast pain? . . . . 81. ☐ ☐

If yes, is this only present around menstruation time (monthly periods)? . . . . 82. ☐ ☐

Have you noticed any changes in your nipples? . . . . 83. ☐ ☐

If yes:
Have they begun to pull in (retract)? . . . . 84. ☐ ☐

Is there a discharge or bleeding from them? . . . . 85. ☐ ☐

Have you noticed any changes in the skin of your breasts? . . . . 86. ☐ ☐

Is yes, have you noticed a dimpling or puckering of the skin? . . . . 87. ☐ ☐

Have you ever had a biopsy of the breast? . . . . 88. ☐ ☐

To your knowledge, have any of your female blood relatives ever had breast
cancer? . . . . 89. ☐ ☐

Has a doctor ever told you that you had breast cancer? . . . . 90. ☐ ☐

Do you carefully examine your breasts each month? . . . . 91. ☐ ☐

APPENDIX D

Breast Cancer Treatment: Summary of Alternative Effective Methods

RISKS, ADVANTAGES, DISADVANTAGES
(January 1983)

INTRODUCTION

You have a treatable disease and are entitled to know about the various medically effective surgical, radiological and chemotherapeutic treatment procedures available.

This brochure has been developed to assist you to understand what these various treatment procedures are, their advantages, disadvantages, and risks.

The treatment of cancer is quite complex. It must be individualized. The choice of therapy may be difficult to make. It is important for you to have this basic information about the methods of treatment so that you may discuss them more fully with your physician as they apply to your case. This will help you understand what treatment programs may be used and what their effects may be in your individual situation. Using this information as a basis for discussion, you and your physician should be able to make an informed choice.

Because cancer is a serious disease, it may be appropriate for either you or your physician to

This summary is required by SB 1893, "The Breast Cancer Informed Consent Law", effective January 1, 1981. Prepared by the California State Department of Health Services based on recommendations of the State Cancer Advisory Council; printed and distributed by the Board of Medical Quality Assurance, California State Department of Consumer Affairs.

seek additional opinions if either of you desires. Your consent is required before any treatment is carried out and you have the right to participate in making the final choice of the treatment procedure(s). Your physician has a corresponding right to withdraw from the case if he chooses.

It is very important to take a reasonable amount of time to obtain enough medical information and consultation to make a final and informed decision. But prolonged delay may interfere with the success of your treatment. Making this choice is an important step. Once you and your physician have reached a decision about your treatment, you will have a positive attitude which will be a tremendous help as you and your physician begin and carry out the treatment of your cancer.

MANAGEMENT OF BREAST CANCER

Management of breast cancer is achieved by the cooperation of appropriate specialists in the field: the primary (personal) physician for general support and coordination; the surgeon for diagnosis by biopsy and specific surgical procedure for removal of the breast tumor; the pathologist for gross and microscopic diagnosis; the radiation oncologist for supervising and administering radiation treatment; the medical

285

oncologist for specialized management of the patient's care and administration of chemotherapy. In actual practice these members proceed fairly independently but maintain liaison by telephone and written reporting.

TREATMENT ALTERNATIVES: ADVANTAGES, DISADVANTAGES, RISKS

If your diagnosis is breast cancer, it is important for you to understand there is enough time to make a careful decision. Prolonged delay and failure to get adequate treatment may result in the deterioration of your situation. In contrast, the benefits of modern breast cancer therapy far outweigh the risks. This is especially true when treatment is undertaken early. The risk may be small or serious, and its occurrence may vary from frequent to rare. There is a wide range of potential benefits and risks from the various treatment procedures for the different stages and kinds of breast cancer. Before deciding on your course of therapy, you should discuss with your physician the particular benefits and risks of the treatment methods suitable for your individual case.

DIAGNOSIS

Diagnosis is the scientific determination of the nature of the lump. It is made by the pathologist who examines the tissue from the breast lump (breast biopsy) under the microscope.

The breast biopsy entails the surgical removal of part or all of the lump under suitable anesthesia. Unless the lump is quite large it is usually removed in one piece (excisional biopsy). (A large lump may be biopsied with a special needle or by surgically removing a small sample.) The tissue removed by biopsy provides material for the definitive test for cancer, namely the examination of tissue under the microscope by the pathologist. If cancerous, part of the fresh tissue may also be studied for receptors for hormones (estrogen and proges-

terone), which could be important if future treatment decisions become necessary. (Only about 20% of breast biopsies are cancerous; the remainder represent less serious conditions.)

The procedure for obtaining the biopsy should be discussed with you since you must make a decision between two courses of action — the one-step or two-step procedure.

In the *one-step* procedure, you and your physician decide beforehand that if the biopsy shows cancer and if surgery will be the treatment of choice, the entire procedure (biopsy, diagnosis by pathologist, and the appropriate surgery) will be completed in one operation.

In the *two-step* procedure, the biopsy is done under local or general anesthesia and no additional operation is performed at this time. After the pathologist examines and reports on the biopsy, the surgeon reviews the pathology report with you and discusses with you the various treatment options available and effective for your particular case. A decision is then made by you and your physician on which procedure is preferred by you for your individual care.

Prior to the procedure you choose, a general medical evaluation which may include any or all of the following diagnostic procedures is usually done to determine your individual situation:

Your medical history (including family history of cancer)

Physical examination

Blood tests evaluating function of various systems, e.g., liver, kidney, immunity, etc.

X-ray films (chest, bones, etc.)

Breast x-ray films (mammography)

Radioisotope scan (bones, liver, brain, etc.)

Computerized tomographic body scans (specialized x-ray views of any or all of internal organs and bones)

Sonograms (pictures of internal organs made with ultra-sound waves)

Treatment recommendations are individualized. They are based primarily on the extent (stage) and type of disease present as well as other factors related to your personal health.

SURGERY

This process involves removal of the tumor, and either a portion of the breast, all of the breast, or all of the breast and some surrounding tissues as well.

Radical (Halsted) mastectomy

The radical (Halsted) mastectomy is not commonly used today except in unusual cases. In this procedure, the entire breast, nipple, some of the overlying skin, underlying chest muscles, nearby soft tissue and lymph nodes extending into the armpit are removed.

Advantages. If cancer has not spread beyond breast or nearby tissue, it can be completely removed. Examination of lymph nodes provides information that is essential in planning future treatment.

Disadvantages. Removes entire breast and underlying chest muscles. Leaves a long scar and a hollow area where the muscles were removed. May result in swelling of the arm, some loss of muscle power in the arm, restricted shoulder motion, and some numbness and discomfort. Reconstructive (plastic) surgery and fitting of breast prosthesis are difficult.

Modified radical mastectomy

Entire breast, nipple, some of overlying skin, nearby soft tissue and lymph nodes in armpit are removed. Chest muscles are left intact, but overlying covering of muscle is removed.

Advantages. Retains the chest muscles and muscle strength of arm. Swelling of arm occurs less frequently and is milder than after radical. Cosmetic appearance is better than with radical. Apparently as effective as radical, but not if cancer is large or has invaded the muscle sheath. Cosmetically effective reconstructive surgery is usually feasible.

Disadvantages. Entire breast and part of overlying skin are removed. In some cases removal of lymph nodes in armpit may be incomplete. Some persons may experience swelling of the arm.

Simple mastectomy

The main breast structure but not overlying skin is removed. Underlying chest muscles and often armpit lymph nodes are left in place. Many surgeons remove some of the armpit lymph nodes through a separate small incision under the arm to determine if cancer has spread to nodes. Often followed by radiation therapy.

Advantages. Chest muscles are not removed and strength of arm is not affected. Swelling of arm occurs infrequently. Reconstructive surgery usually feasible.

Disadvantages. Breast is not preserved. If cancer has spread to armpit lymph nodes, it may remain undiscovered unless these nodes are sampled or removed at the time of surgery; adequate treatment could be delayed.

Segmental mastectomy, partial mastectomy and lumpectomy

If cancer is small and detected early, a segment of the breast containing the tumor is removed. Many surgeons also remove some armpit lymph nodes through a separate incision to check for possible spread of cancer. Most cancer experts feel this type of operation should be followed by radiation therapy and some feel chemotherapy should be used in selected cases as well. These procedures are relatively new and long term results are being documented.

Advantages. Most of the breast remains. Reconstructive surgery is usually easier if needed at all. Loss of muscle strength and swelling of the arm are unlikely to occur. Commonly used as first step for *Radiation Therapy as Primary Treatment in Early Breast Cancer,* especially if preservation of the breast is desired.

Disadvantages. Most cancer specialists feel these procedures may be incomplete unless armpit lymph nodes are removed for pathological examination and person is given radiation therapy or a combination of radiation therapy and chemotherapy. Otherwise, spread of cancer into armpit lymph nodes or undetected areas of cancer present elsewhere in breast may go untreated and chance for cure may be lost.

RADIATION (X-RAY) THERAPY

Radiation treatment of local tissues of the body, known as radiotherapy, can destroy cancer cells while producing less injury to surrounding tissues. Radiation for treatment may come from a number of devices, e.g., super voltage x-ray, linear accelerator, Betatron, Cobalt-60 and radioactive isotopes. The source and type of radiation is chosen to suit the requirements of the individual.

Radiation therapy as primary treatment in early breast cancer

This approach has been used for about 10 years in this country and for about 20 years in Europe for the treatment of early breast cancer. After pathologic diagnosis by biopsy and surgical removal of the local tumor, external radiation therapy is used to treat the remainder of the breast, the lymph nodes, and the chest wall. This is then followed by a radiation "boost" to the biopsy site with radioactive sources temporarily introduced into the area of the excision. Sometimes the boost may be given with more external irradiation (or electron beam).

Advantages. The breast is preserved. It may be mildly to moderately firmer. Usually there is minimal or no visible deformity of surrounding tissues. After completion of the treatment, the skin usually regains normal appearance.

In early breast cancer, lumpectomy or segmental resection, with radiation as the primary treatment, has demonstrated results that currently appear equal to long established surgical procedures.

Disadvantages. A full course of treatment re-

quires daily outpatient visits for four to six weeks. Treatment may produce a skin reaction similar to sunburn and may cause temporary difficulty in swallowing. Radiation therapy can affect bone marrow where blood cells are made. This may limit the dosage and effectiveness of later chemotherapy if it is needed. A small area of scarring, permanently visible on x-ray examination, may develop in the lung, but usually causes no symptoms.

Radiation therapy as a supplement (adjuvant) to surgery

Following surgery, examination of the surgical specimen by the pathologist may show the cancer has spread outside the breast and into armpit lymph nodes or local surrounding areas. Radiation therapy will usually control cancer cells remaining in these areas. The treatment of advanced cancer often requires the consultation and coordinated efforts of the surgeon, radiation oncologist and the medical oncologist (see below).

Advantages. The goal of radiation therapy is to destroy cancer cells in tissue in the radiation treatment area which improves control of or stops the spread of cancer in the treatment area. Modern equipment gives very precise control of the x-ray treatment. Radiation therapy may be used to treat localized metastases.

Disadvantages. The major side effects are the same as those listed under radiation therapy as a primary treatment. When cancer is treated by radiation therapy as a supplement to surgery, there may be wide variations in the extent of the treatments required depending on the problem or site of disease being treated.

CHEMOTHERAPY

Medical oncologist is the specialist who usually plans and administers the chemotherapy and may coordinate the patient's management with other physicians. Chemotherapy is designed to destroy breast cancer cells that cannot be removed surgically or by radiation or their combination.

In recent years important and effective advances in breast cancer treatment have been made in this area, especially advanced cancer. Different drugs or a combination of drugs are administered orally or by injection. This program is adapted to the individual and may continue at intervals for six months to two years or longer depending on the cancer being treated and the drug program being used.

Supplemental (adjuvant) chemotherapy

Chemotherapy supplements primary surgical or radiation treatment when it is likely the patient has a cancer which has spread into or beyond nearby lymph nodes. Such patients have a higher risk of recurrence than those whose lymph nodes are found to be free of cancer. Supplemental chemotherapy may reduce this risk considerably.

Advantages. Increases the effectiveness of surgery or radiation therapy and reduces the risk of breast cancer recurrence. Works to stop its growth at distant sites in the body.

Disadvantages. Most chemotherapy drugs have reversible side effects. Some side effects are minimal while others can cause discomfort, including nausea, temporary loss of hair, bone marrow depression (resulting in temporary susceptibility to infection and bleeding tendency), anemia, loss of appetite and fatigue, and rarely damage to heart muscles. Also may depress reproductive function and cause change of life symptoms. Newer techniques of administration and dosage reduce the side effects of chemotherapy.

Chemotherapy for recurrent breast cancer

Anti-cancer drugs, taken alone or in combination with other modalities, can arrest the disease, help to relieve symptoms, and prolong the life of a patient who experiences recurrence of breast cancer.

Hormonal therapy

Many breast cancers are sensitive to female hormones (estrogen and progesterone) and are partially controlled by them. In many treatment centers, fresh tissue from the tumor (specimen or biopsy) can be tested to measure this hormone sensitivity (estrogen receptor assay). In some breast cancer patients, beneficial effects can be received by adding hormones, removing glands that produce them, or by administering drugs (anti-hormones) that counteract the hormones produced by the body. Hormone therapy often increases significantly the effectiveness of other cancer therapy.

INVESTIGATIVE TREATMENTS FOR BREAST CANCER

Clinical trials are new treatments which are not yet generally available. Laboratory or other reliable studies may indicate a new cancer treatment procedure or therapy program could be better than ones in current use. Research to measure effectiveness is conducted in clinical trials by many major cancer treatment groups. New treatment methods are put to general use only after long-term evaluation by cancer experts shows that the new methods give results as good as, or better than, established treatments.

BREAST FORMS

Breast forms (prostheses) are made with a variety of substances such as silicone, foam rubber, silastic, viscous fluid or glycerin. Fitted individually and worn in brassiere pockets, they can give the form, weight, and appearance of a normal bustline. The right bra for you may very well be the one you've always worn. Your health insurance generally covers a portion of this cost with your physician's prescription.

RECONSTRUCTIVE BREAST PROCEDURES

Reconstructive plastic surgery may effectively restore the form of the breast and adjacent tissues lost at surgery. Implants of breast prosthesis or surgical transfer of body tissues may be used. Usually at least two surgeries are required to achieve desired results, but in some cases advance planning can minimize this. The possibility of reconstructive surgery should be discussed with your physician in advance of a definitive surgical treatment procedure. You should investigate the extent of financial coverage available through your health insurance for this procedure.

FOLLOW-UP

The success of cancer treatment depends not only on early detection and effective treatment, but also on a careful, consistent follow-up program to detect cancer recurrence as early as possible if it should occur. Consistent regular visits to the treating physician and monthly self-examination are essential. New methods of detection and treatment are being continually developed and can be used to your advantage.

Many very helpful and thoughtful women who have been through a similar experience can lend you their support and guidance. They can be contacted through your physician, your hospital, your local unit of the American Cancer Society, or the National Cancer Institute's Cancer Information Service.

SUMMARY

This brochure is intended to make you aware of the effective alternative methods of treating breast cancer available in California, and your role in choosing the method to be used in your care. In order to reach a decision on the treatment method, it is important for you to understand the nature of the disease, the extent of your problem, the treatment needed, the method or methods of providing that treatment suitable to your particular situation, and finally the results that may reasonably be expected.

This is best done by having a complete evaluation followed by a thorough discussion with your physician(s). The brochure should assist you to participate in these discussions by providing essential background information so you can ask questions you need answered, and help you understand what your physician is talking about and how the choice of cancer treatment method will affect you and your circumstances.

Many important details are necessarily left out and you should look to your physician for your complete and current information. Being well informed and having thoroughly discussed the alternatives will make it easier to make a knowledgeable decision about your course of treatment. It will give you justified confidence you have made the best choice possible. This will be a tremendous help to you and your physician as you carry out your treatment and establish your follow-up program.

HEALTH AND SAFETY CODE, SECTION 1704.5

California Physicians and Surgeons are required by law to inform patients of alternative effective methods of treatment for breast cancer. This brochure describes medically viable treatment including surgical, radiological (x-ray), chemotherapeutic (drugs) treatments or combinations thereof. It has been printed in a form which may be reproduced by physicians for distribution to their patients. If physicians wish to obtain printed copies they may be purchased from:

State of California
Publications Section
P.O. Box 1015
North Highlands, CA 95660

The cost of the brochure:
  Twenty-five copies $3.40
  Fifty copies $6.15
  One hundred copies $9.15

References

Books

Alderson, E.M.: The prevention of cancer, 1982, Edw. Arnold, Ltd., 1982.

Ames, B.N.: Carcinogens and anticarcinogens. In Mutagens in our environment: Proceedings of the Ninth European Environment Mutagen Society Conference, New York, 1982, Alan R. Liss, Inc.

Bennett, I., and Simon, M.: The prudent diet, New York, 1973, David White, Inc.

Benson, H.: The relaxation response, New York, 1976, Avon Books.

Bieliauskas, L.A.: Stress and its relationship to health and illness, Boulder, 1982, Westview Press.

Brody, J.: Jane Brody's nutrition book, New York, 1981, W.W. Norton & Co., Inc.

Brody, J.: You can fight cancer and win, New York, 1977, Quadrangle/The New York Times Book Co.

Cairns, J.: Cancer: science and society, San Francisco, 1978, W.H. Freeman & Co. Publishers.

Cohen, J., Cullen, J.W., and Martin, L.R., editors: Psychosocial dimensions of cancer, New York, 1981, Raven Press.

De Vita, V., Hellman, S. and Rosenberg, S.A.: Cancer: principles and practice of oncology, Philadelphia, 1982, J.B. Lippincott Co.

DiSogra, C., and Groll, L.: Nutrition and cancer prevention, Palo Alto, Calif., 1981, Northern California Cancer Program.

Doll, R., and Peto, R.: The causes of cancer, Oxford, 1981, Oxford University Press.

Epstein, S.S.: The politics of cancer, San Francisco, 1978, Sierra Club Books.

Glemser, B.: Mr. Burkitt and Africa, New York, 1970, Alan R. Liss, Inc.

Higginson, J.: Current aspects of cancer etiology, New York, 1980, Hemisphere Publishing Corp.

Hixon, J.: The patchwork mouse: politics and intrigue in the campaign to conquer cancer, New York, 1976, Anchor Press.

Koop, C.E.: A report of the Surgeon General, U.S. Department of Health and Human Services, Office on Smoking and Health, Rockville, Md.

Koop, C.E., and Richmond, J.B.: The health consequences of smoking for women, U.S. Department of Health and Human Services, Office on Smoking and Health, Rockville, Md.

Kushner, R.: Breast cancer, New York, 1975, Harcourt Brace Jovanovich, Inc.

Levitt, P.M., and Guralnick, E.: The cancer reference book, New York, 1979, Paddington Press, Ltd.

Locke, S., and Hornig-Rohan, M.: Mind and immunity: behavioral immunology (1976–1982) — an annotated bibliography. In press, 1983.

McWaters, E.D., Thompson, M., and Renneker, M.: Preventing cancer, Palo Alto, Calif., 1981, Bull Publishing Co.

Pilgrim, I.: The topic of cancer, New York, 1974, Thomas Y. Crowell Co. Publishers.

Proctor, N.: The chemical hazards of the workplace, Philadelphia, 1978, J.B. Lippincott Co.

NOTE: Because of limited space in this book, many of the citations have been omitted; specific authors and investigators who have created a tremendous bulk of knowledge that has been used in this book are listed. Additional references are available on request.

291

Renneker, M., and Leib, S., editors: Understanding cancer, Palo Alto, Calif., 1979, Bull Publishing Co.

Robertson, L., Flinders, C., and Godfrey, B.: Laurel's kitchen, Petaluma, Calif., 1979, Nilgiri Press.

Russell, M.A.H., and others: Addiction Research Unit nicotine titration studies. In Thornton, R.E., editor: Smoking, behavior, physiological and psychological influences, New York, 1978, Churchill Livingstone, pp. 336-348.

Schottenfeld, D., and Fraumeni, J., Jr.: Cancer epidemiology and prevention, Boston, 1982, W.B. Saunders Co.

Schwartz, J.L.: Cigarette smoking. In Chang, R.S., editor: Preventive health care, Boston, 1982, G.K. Hall.

Spletter, M.: A woman's choice: new options in the treatment of breast cancer, Boston, 1982, Beacon Press.

Whelan, E.: Preventing cancer, New York, 1980, W.W. Norton & Co., Inc.

Wynder, E.L., editor: The book of health, New York, 1981, Franklin Watts, Inc.

Wynder, E.L., and others: Cancer among black population: opportunities for prevention of cancer in blacks. In Wynder, E.L., editor-in-chief: The book of health, New York, 1981, Franklin Watts.

Articles

Abbott, T.: The rights of the non-smoker, Outlook 94:763, 1910.

Alter, H.J.: The evolution, implications, and applications of hepatitis B vaccine, J.A.M.A. 247:2272, 1983.

Arien, M.C., and others: Hepatitis B viral markers in patients with primary hepatocellular carcinoma in Taiwan, J. Natl. Cancer Inst. 66:475, 1981.

Ames, B.N.: Identifying environmental chemicals causing mutations and cancer, Science 201(4393):587, 1979.

Bertino, J.R.: Nutrients, vitamins and minerals as therapy, Cancer suppl. 43:2137, 1979.

Bieliauskas, L.A., and Garron, D.C.: Psychological depression and cancer, Gen. Hosp. Psychiatry 4:187, 1982.

Bollag, W.: Vitamin A and retinoids: from nutrition to pharmacotherapy in dermatology and oncology, Lancet, pp. 860-863, 1983.

Borysenko, J.Z.: Behavioral-psychological factors in the development and management of cancer, Gen. Hosp. Psychiatry 4:69, 1982.

Breast Cancer Detection Demonstration Project: 5-year summary report, CA 32:4, 1982.

Breslow, L., and Enstrom, J.: Persistence of health habits and their relationship to mortality, Prev. Med. 9:469, 1980.

Breslow, L., and Somers, A.: The lifetime health-monitoring program, N. Eng. J. Med. 296:601, 1981.

Burkitt, D.: The effect of dietary fiber on stools and transit times and its role in the causation of disease, Lancet, Dec. 30, 1972.

Butterfield, G.: Personal communication, 1982.

Cameron, P., and Robertson, D.: Effect of home environment tobacco smoke on family health, J. Appl. Psychol. 57:141, 1973.

Cassidy, M.M., and others: Effect of chronic intake of dietary fibers on the ultrastructural topography of rat jejunum and colon: a scanning electron microscopy study, Am. J. Clin. Nutr. 34:218, 1981.

Conley, G.R., and others: Seminoma epididymal cysts in a young man with known diethylstilbestrol exposure in utero, J.A.M.A. 249:1325, 1983.

Cummings, S.R.: Kicking the habit: benefits and methods of quitting smoking, West. J. Med. 137:443, 1982.

Dales, L., and others: Evaluating periodic multiphasic health checkups: a controlled trial, J. Chronic Dis. 32:385, 1979.

De Vita, V.T., and Kershner, L.M.: Cancer, the curable diseases, Am. Pharm., April 1980.

Diamond, G.A., and Forrester, J.S.: Clinical traits and statistical verdicts: probable grounds for appeal, Ann. Intern. Med. 98:385, 1983.

Doll, R., and Hill, A.B.: Smoking and carcinoma of the lung, Br. Med. J., Sept. 30, 1950, p. 739.

Epstein, M.A.: Epstein-Barr virus as the cause of a human cancer, Nature, Aug. 24, 1978.

Flamm, W.G.: The need for quantifying risk from exposures to chemical carcinogens, Prev. Med. 5:4, 1976.

Fox, C.H.: The inevitability of cancer, Science 218:108, 1982.

Fraumeni, J.F., and others: Cancer mortality among nuns: the role of marital status in the etiology of neoplastic disease in women, J. Nat. Cancer Inst. 42:455, 1969.

Garfinkel, L.: Time trends in lung cancer mortality among nonsmokers and a note on passive smoking, J. Nat. Cancer Inst. **66**:1061, 1981.

Golden, B.R., and others: Estrogen excretion patterns and plasma levels in vegetarians and omnivorous women, N. Engl. J. Med. **307**:1504, 1982.

Gori, G., and Peters, J.: Etiology and prevention of cancer, Prev. Med. **4**:239, 1975.

Hammond, E.C., and Horn, D.: The relationship between human smoking habits and death rates, J.A.M.A. **155**:1316, 1954.

Hammond, E.C., and others: Smoking and cancer in the United States, Prev. Med. **9**:169, 1980.

Hanke, C., and Williams, P.: A guide to sunscreens for you and your patients, Your Patient and Cancer, July, 1982, p. 37.

Herns, G.: The contribution of diet and childbearing to breast cancer rates, Br. J. Cancer **37**:974, 1978.

Higginson, J.: Cancer and environment: Higginson speaks out, Science **205**:1363, 1979.

Higginson, J.: Proportion of cancer due to occupation, Prev. Med. **9**:180, 1980.

Higginson, J.: Rethinking the environmental causation of human cancer, Toxicology **19**:534, 1981.

Higginson, J., and Muir, C.S.: Environmental carcinogens: misconceptions and limitations to cancer control, J. Nat. Cancer Inst. **63**:1291, 1979.

Higginson, J., and Muir, C.S.: Cancer detection and prevention, Prev. Med. **1**:79, 1976.

Hiroyama, T.: Non-smoking wives of heavy smokers have a risk of lung cancer: a study from Japan, Br. Med. J. **282**:183, 1981.

Ingelfinger, F.J.: Cancer! Alarm! Cancer! N. Engl. J. Med. **293**:1319, 1975.

Jensen, O.M.: Cancer morbidity and causes of death among Danish brewery workers, Int. J. Cancer **23**:454, 1979.

Koop, C.E., and Luoto, J.: The health consequences of smoking: cancer; overview of a report of the Surgeon General, Public Health Rep. **97**(4):318, 1982.

Kozlowski, L.T.: Tar and nicotine delivery of cigarettes, J.A.M.A. **245**(2):158, 1981.

Kozlowski, L.T.: Tar and nicotine ratings may be hazardous to your health, Toronto, 1982, Alcohol and Drug Addiction Research Foundation.

Lee, P.N.: Passive smoking, Food Cosmet. Toxicol. **20**:223, 1982.

Lehman, P.E., and Kalmar, V.: Improving the quality of the work environment. In Healthy people: the Surgeon General's Report on Health Promotion and Disease Prevention, background papers, Washington, D.C., U.S. Department of Health, Education and Welfare. U. S. Government Printing Office.

Leo, M.A., and Lieber, C.S.: Hepatic vitamin A depletion in alcoholic liver injury, N. Engl. J. Med. **307**:592, 1982.

Locke, S.E.: Stress, adaptation and immunity: studies in humans, Gen. Hosp. Psychiatry **4**:49, 1982.

Lubin, J.H., and others: Breast cancer following high dietary fat and protein consumption, Am. J. Epidemiol. **144**:422, 1981.

MacMahon, B., and others: Coffee and cancer of the pancreas, N. Engl. J. Med., March 12, 1981.

The magazines' smoking habit, Columbia J. Rev., Jan./Feb., pp. 29-31, 1978.

Martell, E., and others: Letters to the editor, Radioactivity in cigarette smoke, N. Engl. J. Med. **307**:309, 1982.

Mashberg, A., Garfinkel, L., and Harris, S.: Alcohol as a primary risk factor in oral squamous carcinoma, Ca—A Cancer Journal for Clinicians **31**(3):146, 1981.

Merz, B.: Radiologists revise mammography guidelines, J.A.M.A. **249**:2142, 1983.

Miller, D.G.: If you look for early cancer, you will find it, Your Patient and Cancer, July 1981.

Miller, G.H.: The Pennsylvania study on passive smoking, J. Breathing **41**(5):5, 1978.

Miller, L.H., Ross, R., and Cohen, S.I.: Stress: what can be done? Bostonia Magazine **56**(415):13, 1982.

Newell, G.R.: Overview of cancer prevention, Cancer Bull. **32**:128, 1980.

Newell, G.R., and Ellison, N.N.: Relationship between diet and cancer: a brief review for the practicing physician, Cancer Bull. **32**:157, 1981.

Norr, R.: Cancer by the carton, Reader's Digest, December 1952.

Ochsner, A., and Debakey, Z.: Carcinoma of the lung, Arch. Surg. **42**:209, 1941.

Redmond, D.C.: Tobacco and cancer: the first clinical report, 1761, N. Engl. J. Med. **282**:18, 1979.

Reif, A.E.: The causes of cancer, Am. Sci. **69**(4):437, 1981, p. 437.

Repace, J.L.: The problem of passive smoking, Bull. N.Y. Acad. Med. 57(10):936, 1981.

Repace, J.L., and Lowrey, A.H.: Indoor air pollution, tobacco smoke, and public health, Science 208:464, 1980.

Rogers, M.P., Dubey, D., and Reich, P.: The influence of the psychs and the brain on immunity and disease susceptibility: a critical review, Psychosom. Med. 41:147, 1979.

Rosenberg, L., and others: Breast cancer and alcoholic-beverage consumption, Lancet, p. 267, 1982.

Ross, W.: The dangers of smoking, the benefits of quitting, The American Cancer Society, 1972.

Rossiter, C.E.: Passive smoking, Lancet, 1982, p. 1356.

Rothman, K., and Keller, A.: The effects of joint exposure to alcohol and tobacco on risk of cancer of the mouth and pharynx, J. Chronic Dis. 25:74, 1972.

Russell, M.A.H.: The case for medium-nicotine, low-tar, low-carbon monoxide cigarette? Cold Spring Harbor, New York, 1980, Cold Spring Harbor Laboratory, pp. 297-310.

Russell, M.A.H., and others: Nicotine chewing gum as a substitute for smoking, Br. Med. J. 1(6068): 1060, 1977.

Ryan, K.: Cancer risk and estrogen use in menopause, N. Engl. J. Med. 293:1199, 1975.

Schottenfeld, D.: Cancer risks of medical treatment, CA 32(5):258, 1982.

Schottenfeld, D.: Alcohol as a cofactor in the etiology of cancer, Cancer Suppl. 43(5):258, 1979.

Schottenfeld, D., and Haas, J.F.: Carcinogens in the workplace, Clin. Bull., 1978, pp. 54, 107.

Schranzer, G.N., and others: Cancer mortality correlation studies III: statistical associations with dietary selenium intakes, Bioinorg. Chem. 7:23, 1977.

Shekelle, R.B., and others: Dietary vitamin A and risk of cancer in the Western Electric (Chicago) study, Lancet 2:1185, 1981.

Sigimura, T.: Mutagens, carcinogens, and tumor promoters in our daily food, Cancer 49:1970, 1982.

Stellman, S.P., and Stellman, J.M.: Women's occupations, smoking, and cancer and other diseases, CA 31:29, 1981.

Takashi, S.: Mutagens, carcinogens and tumor promotors in our daily food, Cancer, May 15, 1982.

Tannenbaum, A., and Silverstone, H.: Nutrition and the genesis of tumours. In Raven, R., editor: Cancer, London, 1957, Butterworth Ltd., pp. 306-334.

Thomas, C.B., Duszynski, K.R., and Shaffer, J.W.: Family attitudes reported in youths as potential predictors of cancer, Psychosom. Med. 41:287, 1979.

Weaver, A., Fleming, S.M., and Smith, D.B.: Mouthwash and oral cancer: carcinogen or coincidence? Oral Surg. 37(4):250, 1979.

Whelan, E., and others: Analysis of coverage of tobacco hazards in women's magazines, J. Public Health 2:28, 1981.

White, J.R., and Froeb, H.F.: Small airways dysfunction in non-smokers chronically exposed to tobacco smoke, N. Engl. J. Med. 306:364, 1982.

Winters, T.H., and Di Franza, R.R.: Radioactivity in cigarette smoke, N. Engl. J. Med, 306:364, 1982.

Wynder, E.: Tobacco as a carcinogen, Your Patient and Cancer, August 1981.

Wynder, E.: Dietary habits and cancer epidemiology, Cancer Suppl. 43(5):1955, 1979.

Wynder, E., and Gori, G.B.: Contribution of the environment to cancer incidence: an epidemiologic exercise, J. Natl. Cancer Inst. 48:1749, 1972.

Wynder, E., and Graham, E.A.: Etiologic factors in bronchogenic carcinoma with special reference to industrial exposures—report on 857 proved cases, AMA Arch. Ind. Hyg. Occup. Med. 4:221, 1951.

Wynder, E., and Hoffman, D.: Tobacco and health, N. Engl. J. Med. 300: 894, 1980.

Wynder, E., and Hoffman, D.: Less harmful ways of smoking, J. Natl. Cancer Inst. 48:1749, 1979.

Wynder, E.L., and others: Oral cancer and mouthwash use, J. Natl. Cancer Inst. 70(2):255, 1983.

Wynder, E.L., and others: Tumor promotors and cocarcinogens as related to man and his environment. In Carcinogenesis—a comprehensive survey, Slaga, T.J., Sivak, A., and Boutwell, R.K., editors: vol. 2, New York, 1978, Raven Press.

Yang, C.S.: Research on esophageal cancer in China: a review, Cancer Res. 40:2633, 1980.

Young, V.R.: Nutrients, vitamins and minerals in cancer prevention, Cancer Suppl. 43(5):2125, 1979.

Ziegler, J.L.: Burkitt's lymphoma, CA 32(3):144, 1982.

Other publications

Ames, B.: Diet and Mutagens. From Conference on Cancer and the Environment, Sept. 25, 1982, French Hospital, San Francisco.

Canadian Task Force: The periodic health examination, Can. Med. Assoc. J. **121**:1193, 1979.

Cancer Facts and Figures—1983, New York, 1983, The American Cancer Society.

Cole, P.: Some epidemiological aspects of cancer prevention: cancer in Ontario. Report of the Ontario Cancer Treatment and Research Foundation, 1979.

Dangers of smoking, benefits of quitting and relative risks of reduced exposure, New York, 1980, The American Cancer Society.

Diet, nutrition and cancer. Prepared by the Committee on Diet, Nutrition and Cancer, Assembly of Life Sciences, National Research Council, 1982, National Academy Press.

Dietary Goals for the United States. Prepared by the Staff of the Select Committee on Nutrition and Human Needs—United States Senate, Washington, D.C., 1977, U.S. Government Printing Office.

Directory of stop-smoking clinics in the San Francisco Bay area, ed. 3, September 1982. Prepared by the Regional Cancer Foundation.

Guidelines for the cancer-related checkup, CA **30**:194, 1980.

Hammond, E.C., and the American Cancer Society: The American Cancer Society Cancer Prevention Study: 1959-79, New York, 1979, American Cancer Society.

Newell, G.R.: Cancer prevention and control. Paper presented at the Conference on Cancer Control, Sept. 29-30, 1980, Buffalo, New York.

Richmond, E.J., editor: The health consequences of smoking for women. Report of the Surgeon General, Washington, D.C., 1982, U.S. Department of Health and Human Services, U.S. Government Printing Office.

Science and Cancer, Washington, D.C., 1980, U.S. Department of Health and Human Services, U.S. Government Printing Office.

Shiffman, S.M., and Jarvik, M.E.: Withdrawal symptoms: the first week is the hardest, World Smoking and Health, Winter 1980.

Shimkin, M.B.: Contrary to nature, Washington, D.C., 1979, U.S. Department of Health, Education and Welfare, U.S. Government Printing Office.

Smoking Cessation Newsletter, 9550 North Zionville Rd., P.O. Box 68511, Indianapolis, Ind. 46268 (B.H. Ellis, Jr., subscriptions). (Initial issues complementary.)

Smoking and Health. Prepared by the Cancer Information Clearing House, Office of Cancer Communications, National Cancer Institute, Washington, D.C., 1978, U.S. Department of Health and Human Services, U.S. Government Printing Office.

U.S. Department of Health, Education and Welfare publications: Clearing the air: a guide to quitting smoking, Washington, D.C., 1979, Public Health Service–National Institute of Health.

The smoking digest, Washington, D.C., 1977, Public Health Service–National Institute of Health.

Smoking and health: a report of the surgeon general, Washington, D.C., 1971, Office on Smoking and Health–Public Health Service.

ADDENDUM TO AIDS SECTION

Chapter 10: Life-style and Cancer

Viruses have been suspected as causes of cancer in birds, mice, cats, and cows since the early 1900s. Recently the human T-cell leukemia virus (HTLV) has been linked with human T-cell leukemia and lymphoma. The virus is an RNA tumor virus (retrovirus). It has *not* been proved to be the cause of *human* T-cell lymphoma/leukemia—but thus far there is a strong link or association. It has been isolated in patients in the United States, Israel, Japan, and the Caribbean.

The course of this more aggressive form of disease is being studied all over the world, especially at our National Cancer Institute by Dr. Robert Gallo and associates. It is hoped that the scope of HTLV infections will be better defined, including its disease association, transmission, the mechanism of how it can cause cancer, and how to prevent and treat it.

Most recently, investigators have detected evidence of HTLV infection in a small proportion of patients with AIDS. Whether this virus is a contributing cause of AIDS or is merely a coincidental finding remains to be determined.

I wish to thank Lawrence Mints, M.D., and Lawrence Drew, M.D., Infectious Disease Department, Mount Zion Hospital and Medical Center, for aid, editing, and advice in the section on AIDS.

Index